T0127861

Pediatric Infections

Editors

REBECCA G. SAME
JASON G. NEWLAND

INFECTIOUS DISEASE CLINICS
OF NORTH AMERICA

www.id.theclinics.com

Consulting Editor
HELEN W. BOUCHER

March 2022 • Volume 36 • Number 1

ELSEVIER

1600 John F. Kennedy Boulevard • Suite 1800 • Philadelphia, Pennsylvania, 19103-2899.
http://www.theclinics.com

INFECTIOUS DISEASE CLINICS OF NORTH AMERICA Volume 36, Number 1
March 2022 ISSN 0891-5520, ISBN-13: 978-0-323-83542-8

Editor: Kerry Holland
Developmental Editor: Hannah Almira Lopez

Infectious Disease Clinics of North America (ISSN 0891-5520) is published in March, June, September, and December by Elsevier Inc., 360 Park Avenue South, New York, NY 10010-1710. Periodicals postage paid at New York, NY and additional mailing offices. Subscription prices are $357.00 per year for US individuals, $950.00 per year for US institutions, $100.00 per year for US students, $408.00 per year for Canadian individuals, $979.00 per year for Canadian institutions, $445.00 per year for international individuals, $979.00 per year for international institutions, $100.00 per year for Canadian students, and $200.00 per year for international students. To receive student rate, orders must be accompanied by name of affiliated institution, date of term, and the *signature* of program/residency coordinator on institution letterhead. Orders will be billed at individual rate until proof of status is received. Foreign air speed delivery is included in all *Clinics* subscription prices. All prices are subject to change without notice. **POSTMASTER**: Send address changes to *Infectious Disease Clinics of North America*, Elsevier Health Sciences Division, Subcription Customer Service, 3251 Riverport Lane, Maryland Heights, MO 63043. **Customer Service: 1-800-654-2452 (US). From outside of the US and Canada, call 1-314-447-8871. Fax: 1-314-447-8029. E-mail: JournalsCustomerService-usa@elsevier.com (print support) or JournalsOnlineSupport-usa@elsevier.com (online support).**

Infectious Disease Clinics of North America is also published in Spanish by Editorial Inter-Médica, Junin 917, 1er A 1113, Buenos Aires, Argentina.

Reprints. For copies of 100 or more, of articles in this publication, please contact the Commercial Reprints Department, Elsevier Inc., 360 Park Avenue South, New York, New York 10010-1710. Tel. 212-633-3874, Fax: 212-633-3820, E-mail: reprints@elsevier.com.

Infectious Disease Clinics of North America is covered in *MEDLINE/PubMed (Index Medicus), Current Contents/ Clinical Medicine, Science Citation Alert, SCISEARCH,* and *Research Alert.*

Contributors

CONSULTING EDITOR

HELEN W. BOUCHER, MD, FIDSA, FACP
Director, Infectious Diseases Fellowship Program, Division of Geographic Medicine and Infectious Diseases, Tufts Medical Center, Associate Professor of Medicine, Tufts University School of Medicine, Boston, Massachusetts

EDITORS

REBECCA G. SAME, MD
Assistant Professor, Department of Pediatrics, Division of Pediatric Infectious Diseases, Washington University School of Medicine, St Louis, Missouri

JASON G. NEWLAND, MD, MEd
Professor, Department of Pediatrics, Division of Pediatric Infectious Diseases, Washington University School of Medicine, St Louis, Missouri

AUTHORS

SAMANTHA A. BASCO, PharmD, BCPS
Post-Graduate Year 2 Infectious Diseases Pharmacy Resident, University of Connecticut, Storrs CT and Connecticut Children's, Hartford, Connecticut

JEANETTE BEAUDRY, MD, PhD
Division of Pediatric Infectious Diseases, Johns Hopkins University, Baltimore, Maryland

ALEXIS ELWARD, MD, MPH
Professor, Department of Pediatrics, Division of Pediatric Infectious Diseases, Washington University School of Medicine, St Louis, Missouri

STEPHANIE A. FRITZ, MD, MSCI
Associate Professor, Department of Pediatrics, Division of Pediatric Infectious Diseases, Washington University School of Medicine, St Louis, Missouri

HOLLY FROST, MD
Department of Pediatrics, Center for Health Systems Research, Denver Health and Hospital Authority, University of Colorado School of Medicine, Denver, Colorado

JENNIFER E. GIROTTO, PharmD, BCPPS, BCIDP
Clinical Associate Professor of Pharmacy Practice, University of Connecticut School of Pharmacy, Co-Director of the Antimicrobial Stewardship Program, Connecticut Children's, Hartford, Connecticut

OREN GORDON, MD, PhD
Division of Infectious Diseases, Department of Pediatrics, Johns Hopkins School of Medicine, Baltimore, Maryland

ABBY GREEN, MD
Division of Infectious Diseases, Department of Pediatrics, Washington University, St Louis, Missouri

DEVAN JAGANATH, MD, MPH
Division of Pediatric Infectious Diseases, University of California, San Francisco, San Francisco, California

IBUKUNOLUWA C. KALU, MD
Assistant Professor, Department of Pediatrics, Division of Pediatric Infectious Diseases, Medical Director, Pediatric Infection Prevention, Duke University Medical Center, Durham, North Carolina

CAROL M. KAO, MD
Assistant Professor, Department of Pediatrics, Division of Pediatric Infectious Diseases, Washington University School of Medicine, St Louis, Missouri

JASON LAKE, MD, MPH
Division of Infectious Diseases, Department of Pediatrics, University of Utah School of Medicine, Salt Lake City, Utah

MICHELLE L. MITCHELL, MD
Assistant Professor, Department of Pediatrics, Division of Infectious Diseases, Pediatric Infectious Diseases, Medical College of Wisconsin, Children's Corporate Center, Milwaukee, Wisconsin

WILLIAM R. OTTO, MD
Division of Infectious Diseases, Department of Pediatrics, The Children's Hospital of Philadelphia, Philadelphia, Pennsylvania

NADINE PEART AKINDELE, MD
Department of Pediatrics, Division of Pediatric Infectious diseases, Johns Hopkins University, School of Medicine, Baltimore, Maryland; United States Food and Drug Administration, Silver Spring, Maryland

NICOLE M. POOLE, MD, MPH
Department of Pediatrics, Division of Pediatric Infectious Diseases and Epidemiology, University of Colorado School of Medicine, Children's Hospital Colorado, Aurora, Colorado

PATRICK REICH, MD, MSCI
Assistant Professor, Department of Pediatrics, Division of Pediatric Infectious Diseases, Washington University School of Medicine, St Louis, Missouri

NICOLE SALAZAR-AUSTIN, MD
Division of Pediatric Infectious Diseases, Johns Hopkins University, Baltimore, Maryland

REBECCA G. SAME, MD
Assistant Professor, Department of Pediatrics, Division of Pediatric Infectious Diseases, Washington University School of Medicine, St Louis, Missouri

ANNA C. SICK-SAMUELS, MD, MPH
Assistant Professor of Pediatrics, Division of Infectious Diseases, Department of Pediatrics, Johns Hopkins School of Medicine, Department of Hospital Epidemiology and Infection Control, The Johns Hopkins Hospital, Baltimore, Maryland

DAVID E. VYLES, DO, MS
Assistant Professor, Department of Pediatrics, Section of Pediatric Emergency Medicine, Medical College of Wisconsin, Children's Corporate Center, Milwaukee, Wisconsin

CHARLOTTE WOODS-HILL, MD, MSHP
Assistant Professor of Anesthesiology and Critical Care, Division of Critical Care Medicine, The Children's Hospital of Philadelphia, University of Pennsylvania Perelman School of Medicine, The Leonard Davis Institute of Health Economics, University of Pennsylvania, Philadelphia, Pennsylvania

PHILIP ZACHARIAH, MD, MS, MA
Department of Pediatrics, Columbia University Irving Medical Center, New York, New York

TRACY N. ZEMBLES, PharmD
Lead Antimicrobial Stewardship Pharmacist, Department of Enterprise Safety, Children's Wisconsin, Children's Corporate Center, Milwaukee, Wisconsin

Contents

> Although COVID-19 has impacted many children, severe disease is rare and most recover with supportive care. Manifestations are diverse and often nonrespiratory. Adolescents/children with medical comorbidities are at risk for severe respiratory compromise. The most serious manifestation in previously healthy children is a delayed multisystem inflammatory syndrome with cardiac compromise in severe cases. Anti–SARS-CoV-2 monoclonal antibodies are available for adolescents at risk of progression and not hospitalized. Therapeutic options for severe respiratory disease with hypoxia include remdesivir and glucocorticoids. Therapies for multisystem inflammatory syndrome in children include intravenous immunoglobulin and glucocorticoids. Refractory cases may benefit from additional immunomodulators.

> COVID-19 is a nonspecific viral illness caused by a novel coronavirus, SARS-CoV-2, and led to an ongoing global pandemic. Transmission is primarily human-to-human via contact with respiratory particles containing infectious virus. The risk of transmission to health care personnel is low with proper use of personal protective equipment, including gowns, gloves, N95 or surgical mask, and eye protection. Additional measures affecting the risk of transmission include physical distancing, hand hygiene, routine cleaning and disinfection, appropriate air handling and ventilation, and public health interventions such as universal masking and stay-at-home orders.

> Measles virus is an RNA virus that causes the highly contagious childhood exanthem. Despite the presence of a safe and effective vaccine, in 2018, measles was responsible for more than 140,000 deaths worldwide, most of which were in children less than 5 years of age. Mortality is primarily associated with the complications of secondary bacterial and viral infections causing pneumonia but also diarrhea. Recent outbreaks have reinstilled interest in maintaining herd immunity to prevent continued resurgence of disease and associated comorbidities.

Gram-negative resistance is increasing in serious infections, including in children. There are many mechanisms of resistance, most commonly beta-lactamases. The most concerning beta-lactamases are AmpC, extended spectrum beta-lactamases, and carbapenemases. Efflux pumps and porins are also important in Pseudomonas infections. For some mechanisms of resistance, dose adjustment of antibiotics may help to overcome resistance and effectively treat infections. Therefore, it is important to consider pediatric pharmacokinetic differences when dosing antibiotics to ensure adequate concentrations are reached and maintained. These considerations important for older antibiotics and newer agents.

Antibiotic use in hospitalized children is highly variable and often unnecessary, which puts children at risk of antibiotic-associated harms including adverse drug events, antibiotic resistance, and long-term chronic health problems. Antimicrobial stewardship programs reduce unnecessary antibiotic use through antimicrobial review, the development of guidelines and clinical decision-support tools, diagnostic stewardship, and other targeted interventions. Future directions for inpatient stewardship include increased collaboration with nurses, utilization of implementation science to close the gap between evidence-based recommendations and practice changes, and the extension of stewardship from large academic centers to smaller hospitals.

Antibiotics are overprescribed for children in outpatient settings, primarily for the diagnosis of acute respiratory tract infections. The overuse of antibiotics leads to antibiotic-resistant infections, avoidable adverse drug events, and chronic inflammatory conditions in children. Decreasing unnecessary antibiotic use is therefore a public health priority. In this article, the authors describe the burden of antibiotic prescribing to children in outpatient settings, identify targets for improvement, and use national recommendations as a guide to describe pragmatic methods to measure and improve antibiotic prescribing for children in outpatient settings.

In the pediatric intensive care unit (PICU), clinicians encounter complex decision making, balancing the need to treat infections promptly against the potential harms of antibiotics. Diagnostic stewardship is an approach to optimize microbiology diagnostic test practices to reduce unnecessary antibiotic treatment. We review the evidence for diagnostic stewardship of blood, endotracheal, and urine cultures in the PICU. Clinicians should consider 3 questions applying diagnostic stewardship: (1) Does the patient have signs or symptoms of an infectious process? (2) What is the optimal diagnostic test available to evaluate for this infection? (3) How should the diagnostic specimen be collected to optimize results?

Penicillin allergy is the most commonly reported medication allergy. Reported allergy is associated with increased morbidity and mortality. Risk categorization tools can help determine the optimal testing strategies to delabel patients with reported allergy. Approaches to allergy removal include oral challenge in low-risk patients and skin testing in high-risk patients. Many different locations may be used to test for allergy, including ambulatory care clinics, inpatient units, and emergency departments. Interventions (eg, use of the electronic medical record) are needed to ensure that once the allergy is removed, this information is effectively transmitted to the patient and appropriate providers.

INFECTIOUS DISEASE CLINICS OF NORTH AMERICA

Preface

Pediatric Infections in the Time of COVID-19

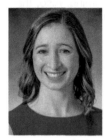
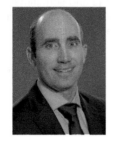

Rebecca G. Same, MD   Jason G. Newland, MD, MEd
Editors

We began planning this issue of *Infectious Diseases Clinics of North America* in February of 2020, at the threshold of the Coronavirus Disease 2019 (COVID-19) pandemic. We felt great anticipation and some anxiety at the time, but we could never have known then how COVID-19 would so drastically change all aspects of our society: politics, education, social justice, and medicine. Compared with adults, children have been relatively spared by the most severe manifestations of severe acute respiratory syndrome coronavirus-2, but they have still suffered significantly from the direct impact of the virus. There have been over 600 childhood deaths in the United States and nearly 6,000 cases of the novel multisystem inflammatory syndrome in children. Perhaps of even greater significance, many children's lives have been forever affected by the prolonged loss of in-person education, COVID-19 deaths among their caregivers and family members, and the exacerbation of the ongoing mental health crisis in children and teenagers. While COVID-19 has monopolized our attention, common childhood infections persist and have also been impacted by our focus on COVID-19 and the strategies we have employed to address the pandemic.

This issue has been significantly delayed due to the pandemic, but we have an outstanding collection of articles that demonstrate the breadth, complexity, and impact of the many infectious diseases that affect children. In this issue, you will have the opportunity to reflect and learn about COVID-19 in children and our ongoing efforts toward infection prevention for emerging diseases, including COVID-19. There is an excellent review on measles, which unfortunately remains relevant due to the problem of waning childhood immunization rates that has been significantly exacerbated by the pandemic. An article about tuberculosis focuses on new approaches to an ancient infection that continues to impact children around the world. Important articles are provided on the treatment and prevention of *Staphylococcus aureus*, the management of hardware-associated infections, and the use of antivirals in the

Infect Dis Clin N Am 36 (2022) xiii–xiv
https://doi.org/10.1016/j.idc.2021.12.003
0891-5520/22/© 2021 Published by Elsevier Inc.

immunocompromised host. As we fight the ongoing rise in antibiotic resistance, one article reviews the latest treatment of multidrug-resistant gram-negative infections, and a group of articles address strategies to optimize antimicrobial use, including inpatient and outpatient antimicrobial stewardship, diagnostic stewardship, and how to approach penicillin allergy.

We are grateful for the opportunity to work with all the authors who contributed their expertise to this endeavor, especially at such a difficult time when the demands of the COVID-19 pandemic were unpredictable and sometimes overwhelming. Also, thank you to the staff of *Infectious Diseases Clinics of North America*, who patiently worked with us during these difficult and extremely busy times.

Rebecca G. Same, MD
Division of Pediatric Infectious Diseases
Department of Pediatrics
MSC 8116-43-10
Washington University School of Medicine
660 South Euclid Avenue
St. Louis, MO 63110, USA

Jason G. Newland, MD, MEd
Division of Pediatric Infectious Diseases
Department of Pediatrics
MSC 8116-43-10
Washington University School of Medicine
660 South Euclid Avenue
St. Louis, MO 63110, USA

E-mail addresses:
rsame@wustl.edu (R.G. Same)
jgnewland@wustl.edu (J.G. Newland)

COVID-19 in Children

Philip Zachariah, MD, MS, MA*

KEYWORDS

- COVID-19 • SARS-CoV-2 • MIS-C • Children • Pediatrics

KEY POINTS

- COVID-19 is less severe in children than in adults and usually only requires supportive therapy.
- The 2 main phenotypes of severe disease are acute respiratory failure in children with co-morbidities and a delayed hyperinflammatory response called multisystem inflammatory syndrome in children with cardiac dysfunction.
- Multisystem inflammatory syndrome in children mostly occurs in previously healthy children.
- Remdesivir and steroids are options for worsening acute respiratory disease and hypoxia.
- Intravenous immune globulin and steroids are first-line agents for multisystem inflammatory syndrome in children.

INTRODUCTION AND EPIDEMIOLOGY

The historic advent of COVID-19 has not spared children. Since March 2020, close to 7 million children have tested positive for severe acute respiratory syndrome coronavirus 2 (SARS-CoV-2) in the United States,[1] infected in the household and rarely other communal settings.[2,3] Current evidence is mixed on the differential susceptibility of children versus adults to be infected once exposed,[4] but more conclusive on the effectiveness of standard infection control strategies (masking, social distancing).[5] Hypotheses to why rates of infection and severe disease are lower in pediatrics include age-specific differences in the expression of the binding receptors for SARS-COV-2 (angiotensin-converting enzyme 2 and TMPRSS2)[6,7] or pre-existing immunity to seasonal coronaviruses.[8] Variability in the immune response once infected compared with adults seems likely.[9] Infected children demonstrate stronger innate immune responses compared with adults with a higher expression of genes associated with interferon signaling and the NLRP3 inflammasome.[7] The striking racial and socio-economic disparities in clinical disease and severe outcomes, well-described in

Department of Pediatrics, Columbia University Irving Medical Center, New York, NY, USA
* 622 West 168th Street, PH4-473, New York, NY, 10031.
E-mail address: pz2177@cumc.columbia.edu
Twitter: @pzach13 (P.Z.)

Infect Dis Clin N Am 36 (2022) 1–14
https://doi.org/10.1016/j.idc.2021.11.002
0891-5520/22/© 2021 Elsevier Inc. All rights reserved.

id.theclinics.com

adults, have been noted in multiple pediatric studies and non-White children are over-represented in many case series.[10–13]

CLINICAL SPECTRUM AND MANIFESTATIONS OF PEDIATRIC COVID-19

The clinical spectrum of pediatric COVID-19 is diverse, arguably more than in adults. The majority of children are asymptomatic or mildly symptomatic. Rates of asymptomatic disease are estimated to be around 30% overall[14] and could be as high as 50% in children.[15] Asymptomatic seroconversion in hospitalized children has been noted.[16]

Among symptomatic patients, distinct syndromes occur at varying time points, with severe disease occurring either early or late in an individual child. Adolescents and medically complex children present early with predominantly respiratory manifestations.[12,17] Infants often have fever without additional manifestations.[18,19] A subset of mostly previously healthy children presents 4 to 6 weeks after an initial mild or inapparent infection with a delayed immune response characterized by higher fever, rising inflammatory markers, with what is now termed multisystem inflammatory syndrome in children (MIS-C).[20,21] The community peak of MIS-C has been noted to be 2 to 5 weeks after the peak of acute COVID-19 in a particular locality.[22] The case definition for MIS-C is broad[23] and includes the presence of fever and laboratory evidence of inflammation, along with evidence of severe multisystem involvement (cardiac, renal, respiratory, hematologic, gastrointestinal, dermatologic, or neurologic). Two groups feature prominently in MIS-C presentations: (i) older children with shock and cardiac dysfunction, gastrointestinal symptoms and highly abnormal laboratory parameters (lymphopenia and elevated markers of cardiac injury) and (ii) younger children with features of Kawasaki disease (KD) with rash and mucocutaneous findings and a higher risk of coronary artery aneurysms.[24] Although MIS-C symptoms overlap with KD, cytopenia in the former is an important distinction.[25] This hyperinflammatory response has been variously attributed to a superantigen-mediated process,[26] activation of specific T-cell subsets,[27] and/or higher antibody levels.[28]

The overall rates of hospitalization for pediatric COVID-19 are low (approximately 2%), but among those hospitalized, rates of intensive care admission are comparable with those of adults and higher for MIS-C.[29] The median duration of hospitalization is typically close to 1 week.[30] Data from the Centers for Disease Control and Prevention on patients with COVID-19 aged 0 to 24 years from March to December 2020 showed 2.5% requiring hospitalization and 0.8% requiring admission to an intensive care unit.[31] The rarity of severe disease in pediatrics continues to be born out with current estimates suggesting that only 0.1% to 2.0% of all child COVID-19 cases result in hospitalizations and that mortality is extraordinarily rare, but can be up to 1% of hospitalizations.[1,22] The circulation of the more transmissible delta variant has significantly increased COVID-19–associated pediatric hospitalization rates, but the proportions of those hospitalized with severe disease has remained similar in the United States.[32]

Respiratory Manifestations

Respiratory manifestations typically include upper respiratory or influenza-like symptoms, with fever variably present.[33] Pathognomonic symptoms such as anosmia and loss of taste are seen in older children.[12] Infants may present with apnea.[34] A higher fever curve and the presence of multisystem findings suggests overlap with MIS-C where respiratory findings are rarely predominant.[24] Around 30% of patients hospitalized in critical care units show evidence of acute respiratory distress syndrome with higher inflammatory markers, pronounced radiographic findings,[35] and pathology that shows type 2 pneumocyte atypia, pulmonary microthrombosis, and exudative diffuse alveolar damage.[36] Viral bronchiolitis or asthma exacerbations are not typical presentations and rates of both initially plummeted during early waves of COVID-19.[37,38] The presence of either of these conditions should raise suspicion for viral coinfections.

Gastrointestinal and Hepatic Manifestations

The prevalence of gastrointestinal symptoms as the index presentation for pediatric COVID-19 has varied across case series.[17] However, gastrointestinal manifestations occur in the majority of cases of MIS-C,[24] and persistent antigenemia from a gastrointestinal source has been linked to pathogenesis.[39] Symptoms range from nausea, vomiting, and diarrhea to more severe phenotypes that may mimic acute appendicitis or intussusception.[12,40] In severe cases, radiographic findings can resemble those of inflammatory bowel disease.[41]

Cardiac Manifestations

The cardiac manifestations of SARS-Cov2 are predominantly seen in severe cases of MIS-C with accompanying evidence of myocardial inflammation, necrosis, and direct viral invasion.[42] In case series of MIS-C, a reduced left ventricular ejection fraction is present in more than one-half of the patients, and the overwhelming majority of children with cardiac manifestations had elevated cardiac troponins.[20,43] In a large case series of 1733 patients, cardiac dysfunction was reported in 484 patients (31.0%), pericardial effusion in 365 (23.4%), myocarditis in 300 (17.3%), and coronary artery dilatation or aneurysms in 258 (16.5%).[43]

Neurologic Manifestations

Neurologic symptoms occur in 20% of children with COVID-19 and more commonly in those with pre-existing neurologic disorders.[44] Infants may present with nonlocalizing neurologic symptoms (eg, new seizures, apneic episodes). Adolescents can have severe headaches, sometimes overlapping with pseudotumor cerebri syndrome.[45] Classic postinfectious sequelae, for example, peripheral neuropathy, demyelination, transverse myelitis, and Guillain–Barre syndrome, all can follow recent SARS-CoV-2 infection, sometimes without additional systemic manifestations.[46,47] Other severe manifestations such as encephalopathy, stroke, demyelination, and cerebral edema are rare.[44] Interestingly, neuropathology does not suggest viral infection of the central nervous system and SARS-CoV-2 is rarely detected in the cerebrospinal fluid.[48]

Dermatologic Manifestations

Transient rash, usually maculopapular in nature, can occur in both acute and late COVID-19.[12,17] SARS-CoV-2 infection can trigger cutaneous vasculitis, causing benign entities like perniosis (COVID toes) to acral gangrene. Petechiae can occur as part of thrombocytopenia-associated syndromes like Henoch–Schoenlein purpura.[49] Mucocutaneous manifestations seen in MIS-C are similar to that in KD, including polymorphous rash and involvement of the oral mucosa.[50]

Other Systemic Manifestations

Clinical thrombotic events are rare in children in comparison with adults with COVID-19; they are more common in older children with MIS-C and in those with pre-existing risk factors for thrombosis (eg, cancer, presence of a central line). These manifestations can include deep vein thrombosis, pulmonary embolism, and strokes.[51] Diabetic ketoacidosis has been reported as a presentation for children hospitalized with MIS-C,[52] as well as a complication in those children with known diabetes.[53] Acute renal failure is noted in up to one-quarter of children hospitalized in the intensive care unit with MIS-C, but usually resolves by discharge.[54]

EVALUATION AND APPROACH

The initial approach to a pediatric patient with suspected COVID-19 should aim to (i) confirm the diagnosis, (ii) identify competing causes, (iii) define the risk of disease progression in an individual child using clinical and/or laboratory risk factors, (iv) choose antiviral and immunomodulatory therapy as applicable, and (v) provide excellent supportive care.

Confirm SARS-Cov2 Infection

Testing for SARS-CoV-2 is ideally done using nucleic acid amplification and antigen tests should be interpreted accounting for pretest probability. Antigen testing has a reduced sensitivity, but usually correlates with nucleic acid amplification results when the viral load and infectiousness are highest and thus can be a useful adjunct. The possibility of false negatives should be considered taking into account the local average positivity rate over the past 7 to 10 days.[55]

Although nasopharyngeal swabs specimens are the gold standard, studies show equivalent performance using midturbinate, anterior nasal, saliva, or a combined anterior nasal/oropharyngeal swabs in symptomatic adults.[56] Prolonged shedding and viral evolution are described particularly in immunocompromised children.[57] SARS-CoV-2 polymerase chain reaction testing is mostly negative in MIS-C[20] and serology testing should be done to confirm exposure.[58]

Increased viral loads have been associated with severity of disease in adults,[59] but data in pediatrics are conflicting.[60,61] Viral loads seem to be similar between adults and children.[7] The routine use of cycle thresholds from polymerase chain reaction tests is not currently part of clinical care, and caution must be exercised when comparing across assays and in light of the potential variability attributable to different sampling practices.[62]

Identify Competing Diagnoses

Because the absolute risk for hospitalizations owing to acute COVID-19 is low in children, a careful assessment for competing causes should be considered in severely ill children. Both common (eg, bacterial enteritis)[63] and uncommon (eg, primary immunodeficiency syndromes)[64] diagnoses have been misidentified as MIS-C, so a comprehensive diagnostic approach with subspecialist input is encouraged for children with diverse symptoms and SARS-CoV-2 positivity. Coinfections have been described in acute COVID-19 and MIS-C including both bacterial (eg, *Staphylococcus aureus*, group A Streptococcus) and viral (eg, Epstein–Bar virus, parvovirus, herpes viruses, and other respiratory viruses) pathogens.[65]

Additional Laboratory Testing to Risk Stratify and Classify Disease

The role of outpatient laboratory testing to triage admission is undefined but higher trends in inflammatory markers (eg, C-reactive protein [CRP]) may predict disease trajectory.[66] For hospitalized children with acute severe COVID-19 or MIS-C, initial investigations usually include complete blood counts, comprehensive metabolic panel, inflammatory markers (CRP, procalcitonin, ferritin) and coagulation parameters. For patients with features of MIS-C, markers for cardiac injury (B-type natriuretic peptide, troponin) are included in initial testing. Cardiac investigations (electrocardiogram and echocardiogram) should be obtained in patients suspected to have MIS-C and are usually repeated during the hospital stay based on institutional protocols.[67]

Accurate risk prediction scores are not available, although it seems clear that severe COVID-19 correlates with an overall derangement of most of these parameters, which are more severe in MIS-C.[68] Elevated CRP is a prognostic marker for critical care admission in pediatric acute COVID-19,[69] whereas CRP, lymphopenia, and B-type natriuretic peptide elevations are the strongest predictors for intensive care admission in MIS-C.[17,68] Genetic screening for immune system defects, usually as a part of research efforts, may be considered, particularly for younger children with no associated comorbidities who present with severe acute COVID-19. Defects in interferon signaling and the presence of interferon antibodies have been described.[70] Immune phenotyping can also help to distinguish between MIS-C and acute COVID-19, with the activation of CD8$^+$ cells[27] and specific cytokine elevations observed in MIS-C.[71]

THERAPEUTIC OPTIONS: RISK STRATIFICATION

The majority of children with acute COVID-19 recover completely with supportive care alone.[1] Comparative data on efficacy for therapeutic agents are mostly derived from studies in adults, so any observed relative risk reduction must be interpreted in light of the lower absolute risk and the larger number needed to treat in pediatrics.[72] Ongoing updated guidance is available from the Pediatric Infectious Diseases Society,[73] National Institutes of Health,[74] and the Infectious Disease Society of America.[75]

Most pediatric patients hospitalized with acute COVID-19 patients have comorbidities.[10,12] Obesity is an independent risk factor for severe disease in adults and most likely in adolescents.[17,35,76] Medical complexity, an amalgam of conditions including neurodevelopmental delay, genetic syndromes, and respiratory technology dependence, is prevalent in most severe COVID-19 case series,[30] but individual risk ratios are not available. The role of immunocompromise is nuanced. Unexpectedly lower rates of morbidity and mortality have been reported in immunocompromised patients, including those with hematologic malignancies, hematopoietic stem cell transplantation, and solid organ transplantation, but these do contribute to disease severity.[77-79] Adults with primary immune deficiency (eg, specific antibody deficiency) have had severe outcomes,[80] but data are scarce in pediatrics.[81] Children and adolescents with COVID-19 and sickle cell disease often present with typical vasoocclusive crisis, but severe outcomes are rarely described.[82] Asthma has been noted to be prevalent in hospitalized children,[76,83] but whether it is an independent risk factor for COVID-19 is unclear.[84] Diabetes mellitus and chronic renal failure despite initial reports[85] have not been shown conclusively to be independent risk factors for severe disease in children.

THERAPEUTIC OPTIONS FOR COVID-19
Outpatient Care: Monoclonal Antibodies

Neutralizing antibodies target conserved epitopes on the SARS-CoV-2 spike protein located on the receptor-binding domain.[86] Currently available products include bamlanivimab/estevimab, casirivimab/imdevimab, and sotrovimab. Administered as a single dose infusion or subcutaneously (casirivimab/imdevimab), these products have been shown to decrease COVID-19–related hospitalizations and mortality in placebo-controlled trials in adults.[87,88] The magnitude of this reduction is sizable (approximately 70% relative reduction) when administered within a short window (72 hours) from diagnosis[86] and also correlates with biological endpoints like decreases in viral load.[74] Adverse events seem mostly limited to rare infusion reactions in adults (approximately 1%). The US Food and Drug Administration has issued an emergency use authorization for these agents in patients 12 years and over, weighing 40 kg or more, who are not hospitalized for COVID-19 and are at high risk for disease progression. Risk factors relevant to adolescents mentioned in these emergency use authorizations include obesity, immunosuppressive disease, chronic cardiac or pulmonary disease, neurodevelopmental delay, technology dependence, sickle cell disease, chronic renal disease, and diabetes.[87] The lower absolute risk, lack of accurate risk factor stratification, and the logistics of administration complicate pediatric use. Most hospitals have chosen a more targeted approach using local data to select subgroups at highest use within the current US Food and Drug Administration criteria.[89] A significant drawback with the use of these products is the evolution of viral variants (eg, those with L452R or E484K substitutions in the spike protein) with decreased susceptibility and clinicians should monitor the local distribution of variants before use.[90]

Inpatient Care: Antivirals—Remdesivir

Remdesivir, an RNA polymerase inhibitor, was previously studied for pediatric use in Ebola.[91] Data for efficacy in COVID-19 are drawn from an randomized controlled trial of 1062 adults where remdesivir decreased time to recovery compared with placebo (10 days vs 15 days; relative risk reduction, 1.29; 95% confidence interval, 1.12–1.49; $P < .001$), but showed no statistically significant difference in mortality by day 29. The benefit was greatest in patients randomized during the first 10 days after symptom onset and those requiring supplemental oxygen but not higher respiratory support (eg, mechanical ventilation) at enrollment (relative risk, 1.45; 95% confidence interval, 1.18–1.79).[92] Currently remdesivir is standard of care for adults who require supplemental oxygen in the United States, but other studies have demonstrated no impact on mortality and it is not currently recommended by the World Health Organization.[93,94] Remdesivir can be considered in children with new or worsening oxygen requirements in addition to supportive care alone, although data regarding efficacy and safety in children are lacking.[73] Equivalency has been demonstrated between 5- and 10-day courses in adults.[95] A pediatric-specific pharmacokinetic study is ongoing, but results are not available yet. Adverse events are rare and include elevated transaminases, transient gastrointestinal symptoms, and elevation of prothrombin levels.[96]

Agents with Presumed But Not Proven Antiviral Activity and Existing Pediatric Indications

Multiple large randomized controlled trials have failed to demonstrate an effect of azithromycin either alone or in combination with hydroxychloroquine to improve outcomes in hospitalized patients or outpatients with COVID-19.[97] Ivermectin and nitazoxanide are also agents with other pediatric indications that have been proposed for use in COVID-19, but have not yet shown any benefit.[74]

Glucocorticoid Therapy for Acute COVID-19

Evidence for glucocorticoid use comes from a large trial of 2104 adults who were randomized to receive dexamethasone 6 mg once per day for 10 days compared with 4321 patients randomized to usual care. Dexamethasone reduced deaths in ventilated patients (rate ratio, 0.65; 95% confidence interval, 0.48–0.88; $P = .0003$) and in patients receiving supplemental oxygen only (rate ratio, 0.80; 95% confidence interval, 0.67–0.96; $P = .0021$), but there was no benefit among those patients who did not require respiratory support.[98] A meta-analysis of the use of steroids for the treatment of acute COVID-19 showed a significant decrease in all-cause mortality (rate ratio, 0.65, 95% confidence interval, 0.50–0.82).[99] Corticosteroid are the primary immunomodulatory therapy in hypoxic children with severe acute COVID-19 requiring noninvasive positive pressure or mechanical ventilation.[67] Dexamethasone is commonly used at a dose of 0.15 mg/kg/dose (maximum of 6 mg) orally or intravenously every 24 hours for 10 days; alternate agents include hydrocortisone or methylprednisone.[98] Caution should be exercised in the setting of uncontrolled concurrent infections, hyperglycemia, delirium, or underlying psychiatric illness.

Glucocorticoid Therapy for Multisystem Inflammatory Syndrome in Children

For MIS-C, glucocorticoids are part of first-line therapy in a majority of centers, although others choose to reserve steroids for severe disease or as intensification therapy in patients with refractory disease.[100] Retrospective comparisons of intravenous immunoglobulin (IVIG) alone (first-line therapy for MIS-C) with IVIG with steroids have shown faster resolution of fever, improvement in cardiac function, and less of a requirement for sequential immunomodulators,[101,102] but outcome this has not been replicated consistently and the impact on long-term outcomes not fully known. The dosing of steroids is conditional on the severity of disease with typical dosing of IV methylprednisolone 1 to 2 mg/kg/d and the highest dosing (eg, methylprednisolone 10–30 mg/kg/d) usually reserved for children presenting with shock.[67]

Intravenous Immune Globulin for Multisystem Inflammatory Syndrome in Children

The use of IVIG as a first-line therapy for MIS-C evolved from its known efficacy in preventing coronary artery aneurysms in KD, the overlapping presentations of MIS-C with KD, and its potential effectiveness in non–SARS CoV-2 myocarditis.[67] The administration of IVIG is the primary treatment modality for MIS-C and is usually administered at a dose of 2 g/kg similar to use in KD.[67,103] Second doses of IVIG, although typically used for unresponsive KD, are not usually recommended for MIS-C.[67]

Second-line Immunomodulatory Therapy

Other immunomodulators can be considered in refractory cases or in the rare instance of contraindications to using steroids. Tocilizumab, an IL-6 inhibitor used to treat cytokine storm, has shown decreased mortality when added to steroids, for adults with rapidly increasing respiratory support and evidence of systemic inflammation.[104] In adults, baricitinib, an oral agent that inhibits Janus kinases 1 and 2, seems to have an impact on time to recovery when used along with remdesivir and can be considered in the rare instances of contraindications to steroid use or as an addition to standard of care.[105,106] Anakinra has not conclusively shown a benefit for adults with COVID-19 pneumonia,[107] but is the most accepted immunomodulatory therapy in MIS-C that is refractory to both IVIG and steroids.[67,103] Based on previous experience with KD, tumor necrosis factor-α blockade with infliximab can be considered as a potential therapeutic agent for those with a MIS-C phenotype that most closely resembles refractory KD.[103]

Supportive Care

Optimum ventilatory strategies for children with COVID-19 have not been defined, but trials of noninvasive support followed by lung-protective strategies that minimize acute respiratory distress syndrome are advised.[108] Consensus guidelines advise systemic anticoagulation with low-dose low-molecular-weight heparin for children hospitalized for COVID-19–related illness (including MIS-C) in the presence of markedly elevated D-dimer levels or other risk factors for hospital associated venous thromboembolism.[109] The rate of secondary infections in adults have been estimated to be

24%,[110] but is likely lower in children and antibiotic use should be minimized in the absence of known bacterial coinfection.

LONG-TERM OUTCOMES

The majority of children recover from COVID-19 without complications. Neonates born to pregnant mothers with COVID-19 have been reported to have small increases in adverse outcomes like respiratory complications, but perinatal transmission is rare.[111] Follow-up for children with MIS-C done at 6 months shows limited residual organ-specific sequalae.[112] Potential long-term effects, collectively known as postacute sequelae of SARS-CoV-2 infection, after an initial mild infection, is described in adults but accurate measures of the incidence of and therapeutic options for this entity in children are undefined and are the focus of ongoing work led by the National Institutes of Health.[113]

SUMMARY

COVID-19 has not spared children, and the manifestations of pediatric COVID-19 are diverse, ranging from mild upper respiratory tract infection to acute respiratory failure and MIS-C. Supportive care remains the mainstay of treatment for acute infection with the addition of antiviral and immunomodulatory therapy for the rare cases of severe infection.

DISCLOSURE

P. Zachariah has salary support from Pfizer.

REFERENCES

1. American Academy of Pediatrics. Children and COVID-19: state-level data report. 2021. Available at: https://services.aap.org/en/pages/2019-novel-coronavirus-covid-19-infections/children-and-covid-19-state-level-data-report/. Accessed November 6, 2021.
2. Pray IW, Gibbons-Burgener SN, Rosenberg AZ, et al. COVID-19 outbreak at an overnight summer school retreat - Wisconsin, July-August 2020. MMWR Morb Mortal Wkly Rep 2020;69(43):1600–4.
3. Falk A, Benda A, Falk P, et al. COVID-19 cases and transmission in 17 K-12 schools - Wood County, Wisconsin, August 31-November 29, 2020. MMWR Morb Mortal Wkly Rep 2021;70(4):136–40.
4. Viner RM, Mytton OT, Bonell C, et al. Susceptibility to SARS-CoV-2 infection among children and adolescents compared with adults: a systematic review and meta-analysis. JAMA Pediatr 2021;175(2):143–56.
5. Hershow RB, Wu K, Lewis NM, et al. Low SARS-CoV-2 transmission in elementary schools - Salt Lake County, Utah, December 3, 2020-January 31, 2021. MMWR Morb Mortal Wkly Rep 2021;70(12):442–8.
6. Bunyavanich S, Do A, Vicencio A. Nasal gene expression of angiotensin-converting enzyme 2 in children and adults. JAMA 2020;323(23):2427–9.
7. Pierce CA, Sy S, Galen B, et al. Natural mucosal barriers and COVID-19 in children. JCI Insight 2021;6(9):e1486911.
8. Poston D, Weisblum Y, Wise H, et al. Absence of SARS-CoV-2 neutralizing activity in pre-pandemic sera from individuals with recent seasonal coronavirus infection. Clin Infect Dis 2020.

9. Steinman JB, Lum FM, Ho PP, et al. Reduced development of COVID-19 in children reveals molecular checkpoints gating pathogenesis illuminating potential therapeutics. Proc Natl Acad Sci U S A 2020;117(40):24620–6.

10. Kim L, Whitaker M, O'Halloran A, et al. Hospitalization rates and characteristics of children aged <18 years hospitalized with laboratory-confirmed COVID-19 - COVID-NET, 14 States, March 1-July 25, 2020. MMWR Morb Mortal Wkly Rep 2020;69(32):1081–8.

11. Goyal MK, Simpson JN, Boyle MD, et al. Racial and/or ethnic and socioeconomic disparities of SARS-CoV-2 infection among children. Pediatrics 2020; 146(4). e2020009951.27.

12. Zachariah P, Johnson CL, Halabi KC, et al. Epidemiology, clinical features, and disease severity in patients with coronavirus disease 2019 (COVID-19) in a children's hospital in New York City, New York. JAMA Pediatr 2020;e202430.

13. DeBiasi RL, Song X, Delaney M, et al. Severe COVID-19 in children and young adults in the Washington, DC metropolitan region. J Pediatr 2020.

14. Center for Disease Control and Prevention. COVID-19 Pandemic Planning Scenarios. 2021. Available at: https://www.cdc.gov/coronavirus/2019-ncov/hcp/planning-scenarios.html. Accessed May 25, 2021.

15. Davies NG, Klepac P, Liu Y, et al. Age-dependent effects in the transmission and control of COVID-19 epidemics. Nat Med 2020;26(8):1205–11.

16. Hains DS, Schwaderer AL, Carroll AE, et al. Asymptomatic seroconversion of immunoglobulins to SARS-CoV-2 in a pediatric dialysis unit. JAMA 2020; 323(23):2424–5.

17. Fernandes DM, Oliveira CR, Guerguis S, et al. SARS-CoV-2 clinical syndromes and predictors of disease severity in hospitalized children and youth. J Pediatr 2020.

18. Zachariah P, Halabi KC, Johnson CL, et al. Symptomatic infants have higher nasopharyngeal SARS-CoV-2 viral loads but less severe disease than older children. Clin Infect Dis 2020;71(16):2305–6.

19. Paret M, Lighter J, Pellett Madan R, et al. Severe acute respiratory syndrome coronavirus 2 (SARS-CoV-2) infection in febrile infants without respiratory distress. Clin Infect Dis 2020;71(16):2243–5.

20. Feldstein LR, Rose EB, Horwitz SM, et al. Multisystem inflammatory syndrome in U.S. children and adolescents. N Engl J Med 2020;383(4):334–46.

21. Dufort EM, Koumans EH, Chow EJ, et al. Multisystem inflammatory syndrome in children in New York State. N Engl J Med 2020;383(4):347–58.

22. Belay ED, Abrams J, Oster ME, et al. Trends in geographic and temporal distribution of US children with multisystem inflammatory syndrome during the COVID-19 pandemic. JAMA Pediatr 2021.

23. Center for Disease Control and Prevention .A. Multisystem inflammatory syndrome in children (MIS-C) associated with coronavirus disease 2019 (COVID-19). 2021.

24. Godfred-Cato S, Bryant B, Leung J, et al. COVID-19-associated multisystem inflammatory syndrome in children - United States, March-July 2020. MMWR Morb Mortal Wkly Rep 2020;69(32):1074–80.

25. Lee PY, Day-Lewis M, Henderson LA, et al. Distinct clinical and immunological features of SARS-CoV-2-induced multisystem inflammatory syndrome in children. J Clin Invest 2020;130(11):5942–50.

26. Noval Rivas M, Porritt RA, Cheng MH, et al. COVID-19-associated multisystem inflammatory syndrome in children (MIS-C): a novel disease that mimics toxic

shock syndrome-the superantigen hypothesis. J Allergy Clin Immunol 2021; 147(1):57–9.

27. Vella LA, Giles JR, Baxter AE, et al. Deep immune profiling of MIS-C demonstrates marked but transient immune activation compared to adult and pediatric COVID-19. Sci Immunol 2021;6(57). eabf7570.47.

28. Rostad CA, Chahroudi A, Mantus G, et al. Quantitative SARS-CoV-2 serology in children with multisystem inflammatory syndrome (MIS-C). Pediatrics 2020; 146(6).

29. Swann OV, Holden KA, Turtle L, et al. Clinical characteristics of children and young people admitted to hospital with covid-19 in United Kingdom: prospective multicentre observational cohort study. BMJ 2020;370:m3249.

30. Shekerdemian LS, Mahmood NR, Wolfe KK, et al. Characteristics and outcomes of children with coronavirus disease 2019 (COVID-19) infection admitted to us and Canadian pediatric intensive care units. JAMA Pediatr 2020;174(9):868–73.

31. Leidman E, Duca LM, Omura JD, et al. COVID-19 trends among persons aged 0-24 years - United States, March 1-December 12, 2020. MMWR Morb Mortal Wkly Rep 2021;70(3):88–94.

32. Delahoy MJ, Ujamaa D, Whitaker M, et al. Hospitalizations associated with COVID-19 among children and adolescents - COVID-NET, 14 States, March 1, 2020-August 14, 2021. MMWR Morb Mortal Wkly Rep 2021;70(36):1255–60.

33. Viner RM, Ward JL, Hudson LD, et al. Systematic review of reviews of symptoms and signs of COVID-19 in children and adolescents. Arch Dis Child 2020.

34. Loron G, Tromeur T, Venot P, et al. COVID-19 associated with life-threatening APNEA in an infant born preterm: a case report. Front Pediatr 2020;8:568.

35. Derespina KR, Kaushik S, Plichta A, et al. Clinical manifestations and outcomes of critically ill children and adolescents with coronavirus disease 2019 in New York City. J Pediatr 2020.

36. Duarte-Neto AN, Caldini EG, Gomes-Gouvea MS, et al. An autopsy study of the spectrum of severe COVID-19 in children: from SARS to different phenotypes of MIS-C. EClinicalMedicine 2021;35:100850.

37. Van Brusselen D, De Troeyer K, Ter Haar E, et al. Bronchiolitis in COVID-19 times: a nearly absent disease? Eur J Pediatr 2021;180(6):1969–73.

38. Sheehan WJ, Patel SJ, Margolis RHF, et al. Pediatric asthma exacerbations during the COVID-19 pandemic: absence of the typical fall seasonal spike in Washington, DC. J Allergy Clin Immunol Pract 2021;9(5):2073–6.

39. Yonker LM, Gilboa T, Ogata AF, et al. Multisystem inflammatory syndrome in children is driven by zonulin-dependent loss of gut mucosal barrier. J Clin Invest 2021.

40. Giovanni JE, Hrapcak S, Melgar M, et al. Global reports of intussusception in infants with SARS-CoV-2 infection. Pediatr Infect Dis J 2021;40(1):e35–6.

41. Miller J, Cantor A, Zachariah P, et al. Gastrointestinal symptoms as a major presentation component of a novel multisystem inflammatory syndrome in children that is related to coronavirus disease 2019: a single center experience of 44 cases. Gastroenterology 2020;159(4):1571–4.e1572.

42. Dolhnikoff M, Ferreira Ferranti J, de Almeida Monteiro RA, et al. SARS-CoV-2 in cardiac tissue of a child with COVID-19-related multisystem inflammatory syndrome. Lancet Child Adolesc Health 2020;4(10):790–4.

43. Valverde I, Singh Y, Sanchez-de-Toledo J, et al. Acute cardiovascular manifestations in 286 children with multisystem inflammatory syndrome associated with COVID-19 infection in Europe. Circulation 2021;143(1):21–32.

44. LaRovere KL, Riggs BJ, Poussaint TY, et al. neurologic involvement in children and adolescents hospitalized in the United States for COVID-19 or multisystem inflammatory syndrome. JAMA Neurol 2021;78(5):536–47.

45. Verkuil LD, Liu GT, Brahma VL, et al. Pseudotumor cerebri syndrome associated with MIS-C: a case report. Lancet (London, England) 2020;396(10250):532.

46. Lin JE, Asfour A, Sewell TB, et al. Neurological issues in children with COVID-19. Neurosci Lett 2021;743:135567.

47. Appavu B, Deng D, Dowling MM, et al. Arteritis and large vessel occlusive strokes in children after COVID-19 infection. Pediatrics 2021;147(3). e202002344049.

48. Thakur KT, Miller EH, Glendinning MD, et al. COVID-19 neuropathology at Columbia University Irving Medical Center/New York Presbyterian Hospital. Brain 2021.

49. Kumar G, Pillai S, Norwick P, et al. Leucocytoclastic vasculitis secondary to COVID-19 infection in a young child. BMJ Case Rep 2021;14(4).

50. Young TK, Shaw KS, Shah JK, et al. Mucocutaneous manifestations of multisystem inflammatory syndrome in children during the COVID-19 pandemic. JAMA Dermatol 2021;157(2):207–12.

51. Whitworth HB, Sartain SE, Kumar R, et al. Rate of thrombosis in children and adolescents hospitalized with COVID-19 or MIS-C. Blood 2021.

52. Naguib MN, Raymond JK, Vidmar AP. New onset diabetes with diabetic ketoacidosis in a child with multisystem inflammatory syndrome due to COVID-19. J Pediatr Endocrinol Metab 2021;34(1):147–50.

53. Alonso GT, Ebekozien O, Gallagher MP, et al. Diabetic ketoacidosis drives COVID-19 related hospitalizations in children with type 1 diabetes. J Diabetes 2021.

54. Deep A, Upadhyay G, du Pre P, et al. Acute kidney injury in pediatric inflammatory multisystem syndrome temporally associated with severe acute respiratory syndrome coronavirus-2 pandemic: experience from PICUs across United Kingdom. Crit Care Med 2020;48(12):1809–18.

55. Center for Disease Control and Prevention. A. Interim Guidance for Antigen Testing for SARS-CoV-2. Available at: https://www.cdc.gov/coronavirus/2019-ncov/lab/resources/antigen-tests-guidelines.html. Accessed November 11, 2021.

56. Hanson KE, Caliendo AM, Arias CA, et al. The Infectious Diseases Society of America guidelines on the diagnosis of COVID-19: molecular diagnostic testing. Clin Infect Dis 2021.

57. Truong TT, Ryutov A, Pandey U, et al. Increased viral variants in children and young adults with impaired humoral immunity and persistent SARS-CoV-2 infection: a consecutive case series. EBioMedicine 2021;67:103355.

58. Centers for Disease Control and Prevention. Information for healthcare providers about multisystem inflammatory syndrome in children (MIS-C). 2021. Available at: https://www.cdc.gov/mis-c/hcp/. Accessed March 26, 2021.

59. Fajnzylber J, Regan J, Coxen K, et al. SARS-CoV-2 viral load is associated with increased disease severity and mortality. Nat Commun 2020;11(1):5493.

60. Kociolek LK, Muller WJ, Yee R, et al. Comparison of upper respiratory viral load distributions in asymptomatic and symptomatic children diagnosed with SARS-CoV-2 infection in pediatric hospital testing programs. J Clin Microbiol 2020; 59(1). e02593–20.

61. Hurst JH, Heston SM, Chambers HN, et al. SARS-CoV-2 infections among children in the biospecimens from respiratory virus-exposed kids (BRAVE Kids) study. Clin Infect Dis 2020.

62. Rhoads D, Peaper DR, She RC, et al. College of American Pathologists (CAP) Microbiology committee perspective: caution must be used in interpreting the cycle threshold (Ct) value. Clin Infect Dis 2021;72(10):e685–6.

63. Dworsky ZD, Roberts JE, Son MBF, et al. Mistaken MIS-C: a case series of bacterial enteritis mimicking MIS-C. Pediatr Infect Dis J 2021;40(4):e159–61.

64. Jin H, Moss R, Reed JC, et al. IFN-gamma receptor 2 deficiency initial mimicry of multisystem inflammatory syndrome in children (MIS-C). J Allergy Clin Immunol Pract 2021;9(2):989–92.e1.

65. Whittaker E, Bamford A, Kenny J, et al. Clinical characteristics of 58 children with a pediatric inflammatory multisystem syndrome temporally associated with SARS-CoV-2. JAMA 2020;324(3):259–69.

66. Carlin RF, Fischer AM, Pitkowsky Z, et al. Discriminating multisystem inflammatory syndrome in children requiring treatment from common febrile conditions in outpatient settings. J Pediatr 2021;229:26–32.e2.

67. Henderson LA, Canna SW, Friedman KG, et al. American College of Rheumatology Clinical guidance for multisystem inflammatory syndrome in children associated with SARS-CoV-2 and hyperinflammation in pediatric COVID-19: version 2. Arthritis Rheumatol 2021;73(4):e13–29.

68. Abrams JY, Oster ME, Godfred-Cato SE, et al. Factors linked to severe outcomes in multisystem inflammatory syndrome in children (MIS-C) in the USA: a retrospective surveillance study. Lancet Child Adolescent Health 2021;5(5):323–31.

69. Graff K, Smith C, Silveira L, et al. Risk factors for severe COVID-19 in children. Pediatr Infect Dis J 2021;40(4):e137–45.

70. Beck DB, Aksentijevich I. Susceptibility to severe COVID-19. Science 2020;370(6515):404–5.

71. Diorio C, Henrickson SE, Vella LA, et al. Multisystem inflammatory syndrome in children and COVID-19 are distinct presentations of SARS-CoV-2. J Clin Invest 2020;130(11):5967–75.

72. Chiotos K, Hayes M, Kimberlin DW, et al. Multicenter interim guidance on use of antivirals for children with COVID-19/SARS-CoV-2. J Pediatr Infect Dis Soc 2020.

73. Chiotos K, Hayes M, Kimberlin DW, et al. Multicenter interim guidance on use of antivirals for children with coronavirus disease 2019/severe acute respiratory syndrome coronavirus 2. J Pediatr Infect Dis Soc 2021;10(1):34–48.

74. National Institutes of Health. COVID-19 guidelines. Available at: https://www.covid19treatmentguidelines.nih.gov/tables/table-3a/. Accessed May 30, 2021.

75. Bhimraj AMR, Shumaker AH, Lavergne V, et al. Infectious Diseases Society of America Guidelines on the Treatment and Management of Patients with COVID-19. Infectious Diseases Society of America 2021; Version 4.3.0. Available at: https://www.idsociety.org/practice-guideline/covid-19-guideline-treatment-and-management/. Accessed May 31, 2021.

76. DeBiasi RL, Song X, Delaney M, et al. Severe coronavirus disease-2019 in children and young adults in the Washington, DC, Metropolitan Region. J Pediatr 2020;223:199–203.e191.

77. Boulad F, Kamboj M, Bouvier N, et al. COVID-19 in children with cancer in New York City. JAMA Oncol 2020;6(9):1459–60.

78. Madhusoodhan PP, Pierro J, Musante J, et al. Characterization of COVID-19 disease in pediatric oncology patients: the New York-New Jersey regional experience. Pediatr Blood Cancer 2020;e28843.

79. Goss MB, Galvan NTN, Ruan W, et al. The pediatric solid organ transplant experience with COVID-19: an initial multi-center, multi-organ case series. Pediatr Transpl 2020;e13868.

80. Meyts I, Bucciol G, Quinti I, et al. Coronavirus disease 2019 in patients with inborn errors of immunity: an international study. J Allergy Clin Immunol 2021; 147(2):520–31.

81. Shields AM, Burns SO, Savic S, et al. COVID-19 in patients with primary and secondary immunodeficiency: the United Kingdom experience. J Allergy Clin Immunol 2021;147(3):870–5.e1.

82. Appiah-Kubi A, Acharya S, Fein Levy C, et al. Varying presentations and favourable outcomes of COVID-19 infection in children and young adults with sickle cell disease: an additional case series with comparisons to published cases. Br J Haematol 2020.

83. Chao JY, Derespina KR, Herold BC, et al. Clinical characteristics and outcomes of hospitalized and critically Ill children and adolescents with coronavirus disease 2019 at a tertiary care medical center in New York City. J Pediatr 2020; 223:14–9.e12.

84. Lovinsky-Desir S, Deshpande DR, De A, et al. Asthma among hospitalized patients with COVID-19 and related outcomes. J Allergy Clin Immunol 2020;146(5): 1027–34.e4.

85. Kompaniyets L, Agathis NT, Nelson JM, et al. Underlying medical conditions associated with severe COVID-19 illness among children. JAMA Netw Open 2021;4(6):e2111182.

86. Weinreich DM, Sivapalasingam S, Norton T, et al. REGEN-COV antibody combination and outcomes in outpatients with Covid-19. N Engl J Med 2021.

87. Food and Drug Administration. Fact sheet for healthcare providers- Emergency use authorization of Sotrovimab. Available at: https://www.fda.gov/media/149534/download. Accessed July 12, 2021.

88. Food and Drug Administration. Fact sheet for healthcare providers. Emergency use authorization of Bamlanivimab and Etesevimab. Available at: https://www.fda.gov/media/145802/download. Accessed October 23, 2021.

89. Wolf J, Abzug MJ, Wattier RL, et al. Initial guidance on use of monoclonal antibody therapy for treatment of COVID-19 in children and adolescents. J Pediatr Infect Dis Soc 2021.

90. Prevention CfDCa. SARS-CoV-2 Variant Classifications and Definitions. 2021. Available at: https://www.cdc.gov/coronavirus/2019-ncov/variants/variant-info.html. Accessed May 30, 2021.

91. Mulangu S, Dodd LE, Davey RT Jr, et al. A randomized, controlled trial of Ebola virus disease therapeutics. N Engl J Med 2019;381(24):2293–303.

92. Beigel JH, Tomashek KM, Dodd LE, et al. Remdesivir for the treatment of Covid-19 - Final report. N Engl J Med 2020;383(19):1813–26.

93. WHO Consortium, Pan H, Peto R, et al. Repurposed antiviral drugs for Covid-19 - Interim WHO solidarity trial results. N Engl J Med 2021;384(6):497–511.

94. Rochwerg B, Agarwal A, Siemieniuk RA, et al. A living WHO guideline on drugs for covid-19. BMJ 2020;370:m3379.

95. Goldman JD, Lye DCB, Hui DS, et al. Remdesivir for 5 or 10 days in patients with severe Covid-19. N Engl J Med 2020;383(19):1827–37.

96. Administration FaD. Factsheet for healthcare providers on remdesivir for pediatric patients 2021.

97. Group RC. Azithromycin in patients admitted to hospital with COVID-19 (RE-COVERY): a randomised, controlled, open-label, platform trial. Lancet (London, England) 2021;397(10274):605–12.

98. Group RC, Horby P, Lim WS, et al. Dexamethasone in hospitalized patients with Covid-19. N Engl J Med 2021;384(8):693–704.

99. Group WHOREAfC-TW, Sterne JAC, Murthy S, et al. Association between administration of systemic corticosteroids and mortality among critically ill patients with COVID-19: a meta-analysis. JAMA 2020;324(13):1330–41.

100. Dove ML, Jaggi P, Kelleman M, et al. Multisystem inflammatory syndrome in children: survey of protocols for early hospital evaluation and management. J Pediatr 2021;229:33–40.

101. Ouldali N, Toubiana J, Antona D, et al. Association of intravenous immunoglobulins plus methylprednisolone vs immunoglobulins alone with course of fever in multisystem inflammatory syndrome in children. JAMA 2021;325(9):855–64.

102. Son MBF, Murray N, Friedman K, et al. Multisystem inflammatory syndrome in children - initial therapy and outcomes. N Engl J Med 2021;385(1):23–34.

103. Harwood R, Allin B, Jones CE, et al. A national consensus management pathway for paediatric inflammatory multisystem syndrome temporally associated with COVID-19 (PIMS-TS): results of a national Delphi process. Lancet Child Adolescent Health 2021;5(2):133–41.

104. Investigators R-C, Gordon AC, Mouncey PR, et al. Interleukin-6 receptor antagonists in critically ill patients with Covid-19. N Engl J Med 2021;384(16):1491–502.

105. Kalil AC, Patterson TF, Mehta AK, et al. Baricitinib plus remdesivir for hospitalized adults with Covid-19. N Engl J Med 2021;384(9):795–807.

106. Marconi VC, Ramanan AV, de Bono S, et al. Efficacy and safety of baricitinib for the treatment of hospitalised adults with COVID-19 (COV-BARRIER): a randomised, double-blind, parallel-group, placebo-controlled phase 3 trial. Lancet Respir Med 2021.

107. group C-C. Effect of anakinra versus usual care in adults in hospital with COVID-19 and mild-to-moderate pneumonia (CORIMUNO-ANA-1): a randomised controlled trial. Lancet Respir Med 2021;9(3):295–304.

108. Blumenthal JA, Duvall MG. Invasive and noninvasive ventilation strategies for acute respiratory failure in children with coronavirus disease 2019. Curr Opin Pediatr 2021;33(3):311–8.

109. Goldenberg NA, Sochet A, Albisetti M, et al. Consensus-based clinical recommendations and research priorities for anticoagulant thromboprophylaxis in children hospitalized for COVID-19-related illness. J Thromb Haemost 2020;18(11):3099–105.

110. Musuuza JS, Watson L, Parmasad V, et al. Prevalence and outcomes of co-infection and superinfection with SARS-CoV-2 and other pathogens: a systematic review and meta-analysis. PLoS One 2021;16(5):e0251170.

111. Norman M, Naver L, Soderling J, et al. Association of maternal SARS-CoV-2 infection in pregnancy with neonatal outcomes. JAMA 2021;325(20):2076–86.

112. Penner J, Abdel-Mannan O, Grant K, et al. 6-month multidisciplinary follow-up and outcomes of patients with paediatric inflammatory multisystem syndrome (PIMS-TS) at a UK tertiary paediatric hospital: a retrospective cohort study. Lancet Child Adolescent Health 2021.

113. National Institutes of Health. RECOVER: researching COVID to Enhance Recovery. Available at: https://recovercovid.org/. Accessed November 7, 2021.

Infection Prevention during the Coronavirus Disease 2019 Pandemic

Patrick Reich, MD, MSCI*, Alexis Elward, MD, MPH

KEYWORDS

- COVID-19 • SARS-CoV-2 • Coronavirus • Infection prevention • Epidemiology
- Transmission • Personal protective equipment • Public health

KEY POINTS

- Cases of COVID-19, a nonspecific viral infection caused by the novel coronavirus SARS-CoV-2, were first identified in Wuhan, China, in December 2019 and led to an ongoing global pandemic.
- Transmission is primarily human-to-human via contact with respiratory particles containing infectious virus.
- The risk of transmission to health care personnel is low with proper use of personal protective equipment, including gowns, gloves, N95 or surgical mask, and eye protection.
- Additional important measures to decrease the risk of transmission include physical distancing, hand hygiene, routine cleaning and disinfection, and appropriate air handling and ventilation.
- Public health interventions, including universal masking, stay-at-home orders, and other mitigation strategies, are effective at decreasing transmission rates.

BACKGROUND AND EPIDEMIOLOGY

In December 2019 a cluster of cases of pneumonia of unclear etiology was identified in Wuhan, Hubei Province, China. Evidence from the initial cases suggested a link with exposures at a local seafood market; however, this association waned over time and clear evidence of person-to-person transmission emerged.[1,2] The etiologic agent was identified to be a novel human betacoronavirus subsequently named severe acute respiratory syndrome coronavirus 2 (SARS-CoV-2) and the clinical disease was named coronavirus disease 2019 (COVID-19).[3,4] Other epidemic coronaviruses have contributed to significant outbreaks in the recent past, although on a much smaller scale compared with SARS-CoV-2. The initial severe acute respiratory syndrome

Department of Pediatrics, Division of Pediatric Infectious Diseases, Washington University School of Medicine, 660 S. Euclid Avenue, Campus Box 8116, St Louis, MO 63110-1093, USA
* Corresponding author.
E-mail address: patrickjreich@wustl.edu

Infect Dis Clin N Am 36 (2022) 15–37
https://doi.org/10.1016/j.idc.2021.12.002
0891-5520/22/© 2021 Elsevier Inc. All rights reserved.
id.theclinics.com

(SARS) outbreak caused by SARS-associated coronavirus (SARS-CoV) occurred from 2002 to 2003 and caused 8096 cases in 29 countries, with an overall case fatality ratio of 9.6%. Early on during the COVID-19 pandemic, many recommendations were extrapolated from experience from the SARS pandemic and other epidemic respiratory viral infections.[5,6] Cases of Middle East respiratory syndrome coronavirus (MERS-CoV) have been identified in 27 countries since 2012, with an overall case fatality ratio of 35%.[7] The SARS-CoV-2 outbreak quickly developed into a widespread global pandemic, with more than 250,000,000 cases and 5 million deaths worldwide.[8]

CLINICAL MANIFESTATIONS AND OUTCOMES

Despite accounting for approximately 22% of the population in the United States, children younger than 18 represent a minority of COVID-19 cases (12.4%), hospitalizations (1.6%), and related deaths (0.1%) diagnosed in the United States.[9–11] COVID-19–associated hospitalization rates are lower in pediatric patients than adults; approximately 2.5% of children and young adults with COVID-19 require hospitalization compared with 16.6% of adults.[12] The most common comorbidities in hospitalized patients with COVID-19 include hypertension, obesity, diabetes, chronic lung disease, and prematurity.[12–15] The estimated case fatality ratio is as high as 1.8% to 7.2%, with increasing mortality rates in increasing age brackets.[14–16] COVID-19–related deaths are rare in children (<0.1% of COVID-19 cases) compared with 5% in adults, with increasing mortality rates in adults every decade after age 25.[10,12,17]

Perinatal infection is rare, indeed 2.6% of infants born to mothers with laboratory-confirmed COVID-19 at the time of delivery who were tested had positive SARS-CoV-2 testing.[18] To date, definitive evidence of intrauterine transmission of SARS-CoV-2 from mother to infant has not been confirmed.[19]

Multisystem inflammatory syndrome in children (MIS-C) is a hyper inflammatory condition with features similar to Kawasaki disease and toxic shock syndrome, which has been seen approximately 2 to 4 weeks after acute COVID-19 infection in children. Presenting features include shock, cardiac dysfunction, gastrointestinal symptoms (abdominal pain, vomiting, diarrhea), elevated inflammatory markers, rash, mucocutaneous involvement, and positive polymerase chain reaction (PCR) or antibody testing for SARS-CoV-2. Treatment typically includes intravenous immune globulin with or without antiplatelet/anticoagulant medications and additional immunomodulatory agents.[20]

Meta-analyses demonstrated that 16% to 19% of pediatric patients and 17% of adults with COVID-19 are asymptomatic.[21–23] A meta-analysis including 67 studies with 8302 adult and pediatric patients demonstrated that fever and cough are the most common manifestations in pediatric and adult patients (**Table 1**); however, symptoms differed in adults and children, with fever (69% vs 44%), cough (53% vs 33%), and dyspnea (20% vs 4%) more common among adult patients compared with pediatric patients.[24]

REPRODUCTIVE NUMBER AND SECONDARY ATTACK RATE FOR SEVERE ACUTE RESPIRATORY SYNDROME CORONAVIRUS 2

The estimated reproductive number (R_0) represents the average number of secondary infections from an index case in a susceptible population.[4] The R_0 from analysis of the first 425 patients with confirmed COVID-19 in Wuhan, China, was 2.2 and review of 12 studies estimated the mean R_0 to be 3.28 and the median 2.79.[2,25] These estimates reflect transmission early on during the pandemic (through January 2020) before detection of variants of concern. In comparison, the median R_0 for seasonal influenza

Table 1		
Clinical manifestations of adult and pediatric patients with coronavirus disease 2019		
Manifestation	**Pediatric, %[21,23,24]**	**Adult, %[22,24]**
Asymptomatic	16–19	17
Fever	44–57	69
Cough	33–44	53
Dyspnea	4–15	20
Rhinorrhea	13–16	13
Diarrhea	10–12	9
Nausea/vomiting	9–11	8
Headache	10–13	19
Sore throat	8–14	18
Nasal congestion	9	26
Abdominal pain	6–8	Not reported
Fatigue	6–9	31
Myalgias	5–14	Not reported
Anosmia	4	38

Data from Refs.[21–24]

is 1.28, 1.46 for the 2009 H1N1 influenza epidemic, and 1.80 for the 1918 influenza pandemic.[26]

In the pre-vaccine era, the secondary attack rate, or proportion of susceptible individuals who acquire COVID-19 after exposure, varied with the setting. A systematic review and meta-analysis including 43 studies found a pooled secondary attack rate among household contacts of 18.1%, ranging from 3.9% to 54.9%.[27] Variable attack rates were seen in nonhousehold, non–health care settings, ranging from 0% to 5.8% in larger studies (with >1000 contacts).[27] In comparison the estimated household secondary attack rates for 2009 H1N1 influenza epidemic ranged from 8% to 19%.[28] Secondary attack rates for selected pathogens transmitted via an airborne route include 90% for measles and 85% for varicella.[29,30]

TRANSMISSION

The median incubation period for SARS-CoV-2 is estimated to be 5 days. More than 95% of people develop symptoms within approximately 12 days after exposure and there is a low likelihood of symptomatic infections developing after 14 days.[2,31]

The first documented case of person-to-person transmission of SARS-CoV-2 in the United States involved the spouse of a returning traveler from Wuhan, China.[1] Initial concepts regarding transmission of SARS-CoV-2 were drawn from experience during the original 2003 SARS epidemic, where peak infectiousness occurred 7 to 10 days after symptom onset.[32] However, reports of asymptomatic and more commonly pre-symptomatic transmission quickly emerged,[32–34] including evidence of person-to-person transmission during the pre-symptomatic phase and from fully asymptomatic individuals.[35,36] Approximately 44% of secondary cases were attributed to exposures during the pre-symptomatic stage of index cases, with the period of peak infectiousness extending from 2 days before symptom onset through 1 day after symptom onset.[32] High viral loads have been detected in the nasopharynx/oropharynx during the first week of symptoms, with peak viral loads demonstrated on day 4 of symptoms, and a decline over time.[37–39]

AIRBORNE VERSUS DROPLET

The classic distinction is between large (>5 μm) respiratory droplets, which travel up to 3 to 6 feet from the source and then fall to the ground or another surface and airborne particles known as aerosols, which are tiny (≤5 μm), and may remain suspended in the air for extended periods of time and travel greater distances.[40] Examples of pathogens transmitted primarily via large respiratory droplets include influenza, seasonal human coronaviruses, and many other respiratory viral pathogens. Measles and varicella are classic examples of viruses transmitted via an airborne route. The distinction between these 2 forms of transmission is critical to inform appropriate personal protective equipment (PPE) recommendations for health care personnel (HCP); specifically N95 respirators or equivalent are recommended to prevent transmission of airborne pathogens because tiny aerosols are not adequately filtered by isolation/surgical masks. In addition, 3 to 6 feet of physical distancing and/or surgical masks would not prevent transmission of aerosols via an airborne route, but would interrupt transmission of large respiratory droplets.[41–43] However, individuals generate droplets and aerosols of varying sizes that can travel distances greater than 6 feet, and transmission risk may be higher in crowded indoor environments, particularly those with poor ventilation.[43]

This dichotomy between respiratory droplet and aerosol/airborne transmission likely represents an oversimplification and does not solely define or adequately explain viral transmission risk.[44] Contributing to confusion surrounding this subject, terminology including airborne particles, aerosols, and droplets may be interpreted differently by infection prevention specialists and aerobiologists.[44] Additional factors determining transmission risk to an individual after exposure include the viral burden in the source, environment including ventilation, conditions surrounding the exposure including route and duration, inoculum size, host factors, and PPE use.[41,44]

SARS-CoV-2 has been detected by PCR in air samples from patient rooms and other areas of acute care hospitals during the COVID-19 pandemic,[45–47] raising the possibility of airborne transmission. In experimental models, SARS-CoV-2 remained stable in generated aerosols for 3 hours.[48] Increased transmission risk of SARS has been associated with selected aerosol-generating procedures (AGPs), including tracheal intubation, noninvasive ventilation, tracheotomy, and manual ventilation before intubation, with tracheal intubation consistently identified across multiple studies.[49] Thus AGPs carry additional risk of airborne transmission of aerosols containing SARS-CoV-2.

List of AGPs adapted from Centers for Disease Control and Prevention (CDC) and World Health Organization (WHO) guidance:

- Open suctioning of airways
- Sputum induction (using nebulized hypertonic saline)
- Cardiopulmonary resuscitation
- Endotracheal intubation and extubation
- Noninvasive ventilation (eg, bilevel positive airway pressure, continuous positive airway pressure)
- Bronchoscopy
- Manual ventilation (including before intubation)
- Tracheotomy
- Autopsy procedures

- Based on available data, it is unclear whether aerosols generated from the following procedures are infectious:
  - Nebulizer administration
  - High flow oxygen delivery[50,51]

SPECIFIC SCENARIOS OF CONCERN
Restaurant with Poor Ventilation

Nine individuals from 3 families who dined at adjacent tables in the same restaurant developed COVID-19. No infections were identified in restaurants staff or diners at other tables in the restaurant. All 5 secondary cases in the other 2 families were separated from the index case by more than 1 m, and poor ventilation in the restaurant (0.56–0.77 air changes per hour) was identified as a potential contributing factor.[52]

Cruise Ships

Outbreaks on cruise ships were associated with high transmission rates; 19.2% of passengers and crew on the Diamond Princess had positive SARS-CoV-2 testing, 16.6% on the Grand Princess.[53]

Singing/Choir Practice

Of 61 individuals who attended a 2.5-hour choir practice where 1 person was known to be symptomatic, 33 confirmed cases and 20 probable cases were identified. This represents a secondary attack rate of 53.3% for confirmed cases and 86.7% for confirmed and suspected cases, suggesting the possibility of a superspreader event at the choir practice.[54]

Religious Services

Following exposure at various church events over a 6-day period, 38% of the 92 attendees developed COVID-19.[55]

Homeless Shelters

High SARS-CoV-2 prevalence has been identified among residents of homeless shelters. In 1 study from 19 homeless shelters in 4 US cities, 25% of residents tested positive, with a range of 4% to 66% at each individual shelter.[56]

Overnight Camp

Of 597 campers and staff who attended an overnight summer camp in Georgia where masking was not required for campers and building windows and doors were not opened for ventilation, the attack rate was 44%.[57]

IMPACT OF SUPPLY CHAIN

Global shortages of medical supplies, including PPE such as N95s, necessitated the development of allocation and prioritization strategies for the judicious use of scarce resources.[58] Many hospitals experienced critical shortages of respirators, surgical masks, gowns, gloves, and eye coverings, and therefore implemented extended use of masks/respirators, reprocessing of respirators, extended use or reuse of gowns, and sometimes self-production of PPE, such as eye protection, masks, and gowns. Ethical guidance regarding PPE optimization strategies, COVID-19 therapeutics, patient triaged, and visitor policies were provided to many health care facilities by local institutions, states, and professional organizations.[59]

Based on the scarce supply and availability of N95 or equivalent respirators, the CDC provided recommendations, including extended use and limited reuse of N95 respirators beyond the manufacturer recommendations. In addition, in the setting of critical supply shortages, the CDC recommends prioritization of N95 respirators or equivalent for HCP with the highest risk potential exposures, specifically being present in the room with a patients with COVID-19 undergoing an AGP. Engineering controls, such as the addition of portable high-efficiency particulate air (HEPA) filtration devices, also can be considered.[60]

As a result, many health care institutions implemented a risk-stratified approach for patients with known or suspected COVID-19 whereby N95 respirators or equivalent were recommended during care of patients with confirmed or suspected COVID-19 undergoing AGP, whereas surgical masks or N95 respirators or the equivalent were appropriate for patients not undergoing AGP.[42,59] Most health care facilities that responded to a survey through the Society for Healthcare Epidemiology of America Research Network recommended that HCP wear an N95 respirator or equivalent for patients with confirmed or suspected COVID-19 undergoing higher-risk AGP, including intubation and extubation, as well as for ear, nose, and throat procedures and other procedures of the airway/respiratory tract.[59]

TRANSMISSION TO HEALTH CARE PROVIDERS

Across varying populations, the overall risk of SARS-CoV-2 transmission was low, ranging from 0.9% to 7.0% (**Table 2**). A systematic review and meta-analysis including 18 studies found an estimated secondary attack rate of 0.7% in the health care setting.[27]

EXPOSURE SOURCE AND SETTING

Identified HCP exposure sources were variable, with 55% to 59% in the health care setting, 13% to 27% in the community/household setting, and 5% to 13% with exposures in multiple settings.[62,68] Among health care setting exposures, contact with patients (63%) or colleagues with COVID-19 (31%) were the most common identified sources.[61] HCP with SARS-CoV-2 exposures from household or social contacts had the highest positivity rate. Higher-risk exposures and HCP COVID-19 infections were seen most commonly among nursing assistants/patient care aides (32%–40%) and nursing staff (30%), and occurred most often during direct patient care (66%).[65,69] Factors associated with transmission to HCPs included performing physical examinations and presence in the room during AGPs; longer estimated time in the patient's room may also play a role.[70] HCPs working in congregate living, long-term care, or nursing/residential care facilities were more likely to acquire COVID-19 than HCPs working in an acute care setting.[65,69] However, this may in part be impacted by relative PPE use because HCPs in the acute and ambulatory care setting were more likely than those in the congregate living or long-term care setting to wear masks (83% vs 62%) and eye protection (26% vs 16%).[65]

Interestingly, in a study among 336 active duty military personnel deployed to a field hospital with strict infection prevention measures in place, 1.7% developed COVID-19; infection rates were lower in those who provided direct care to COVID-19 patients (0.9%). The military personnel had continual donning and doffing observation with assistance and wore N95 respirators, eye protection, gowns, gloves, and gowns during patient care. The military personnel stayed in single-occupancy rooms at local hotels and were encouraged by the military chain of command to remain in their hotel room as much as possible.[64] Taken as a whole, these data suggest that the risk of

Table 2
Severe acute respiratory syndrome coronavirus 2 attack rate in health care personnel

Study	Dates	Setting	Sample Size	Attack Rate, %	Miscellaneous
Wang et al,[61] 2020	December 2019–March 2020	China	5442	2.2	All enrolled and tested
Lai et al,[62] 2020	January–February 2020	China	9684	1.1	0.7% of 335 randomly selected asymptomatic HCP tested positive
Kluytmans-van den Bergh et al,[63] 2020	March 2020	Netherlands	9705	1	6.4% of 1353 tested due to development of symptoms tested positive
Clifton et al,[64] 2021	March–April 2020	US army personnel	336	1.7	All enrolled and tested, 2 PCR+, 5 Ab+, 1 both+
Fell et al,[65] 2020	March–July 2020	US	5374	7%	All with higher-risk exposures (household/ workplace)
Self et al,[66] 2020	April–June 2020	US seroprevalence study	3248	6	All enrolled and tested (serology)
Shah et al,[67] 2021	May–November 2020	United States	345	2.3	All with significant occupational exposure to a COVID-19 patient
Koh et al,[27] 2020	January–July 2020	China, United States, Germany, India, Japan, Singapore, Switzerland	4163	0.7	Systematic review and meta-analysis of 18 studies

Abbreviations: Ab, antibody; COVID-19, coronavirus disease 2019; HCP, health care provider; PCR, polymerase chain reaction.
Data from Refs.[27,61–67]

SARS-CoV-2 transmission to HCPs wearing appropriate PPE during patient care is low, and that exposures outside the workplace also play an important role in transmission risk to HCP.

PERSONAL PROTECTIVE EQUIPMENT EFFICACY
Experimental Data

Experimental studies have demonstrated that face coverings are highly effective forms of source control, specifically hospital-grade surgical masks provide a 94% reduction in respiratory droplet particle concentration when used as source control, N95 respirators provide a 95% reduction, and cloth face coverings provide a 77% reduction.[71]

Health Care Setting: Other Viruses

A systematic review of interventions to reduce or prevent transmission of respiratory viral pathogens demonstrated that frequent hand hygiene, wearing masks including N95s, wearing gowns, and wearing gloves were all associated with decreased risk of SARS transmission with a 91% effectiveness and number needed to treat of 3 for the combination of hand hygiene, masks, gowns, and gloves.[72]

A meta-analysis of 4 randomized controlled trials comparing the protective effect of medical masks to N95 respirators in HCPs, which included influenza, SARS, and seasonal human coronaviruses, but not SARS-CoV-2, showed no difference in the incidence of laboratory-confirmed viral respiratory infections or clinical respiratory illnesses.[73]

Health Care Setting: Severe Acute Respiratory Syndrome Coronavirus 2

In a systematic review and meta-analysis including 44 comparator studies evaluating the risk of person-to-person transmission of SARS-CoV-2, SARS, and MERS, physical distancing of at least 1 m, wearing face masks, and wearing eye protection were all independently associated with a decreased risk of transmission. Of note, only 7 of these studies evaluated SARS-CoV-2 transmission, the remainder evaluated SARS or MERS transmission.[74]

A systematic review and meta-analysis evaluating airborne transmission and the role of face masks for prevention of SARS-CoV-2 transmission identified 4 studies with 7688 participants in demonstrated decreased risk of SARS-CoV-2 infection with face masks, including N95s (RR 0.12).[75]

A retrospective study from January 2020 at a single center in Wuhan, China, found that HCPs working in units where no masks were worn and standard hand hygiene practices occurred were more likely to develop COVID-19 than HCPs working in units where N95 respirators were worn and frequent hand hygiene was performed (adjusted odds ratio [aOR] 464.8).[76]

In review of HCP infections that occurred early on during the pandemic in Hubei Province, China, during a time when many HCPs were not yet wearing recommended PPE when caring for patients with possible COVID-19, the relative risk of HCP infection was 36.9 times higher in those who did not wear appropriate PPE compared with those who did. Only 0.08% (1 of 1287) staff members became infected while wearing appropriate PPE.[61]

In a review of 345 HCPs with an occupational exposure to a patient with COVID-19, lack of eye protection during the exposure was associated with an increased risk of SARS-CoV-2 transmission to the HCP (Risk Ratio 14.1, 95% confidence interval 1.3–150.1).[67]

Non–Health Care Settings

Real-world scenarios have also demonstrated the efficacy of masks/face coverings in preventing SARS-CoV-2 transmission both through source control and protection to the wearer. A well-reported example describes the experience of 2 hairstylists who both worked with symptomatic COVID-19. Despite transmission from one hairstylist to the other and to close contacts in their household where there were unmasked exposures, no secondary cases resulted from encounters with any of the 139 clients during which the hairstylists and clients were masked.[77]

A retrospective case-control study from Thailand comparing 211 exposed individuals who developed COVID-19 with 839 exposed individuals who did not develop COVID-19 showed that wearing masks all the time during the contact period was independently associated with decreased risk of COVID-19 infection (aOR 0.23). Maintaining of physical distance of greater than 1 m from the exposure source (aOR 0.15), duration of close contact $\leq$15 minutes (aOR 0.24), and frequent hand hygiene (aOR 0.33) were also associated with a decreased risk of infection.[78]

CENTERS FOR DISEASE CONTROL AND PREVENTION RECOMMENDATIONS FOR HEALTH CARE FACILITIES DURING THE CORONAVIRUS DISEASE 2019 PANDEMIC
Universal Masking

Well-fitting surgical masks, isolation masks, cloth masks, or respirators that cover the mouth and nose are recommended as a form of universal source control as well as protection to the wearer within health care facilities. Masks are not recommended for children younger than 2 or any individuals with an underlying disability or medical condition that prevents them from safely wearing a face mask.

Physical Distancing

When possible, physical distancing of at least 6 feet between people is an important measure in preventing transmission of SARS-CoV-2. Important considerations that enable physical distancing include limiting visitors to health care facilities, scheduling appointments to limit the number of individuals in waiting rooms, arranging seating in waiting rooms and other common area as so individuals may remain 6 feet apart, and modifying in-person visits through the use of virtual communication devices.

Attention to Non–Patient-Care Areas

Importantly, clusters of transmission between HCPs have been described, particularly related to the lack of universal masking and/or physical distancing between colleagues. It is critical that measures including universal masking and physical distancing are followed in non–patient care workspaces throughout health care facilities. Dedicated areas for HCPs to remain physically distanced during breaks or when eating and/or drinking should be identified to promote a safe working environment and minimize exposure risk during these times when HCPs are unmasked.

Exposure Follow-Up and Contact Tracing

In partnership with occupational health and infection prevention experts, health care facilities should design a process to follow up COVID-19 cases, identify potential exposures, and perform contact tracing and other associated follow-up. This should occur promptly after a case is identified and ensures the privacy of patients, visitors, and HCPs. This process should also incorporate notification of the local public health department.

PERSONAL PROTECTIVE EQUIPMENT AND PATIENT CARE

In addition to universal masking, standard precautions, and transmission-based precautions, the CDC recommends the following in areas of moderate to high SARS-CoV-2 transmission during all patient care:

- N95 or equivalent respirators should be used during all AGPs.
- Eye protection should be worn during patient care to protect the eyes from possible exposure to respiratory secretions.

The CDC recommends the following Infection Prevention practices during the care of a patient with suspected or confirmed COVID-19:

- The patient should be cared for in a single-occupancy room with a dedicated bathroom when possible.
- Airborne infection isolation rooms with the door closed are recommended for patients with suspected or confirmed COVID-19 who are undergoing AGP.
  - Facilities should monitor the negative pressure relationship of these rooms.
- Dedicated HCPs on a dedicated unit should be considered for the care of patients with suspected or confirmed COVID-19 as a measure to limit personnel exposures and conserve PPE.
- Patient transports and other movement throughout the health care facility should be minimized, and patients should wear a face covering during transport.
- HCPs should perform hand hygiene before donning PPE, before and after patient contact, after doffing PPE, and during the other recommended scenarios as described in WHO's 5 moments of hand hygiene.[79]
- Training on the indications for PPE use as well as appropriate donning and doffing instruction should be provided to all personnel to maximize protection and minimize the risk of self-contamination.

The CDC recommends that HCPs and other personnel entering the room of patients with suspected or confirmed COVID-19 should don the following PPE:

- N95 or equivalent respirator (during N95 or equivalent respirator shortages, respirators should be prioritized for patients requiring airborne precautions[80])
- Gown
- Gloves
- Eye protection

INFECTIOUS DISEASES SOCIETY OF AMERICA RECOMMENDATIONS

Infectious Diseases Society of America guidelines on infection prevention for HCPs caring for patients with confirmed or suspected COVID-19 recommend N95 respirators or equivalent (in addition to gowns, gloves, and eye protection) for patients undergoing AGPs. A surgical mask or N95 or equivalent respirator is recommended for patients with COVID-19 who are not undergoing an AGP.[81]

Duration of Isolation Precautions

Early on during the pandemic, a test-based strategy was recommended to discontinue transmission-based precautions for patients with COVID-19. However, despite prolonged detection of SARS-CoV-2 virus by PCR, isolation of live, replication-competent virus has not been detected after 8 to 10 days and has been rarely detected up to 20 days in immunocompromised individuals or in individuals with severe infections.[38,82,83] Exposure to an index case after day 5 of symptoms was not associated with SARS-CoV-2 transmission in a large contact-tracing study.[84] In addition, in a study of persistently positive patients, no secondary infections were identified among close contacts, and viable virus was not detected in culture for patients with repeat positive PCR tests.[85]

Based on these data and other emerging evidence, use of a symptom-based strategy to discontinue transmission-based precautions was subsequently recommended. Current CDC guidance recommends the following criteria to discontinue precautions for patients with COVID-19 in health care settings.

For patients with mild to moderate illness who are not severely immunocompromised:

- At least 10 days have passed since symptoms first appeared, and
- At least 24 hours have passed since the last fever without the use of antipyretics, and
- Symptoms have improved

For asymptomatic patients who are not severely immunocompromised:

- At least 10 days have passed since the collection date of the first positive viral test

For patients with severe to critical illness or who are severely immunocompromised:

- At least 10 days and up to 20 days have passed since symptoms first appeared, and
- At least 24 hours have passed since the last fever without the use of antipyretics, and
- Symptoms have improved, and
- Consider consultation with infection prevention experts[86,87]

HAND HYGIENE, ENVIRONMENT OF CARE/CLEANING, AND ENGINEERING CONTROLS

Experimental data have demonstrated that SARS-CoV-2 is effectively inactivated by WHO-recommended alcohol-based hand rub formulations.[88,89] In addition, evidence has shown that frequent hand hygiene in conjunction with other prevention strategies is associated with a decreased transmission risk of SARS-CoV-2 and other similar respiratory viruses to HCPs.[72,76]

Other coronaviruses have been found to persist on environmental surfaces for up to 9 days.[90] In experimental models, SARS-CoV-2 remained viable on hard surfaces for up to 72 hours after being applied,[48] and SARS-CoV-2 has been recovered after sampling environmental surfaces in COVID-19 patient rooms.[45] Experimental evidence has demonstrated that SARS-CoV-2 is inactivated with routine cleaning and disinfection measures, including quaternary ammonium–containing products.[89] In one study, environmental surfaces in COVID-19 patient rooms that were sampled after routine cleaning showed no detection of SARS-CoV-2, compared with 87% of surfaces sampled before routine cleaning with positive SARS-CoV-2 testing.[91]

Because typical cleaning and disinfection measures are effective against the SARS-CoV-2 virus, the CDC recommends following routine practices for patient room cleaning, laundry, food service, and waste removal. Appropriate PPE should be worn by environmental services and other personnel during cleaning. Terminal cleaning after discharge should be delayed until an adequate number of air changes have occurred. Dedicated medical equipment should be used for the care of patients with suspected or confirmed COVID-19 when possible. Any nondedicated equipment should be cleaned per manufacturer instructions for use and hospital policy.[80]

Engineering controls should be considered to minimize exposure within health care facilities. Examples include erecting physical barriers, establishing pathways to guide individuals through common areas, and minimizing the use of semiprivate rooms or open-bay lay-out patient care areas. In conjunction with facilities and engineering experts, steps to optimize air quality should be considered. For example, permanent air handling systems to control air pressure relationships, filtration, and air exchanges should be used where possible. The addition of portable solutions, such as HEPA filters, can be considered in areas where permanent air handling solutions are not possible. Ensuring appropriate room pressure relationships are present in patient care areas is also critical.[50,80]

SCREENING AND VISITATION

The CDC recommends limiting and monitoring entry points to health care facilities. Basic prevention measures include posting visual alerts with instructions about wearing masks or other face coverings, and the importance of hand hygiene. Alcohol-based hand sanitizer with at least 60% alcohol content should be readily available for use. The CDC also recommends screening all individuals, including HCPs, patients, and visitors, entering a health care facility for signs and symptoms of COVID-19, as well as exposures to anyone with COVID-19 in the past 14 days. Admitted patients also should be screened daily for fever and symptoms compatible with COVID-19. Once identified, basic source control measures should be enacted for individuals with suspected or confirmed COVID-19, including ensuring that the individual is wearing a mask, placing the patient in a private room with the door closed, restricting visitors from entering the facility, and excluding HCPs from work. Limitations of screening include not being able to identify asymptomatic or pre-symptomatic individuals, or individuals without known exposures. Unintended consequences of screening and restricting HCPs and visitors include excluding individuals with symptoms due to another cause, for example, an underlying health condition or allergic rhinitis.[80] During the pandemic, the vast majority of health care facilities instituted screening for visitors and HCPs to detect the presence of fever and other symptoms of illness.[59,92,93]

PRE-PROCEDURAL TESTING

The CDC recommends that pre-admission and/or pre-procedure screening SARS-CoV-2 testing can be considered as an adjunctive measure to universal PPE and source control in health care settings. Important considerations include guidance from the local health department, testing availability and turnaround time, and local disease prevalence. Limitations of screening testing include identifying positive results in patients with prior infections who are no longer infectious but have prolonged PCR positivity, and potentially negative results due to testing during the incubation period or false negative results in the setting of an active infection due to limitations of the testing methodology.[80]

Many health care facilities routinely tested asymptomatic patients undergoing selected procedures, most commonly upper and lower airway procedures, labor and delivery, endoscopy, AGP, and sedation.[59] Although PCR testing has most often been described for this indication, antigen testing may have a role as well. In a study of 386 asymptomatic adult patients undergoing pre-procedural testing, the negative predictive value of antigen testing compared with PCR was 99.2%.[94]

Across a variety of settings and patient populations, the prevalence of SARS-CoV-2 in patients tested for pre-procedural indications was low, ranging from 0.1% to 3.8% (**Table 3**). SARS-CoV-2 prevalence was lower in patients tested for pre-procedural indications compared with those who were tested due to exposure or clinical symptoms.[96] In addition, percent positivity was lower in asymptomatic, vaccinated individuals undergoing pre-procedural testing compared with unvaccinated individuals.[102]

Challenges with pre-procedural testing have also been identified. In one study, approximately half of patients either declined pre-procedural testing or could not be reached to arrange testing; barriers identified included lack of interest in testing, distance from testing facility, transport issues, and the patient's perception of not being at risk for COVID-19.[99] Positive pre-procedural SARS-CoV-2 testing was associated with delaying of the procedure by 29 days on average, with no COVID-19–related complications identified in any of the patients whether or not their procedure was delayed.[101] Utility of a risk screening questionnaire to identify patients with positive pre-procedural SARS-CoV-2 testing remains unclear; in one study of 1000 patients undergoing endoscopy the negative predictive value of a validated risk screening questionnaire was 99.4%; however, the positive predictive value was only 2.5%.[100]

VISITATION

During the pandemic, the CDC recommended limiting visitation to those who are essential for the patient's well-being and care, for example, parents and care partners. The use of virtual options for communication is encouraged. For patients with COVID-19, additional considerations surrounding visitation include evaluating the risk to the visitor, providing instruction on hand hygiene and use of PPE, restricting visitation during AGP, and restricting visitors to the patient's room.[80]

Most health care facilities permitted visitors for patients with suspected or confirmed COVID-19, at least under certain circumstances, especially during end-of-life care. Of those who permitted visitors for patients with confirmed or suspected COVID-19, 69% to 91% required visitors to wear PPE.[59,92] For pediatric patients, 67% to 85% of health care facilities allowed 1 visitor per pediatric patient, and the remainder allowed 2.[59,92] The vast majority (86%) did not permit visitors to leave the patient's room. Most (74%) restricted visitors under a certain age, typically those younger than 18 years.[92]

Visitor restrictions and other hospital-based measures implemented to minimize transmission risk in the health care setting posed unique challenges for pediatrics where parents/caregivers are critical members of the patient's care team. For example, pandemic-related restrictions contributed to decreased parental presence at the bedside and participation in rounds in the neonatal intensive care unit setting. Important ancillary services, including therapy services, lactation, and social work support were also at least temporarily less widely available during the pandemic.[93]

PUBLIC HEALTH MEASURES

The initial public health response included screening returning travelers from Wuhan, China, and on January 31, 2020, a presidential proclamation temporarily suspended entry for individuals who have visited China in the past 14 days.[103] However, the yield of airport screening in identifying COVID-19 cases was low, with 0.001% or 1 case per 85,000 travelers screened testing positive for SARS-CoV-2.[104]

Local masking mandates were associated with an increase in masking compliance in those areas,[105] and decreased SARS-CoV-2 transmission rates, associated

Table 3
Pre-procedural testing

Study	Dates	Setting/Population	Sample Size (Patients)	Percent Positivity, %	Miscellaneous
Lin et al,[95] 2020	March–April 2020	US/Pediatric pre-procedural testing	1295	0.9	Range of 0.2% to 2.7% across 3 hospitals
Otto et al,[96] 2020	March–June 2020	US/Pediatric pre-procedural and pre-admission testing	1410	3.8	
Aslam et al,[97] 2020	March–August 2020	US/Cancer center pre-procedural testing	11,540	0.6	Fell below 0.3% after April 2020
Bence et al,[98] 2021	March–October 2020	US/Pediatric pre-procedural testing	11,150	1.4	
Haidar et al,[99] 2021	April–June 2020	US/Pre-procedural testing	10,539	0.1	
Bowyer et al,[100] 2021	May–June 2020	US/Ambulatory pre-procedural testing before endoscopy	1000	0.8	
Larsen et al,[101] 2021	May–July 2020	US/Ambulatory pre-procedural testing	3709	1	
Tande et al,[102] 2021	December 2020–February 2021	US/Pre-procedural testing	39,156	3.1	

Data from Refs.[95–102]

hospitalizations, and deaths.[106–109] Masking compliance varies based on age, sex, geographic setting, location of activity, and political affiliation.[105,110–112]

Stay-at-home orders and other public health mitigation strategies are also effective at decreasing local SARS-CoV-2 transmission rates,[108,113,114] with evidence of decreased mortality rates in areas with more stringent mitigation policies.[115]

Although efficient and early contact tracing can be an effective component in controlling SARS-CoV-2 outbreaks,[84] challenges in identifying and notifying contacts in a timely manner, particularly after increasing caseloads,[116,117] resulted in discontinuation of contact-tracing efforts by a local health department agencies.

Before widespread vaccine availability, recommended public health strategies to prevent ongoing SARS-CoV-2 transmission included the following:

- Universal face covering
- Physical distancing
- Limiting contacts with persons outside your bubble
- Avoiding nonessential indoor spaces and crowded outdoor settings
- Increasing testing to promptly diagnosis and initiate isolation
- Prompt case investigation and contact tracing
- Protecting essential workers and persons at high risk for severe illness, complications, and death
- Postponing travel
- Increasing room air ventilation
- Increased hand hygiene and cleaning/disinfection
- Widespread vaccine coverage[118]

CLINICS CARE POINTS

- SARS-Cov-2 transmission risk in the healthcare setting can be mitigated by proper use of personal protective equipment, including gowns, gloves, N95 or surgical mask, and eye protection.
- Additional strategies such as physical distancing, hand hygiene, routine cleaning and disinfection, appropriate air handling and ventilation, and public health interventions are also important tools to minimize transmission risk of SARS-CoV-2 and other emerging infectious diseases.

DISCLOSURE

P. Reich, author, has no commercial or financial conflicts, or other relevant disclosures. A. Elward, author, is a sub investigator on a clinical trial funded by Moderna. Funding from Moderna is received by the university and not by Dr. Elward.

REFERENCES

1. Ghinai I, McPherson TD, Hunter JC, et al. First known person-to-person transmission of severe acute respiratory syndrome coronavirus 2 (SARS-CoV-2) in the USA. Lancet 2020;395(10230):1137–44. https://doi.org/10.1016/S0140-6736(20)30607-3.
2. Li Q, Guan X, Wu P, et al. Early transmission dynamics in Wuhan, China, of novel coronavirus-infected pneumonia. N Engl J Med 2020;382(13):1199–207. https://doi.org/10.1056/NEJMoa2001316.

3. Sohrabi C, Alsafi Z, O'Neill N, et al. World Health Organization declares global emergency: a review of the 2019 novel coronavirus (COVID-19). Int J Surg 2020; 76:71–6. https://doi.org/10.1016/j.ijsu.2020.02.034.

4. Vaccines WHO. Background paper on COVID-19 disease and vaccines 2020. Available at: WHO/2019-nCoV/vaccines/SAGE_background/2020.1. 12/22/2020.

5. Severe Acute Respiratory Syndrome (SARS). 2021. Available at: https://www.cdc.gov/sars/index.html. Accessed June 15, 2021.

6. Summary of probable SARS cases with onset of illness from 1 November 2002 to 31 July 2003. 2021. Available at: https://www.who.int/publications/m/item/summary-of-probable-sars-cases-with-onset-of-illness-from-1-november-2002-to-31-july-2003. Accessed June 15, 2021.

7. Middle East respiratory syndrome coronavirus (MERS-CoV). 2021. Available at: https://www.who.int/health-topics/middle-east-respiratory-syndrome-coronavirus-mers#tab=tab_1. Accessed 6/15/21.

8. WHO Coronavirus (COVID-19) Dashboard. 2021. Available at: https://covid19.who.int/?adgroupsurvey={adgroupsurvey}&gclid=CjwKCAjwqcKFBhAhEiwA-fEr7zcPRhsL6jDD51Um33KtwAZ3TEKtI1NLk0s1etQHwNiUDygkgkwvmOBoCf-dUQAvD_BwE Accessed November 12, 2021

9. Information for pediatric healthcare providers. 2021. Available at: https://www.cdc.gov/coronavirus/2019-ncov/hcp/pediatric-hcp.html. Accessed June 15, 2021.

10. Demographic trends of COVID-19 cases and deaths in the US reported to CDC. 2021. Available at: https://covid.cdc.gov/covid-data-tracker/?CDC_AA_refVal=https%3A%2F%2Fwww.cdc.gov%2Fcoronavirus%2F2019-ncov%2Fcases-updates%2Fcases-in-us.html#demographics. Accessed June 15, 2021.

11. COVID-NET Laboratory-confirmed COVID-19 hospitalizations. 2021. Available at: https://covid.cdc.gov/covid-data-tracker/?CDC_AA_refVal=https%3A%2F%2Fwww.cdc.gov%2Fcoronavirus%2F2019-ncov%2Fcases-updates%2Fcases-in-us.html#covidnet-hospitalization-network. Accessed June 15, 2021.

12. Leidman E, Duca LM, Omura JD, et al. COVID-19 trends among persons aged 0-24 years - United States, March 1-December 12, 2020. MMWR Morb Mortal Wkly Rep 2021;70(3):88–94. https://doi.org/10.15585/mmwr.mm7003e1.

13. Kim L, Whitaker M, O'Halloran A, et al. Hospitalization rates and characteristics of children aged <18 years hospitalized with laboratory-confirmed COVID-19 - COVID-NET, 14 States, March 1-July 25, 2020. MMWR Morb Mortal Wkly Rep 2020;69(32):1081–8. https://doi.org/10.15585/mmwr.mm6932e3.

14. Richardson S, Hirsch JS, Narasimhan M, et al. Presenting characteristics, co-morbidities, and outcomes among 5700 patients hospitalized with COVID-19 in the New York City Area. JAMA 2020;323(20):2052–9. https://doi.org/10.1001/jama.2020.6775.

15. Wu Z, McGoogan JM. Characteristics of and important lessons from the coronavirus disease 2019 (COVID-19) outbreak in China: summary of a report of 72314 cases from the Chinese center for disease control and prevention. JAMA 2020; 323(13):1239–42. https://doi.org/10.1001/jama.2020.2648.

16. Onder G, Rezza G, Brusaferro S. Case-fatality rate and characteristics of patients dying in relation to COVID-19 in Italy. JAMA 2020;323(18):1775–6. https://doi.org/10.1001/jama.2020.4683.

17. Ahmad FB, Cisewski JA, Minino A, et al. Provisional mortality data - United States, 2020. MMWR Morb Mortal Wkly Rep 2021;70(14):519–22. https://doi.org/10.15585/mmwr.mm7014e1.

18. Woodworth KR, Olsen EO, Neelam V, et al. Birth and infant outcomes following laboratory-confirmed SARS-CoV-2 infection in pregnancy - SET-NET, 16 jurisdictions, March 29-October 14, 2020. MMWR Morb Mortal Wkly Rep 2020;69(44): 1635–40. https://doi.org/10.15585/mmwr.mm6944e2.

19. Chen H, Guo J, Wang C, et al. Clinical characteristics and intrauterine vertical transmission potential of COVID-19 infection in nine pregnant women: a retrospective review of medical records. Lancet 2020;395(10226):809–15. https://doi.org/10.1016/S0140-6736(20)30360-3.

20. Godfred-Cato S, Bryant B, Leung J, et al. COVID-19-associated multisystem inflammatory syndrome in children - United States, March-July 2020. MMWR Morb Mortal Wkly Rep 2020;69(32):1074–80. https://doi.org/10.15585/mmwr.mm6932e2.

21. Assaker R, Colas AE, Julien-Marsollier F, et al. Presenting symptoms of COVID-19 in children: a meta-analysis of published studies. Br J Anaesth 2020;125(3): e330–2. https://doi.org/10.1016/j.bja.2020.05.026.

22. Byambasuren O, Bell K, et al. Estimating the extend of asymptomatic COVID-19 and its potential for community transmission: systematic review and meta-analysis. J Assoc Med Microbiol Infect Dis Can 2020. https://doi.org/10.3138/jammi-2020-0030.

23. Toba N, Gupta S, Ali AY, et al. COVID-19 under 19: a meta-analysis. Pediatr Pulmonol 2021;56(6):1332–41. https://doi.org/10.1002/ppul.25312.

24. Mair M, Singhavi H, Pai A, et al. A meta-analysis of 67 studies with presenting symptoms and laboratory tests of COVID-19 patients. Laryngoscope 2021; 131(6):1254–65. https://doi.org/10.1002/lary.29207.

25. Liu Y, Gayle AA, Wilder-Smith A, et al. The reproductive number of COVID-19 is higher compared to SARS coronavirus. J Trav Med. 2020;27(2). https://doi.org/10.1093/jtm/taaa021.

26. Biggerstaff M, Cauchemez S, Reed C, et al. Estimates of the reproduction number for seasonal, pandemic, and zoonotic influenza: a systematic review of the literature. BMC Infect Dis 2014;14:480. https://doi.org/10.1186/1471-2334-14-480.

27. Koh WC, Naing L, Chaw L, et al. What do we know about SARS-CoV-2 transmission? A systematic review and meta-analysis of the secondary attack rate and associated risk factors. PLoS One 2020;15(10):e0240205. https://doi.org/10.1371/journal.pone.0240205.

28. 2009 H1N1 early outbreak and disease characteristics. 2021. Available at: https://www.cdc.gov/h1n1flu/surveillanceqa.htm. Accessed June 15, 2021.

29. Measles. 2021. Available at: https://www.cdc.gov/vaccines/pubs/pinkbook/meas.html. Accessed June 15, 2021.

30. Marin MLA. Varicella (chickenpox). 2021. Available at: https://wwwnc.cdc.gov/travel/yellowbook/2020/travel-related-infectious-diseases/varicella-chickenpox. Accessed June 15, 2021.

31. Lauer SA, Grantz KH, Bi Q, et al. The incubation period of coronavirus disease 2019 (COVID-19) from publicly reported confirmed cases: estimation and application. Ann Intern Med 2020;172(9):577–82. https://doi.org/10.7326/M20-0504.

32. He X, Lau EHY, Wu P, et al. Temporal dynamics in viral shedding and transmissibility of COVID-19. Nat Med 2020;26(5):672–5. https://doi.org/10.1038/s41591-020-0869-5.

33. Kimball A, Hatfield KM, Arons M, et al. Asymptomatic and presymptomatic SARS-CoV-2 infections in residents of a long-term care skilled nursing facility

- King County, Washington, March 2020. MMWR Morb Mortal Wkly Rep 2020; 69(13):377–81. https://doi.org/10.15585/mmwr.mm6913e1.

34. Wei WE, Li Z, Chiew CJ, et al. Presymptomatic transmission of SARS-CoV-2 - Singapore, January 23-March 16, 2020. MMWR Morb Mortal Wkly Rep 2020; 69(14):411–5. https://doi.org/10.15585/mmwr.mm6914e1.

35. Bai Y, Yao L, Wei T, et al. Presumed asymptomatic carrier transmission of COVID-19. JAMA 2020;323(14):1406–7. https://doi.org/10.1001/jama.2020.2565.

36. Rothe C, Schunk M, Sothmann P, et al. Transmission of 2019-nCoV infection from an asymptomatic contact in Germany. N Engl J Med 2020;382(10):970–1. https://doi.org/10.1056/NEJMc2001468.

37. To KK, Tsang OT, Leung WS, et al. Temporal profiles of viral load in posterior oropharyngeal saliva samples and serum antibody responses during infection by SARS-CoV-2: an observational cohort study. Lancet Infect Dis 2020;20(5): 565–74. https://doi.org/10.1016/S1473-3099(20)30196-1.

38. Wolfel R, Corman VM, Guggemos W, et al. Virological assessment of hospitalized patients with COVID-2019. Nature 2020;581(7809):465–9. https://doi.org/10.1038/s41586-020-2196-x.

39. Zou L, Ruan F, Huang M, et al. SARS-CoV-2 viral load in upper respiratory specimens of infected patients. N Engl J Med 2020;382(12):1177–9. https://doi.org/10.1056/NEJMc2001737.

40. Air: guidelines for environmental infection control in health-care facilities (2003). 2021. Available at: https://www.cdc.gov/infectioncontrol/guidelines/environmental/background/air.html. Accessed June 15, 2021.

41. Klompas M, Baker MA, Rhee C. Airborne transmission of SARS-CoV-2: theoretical considerations and available evidence. JAMA 2020;324(5):441–2. https://doi.org/10.1001/jama.2020.12458.

42. Saiman L, Acker KP, Dumitru D, et al. Infection prevention and control for labor and delivery, well baby nurseries, and neonatal intensive care units. Semin Perinatol 2020;44(7):151320. https://doi.org/10.1016/j.semperi.2020.151320.

43. Samet JM, Prather K, Benjamin G, et al. Airborne transmission of SARS-CoV-2: what we know. Clin Infect Dis 2021. https://doi.org/10.1093/cid/ciab039.

44. Tang JW, Bahnfleth WP, Bluyssen PM, et al. Dismantling myths on the airborne transmission of severe acute respiratory syndrome coronavirus-2 (SARS-CoV-2). J Hosp Infect 2021;110:89–96. https://doi.org/10.1016/j.jhin.2020.12.022.

45. Chia PY, Coleman KK, Tan YK, et al. Detection of air and surface contamination by SARS-CoV-2 in hospital rooms of infected patients. Nat Commun 2020;11(1): 2800. https://doi.org/10.1038/s41467-020-16670-2.

46. Liu Y, Zhi N, Chen Y, et al. Aerodynamic characteristics and RNA concentration of SARS-CoV-2 aerosol in Wuhan Hospitals during COVID-19 Outbreak. bioRxiv 2020. https://doi.org/10.1101/2020.03.08.982637.

47. Noorimotlagh Z, Jaafarzadeh N, Martinez SS, et al. A systematic review of possible airborne transmission of the COVID-19 virus (SARS-CoV-2) in the indoor air environment. Environ Res 2021;193:110612. https://doi.org/10.1016/j.envres.2020.110612.

48. van Doremalen N, Bushmaker T, Morris DH, et al. Aerosol and surface stability of SARS-CoV-2 as compared with SARS-CoV-1. N Engl J Med 2020;382(16): 1564–7. https://doi.org/10.1056/NEJMc2004973.

49. Tran K, Cimon K, Severn M, et al. Aerosol generating procedures and risk of transmission of acute respiratory infections to healthcare workers: a systematic

review. PLoS One 2012;7(4):e35797. https://doi.org/10.1371/journal.pone. 0035797.

50. Clinical questions about COVID-19: questions and answers. 2021. Available at: https://www.cdc.gov/coronavirus/2019-ncov/hcp/faq.html. Accessed June 15, 2021.

51. Infection prevention and control during health care when coronavirus disease (COVID-19) is suspected or confirmed: interim guidance. 2021. Available at: https://www.who.int/publications/i/item/WHO-2019-nCoV-IPC-2020.4. Accessed June 15, 2021.

52. Li Y, Qian H, Hang J, et al. Probable airborne transmission of SARS-CoV-2 in a poorly ventilated restaurant. Build Environ 2021;196:107788. https://doi.org/10. 1016/j.buildenv.2021.107788.

53. Moriarty LF, Plucinski MM, Marston BJ, et al. Public health responses to COVID-19 outbreaks on cruise ships - worldwide, February-March 2020. MMWR Morb Mortal Wkly Rep 2020;69(12):347–52. https://doi.org/10.15585/mmwr. mm6912e3.

54. Hamner L, Dubbel P, Capron I, et al. High SARS-CoV-2 attack rate following exposure at a choir practice - Skagit County, Washington, March 2020. MMWR Morb Mortal Wkly Rep 2020;69(19):606–10. https://doi.org/10.15585/ mmwr.mm6919e6.

55. James A, Eagle L, Phillips C, et al. High COVID-19 attack rate among attendees at events at a church - Arkansas, March 2020. MMWR Morb Mortal Wkly Rep 2020;69(20):632–5. https://doi.org/10.15585/mmwr.mm6920e2.

56. Mosites E, Parker EM, Clarke KEN, et al. Assessment of SARS-CoV-2 infection prevalence in homeless shelters - four U.S. cities, March 27-April 15, 2020. MMWR Morb Mortal Wkly Rep 2020;69(17):521–2. https://doi.org/10.15585/ mmwr.mm6917e1.

57. Szablewski CM, Chang KT, Brown MM, et al. SARS-CoV-2 transmission and infection among attendees of an overnight camp - Georgia, June 2020. MMWR Morb Mortal Wkly Rep 2020;69(31):1023–5. https://doi.org/10.15585/ mmwr.mm6931e1.

58. Emanuel EJ, Persad G, Upshur R, et al. Fair allocation of scarce medical resources in the time of Covid-19. N Engl J Med 2020;382(21):2049–55. https:// doi.org/10.1056/NEJMsb2005114.

59. Calderwood MS, Deloney VM, Anderson DJ, et al. Policies and practices of SHEA Research Network hospitals during the COVID-19 pandemic. Infect Control Hosp Epidemiol 2020;41(10):1127–35. https://doi.org/10.1017/ice.2020.303.

60. Strategies for optimizing the supply of N95 respirators. 2021. Available at: https://www.cdc.gov/coronavirus/2019-ncov/hcp/respirators-strategy/. Accessed August 15, 2021.

61. Wang Q, Bai Y, et al. Epidemiologic characteristics of COVID-19 in medical staff members of neurosurgery departments in Hubei province: a multicentre descriptive study. medRxiv 2020. https://doi.org/10.1101/2020.04.20.20064899.

62. Lai X, Wang M, Qin C, et al. Coronavirus disease 2019 (COVID-2019) infection among health care workers and implications for prevention measures in a tertiary hospital in Wuhan, China. JAMA Netw Open 2020;3(5):e209666. https:// doi.org/10.1001/jamanetworkopen.2020.9666.

63. Kluytmans-van den Bergh MFQ, Buiting AGM, Pas SD, et al. Prevalence and clinical presentation of health care workers with symptoms of coronavirus disease 2019 in 2 dutch hospitals during an early phase of the pandemic. JAMA

Netw Open 2020;3(5):e209673. https://doi.org/10.1001/jamanetworkopen.2020. 9673.

64. Clifton GT, Pati R, Krammer F, et al. SARS-CoV-2 infection risk among active duty military members deployed to a field hospital - New York City, April 2020. MMWR Morb Mortal Wkly Rep 2021;70(9):308–11. https://doi.org/10.15585/mmwr. mm7009a3.

65. Fell A, Beaudoin A, D'Heilly P, et al. SARS-CoV-2 exposure and infection among health care personnel - Minnesota, March 6-July 11, 2020. MMWR Morb Mortal Wkly Rep 2020;69(43):1605–10. https://doi.org/10.15585/mmwr.mm6943a5.

66. Self WH, Tenforde MW, Stubblefield WB, et al. Seroprevalence of SARS-CoV-2 among frontline health care personnel in a multistate hospital network - 13 academic medical centers, April-June 2020. MMWR Morb Mortal Wkly Rep 2020; 69(35):1221–6. https://doi.org/10.15585/mmwr.mm6935e2.

67. Shah VP, Breeher LE, Hainy CM, et al. Evaluation of healthcare personnel exposures to patients with severe acute respiratory coronavirus virus 2 (SARS-CoV-2) associated with personal protective equipment. Infect Control Hosp Epidemiol 2021;1–5. https://doi.org/10.1017/ice.2021.219.

68. Team CC-R. Characteristics of health care personnel with COVID-19 - United States, February 12-April 9, 2020. MMWR Morb Mortal Wkly Rep 2020;69(15): 477–81. https://doi.org/10.15585/mmwr.mm6915e6.

69. Hughes MM, Groenewold MR, Lessem SE, et al. Update: characteristics of health care personnel with COVID-19 - United States, February 12-July 16, 2020. MMWR Morb Mortal Wkly Rep 2020;69(38):1364–8. https://doi.org/10. 15585/mmwr.mm6938a3.

70. Heinzerling A, Stuckey MJ, Scheuer T, et al. Transmission of COVID-19 to health care personnel during exposures to a hospitalized patient - Solano County, California, February 2020. MMWR Morb Mortal Wkly Rep 2020;69(15):472–6. https://doi.org/10.15585/mmwr.mm6915e5.

71. Li L, Niu M, Zhu Y. Assessing the effectiveness of using various face coverings to mitigate the transport of airborne particles produces by coughing indoors. Aerosol Sci Technol 2020. https://doi.org/10.1080/02786826.2020.1846679.

72. Jefferson T, Foxlee R, Del Mar C, et al. Physical interventions to interrupt or reduce the spread of respiratory viruses: systematic review. BMJ 2008; 336(7635):77–80. https://doi.org/10.1136/bmj.39393.510347.BE.

73. Bartoszko JJ, Farooqi MAM, Alhazzani W, et al. Medical masks vs N95 respirators for preventing COVID-19 in healthcare workers: a systematic review and meta-analysis of randomized trials. Influenza Other Respir Viruses 2020;14(4): 365–73. https://doi.org/10.1111/irv.12745.

74. Chu DK, Akl EA, Duda S, et al. Physical distancing, face masks, and eye protection to prevent person-to-person transmission of SARS-CoV-2 and COVID-19: a systematic review and meta-analysis. Lancet 2020;395(10242):1973–87. https:// doi.org/10.1016/S0140-6736(20)31142-9.

75. Tabatabaeizadeh SA. Airborne transmission of COVID-19 and the role of face mask to prevent it: a systematic review and meta-analysis. Eur J Med Res 2021;26(1):1. https://doi.org/10.1186/s40001-020-00475-6.

76. Wang X, Pan Z, Cheng Z. Association between 2019-nCoV transmission and N95 respirator use. J Hosp Infect 2020;105(1):104–5. https://doi.org/10.1016/j. jhin.2020.02.021.

77. Hendrix MJ, Walde C, Findley K, et al. Absence of apparent transmission of SARS-CoV-2 from two stylists after exposure at a hair salon with a universal

Infection Prevention During COVID-19

face covering policy - Springfield, Missouri, May 2020. MMWR Morb Mortal Wkly Rep 2020;69(28):930–2. https://doi.org/10.15585/mmwr.mm6928e2.

78. Doung-ngern P, Panjangampatthana A, et al. Associations between wearing masks, washing hands, and social distancing practices, and risk of COVID-19 infection in public: a cohort-based case-control study in Thailand. Lancet 2020.

79. WHO save lives: clean your hands in the context of COVID-19. 2021. Available at: https://cdn.who.int/media/docs/default-source/integrated-health-services-(ihs)/infection-prevention-and-control/who-hh-community-campaign-finalv3.pdf?sfvrsn=322df98f_2. Accessed June 15, 2021.

80. Interim infection prevention and control recommendations for healthcare personnel during the coronavirus disease 2019 (COVID-19) Pandemic. 2021. Available at: https://www.cdc.gov/coronavirus/2019-ncov/hcp/infection-control-recommendations.html. Accessed June 15, 2021.

81. Lynch JB, Davitkov P, Anderson DJ, et al. Infectious Diseases Society of America Guidelines on infection prevention for health care personnel caring for patients with suspected or known COVID-19. Clin Infect Dis 2020. https://doi.org/10.1093/cid/ciaa1063.

82. Bullard J, Dust K, Funk D, et al. Predicting infectious severe acute respiratory syndrome coronavirus 2 from diagnostic samples. Clin Infect Dis 2020;71(10):2663–6. https://doi.org/10.1093/cid/ciaa638.

83. van Kampen JJA, van de Vijver D, Fraaij PLA, et al. Duration and key determinants of infectious virus shedding in hospitalized patients with coronavirus disease-2019 (COVID-19). Nat Commun 2021;12(1):267. https://doi.org/10.1038/s41467-020-20568-4.

84. Cheng HY, Jian SW, Liu DP, et al. Contact tracing assessment of COVID-19 transmission dynamics in Taiwan and risk at different exposure periods before and after symptom onset. JAMA Intern Med 2020;180(9):1156–63. https://doi.org/10.1001/jamainternmed.2020.2020.

85. Infectivity of persons with repeated positive SARS-CoV-2 RT-PCR tests. 2020. Available at: https://www.cdc.go.kr/board/board.es?mid=a30402000000&bid=0030. Accessed May 20, 2020.

86. Discontinuation of transmission-based precautions and disposition of patients with SARS-CoV-2 infection in healthcare settings. 2021. Available at: https://www.cdc.gov/coronavirus/2019-ncov/hcp/disposition-hospitalized-patients.html. Accessed June 15, 2021.

87. Interim guidance on ending isolation and precautions for adults with COVID-19. 2021. Available at: https://www.cdc.gov/coronavirus/2019-ncov/hcp/duration-isolation.html?CDC_AA_refVal=https%3A%2F%2Fwww.cdc.gov%2Fcoronavirus%2F2019-ncov%2Fcommunity%2Fstrategy-discontinue-isolation.html. Accessed June 15, 2021.

88. Kratzel A, Todt D, V'Kovski P, et al. Inactivation of severe acute respiratory syndrome coronavirus 2 by WHO-recommended hand rub formulations and alcohols. Emerg Infect Dis 2020;26(7):1592–5. https://doi.org/10.3201/eid2607.200915.

89. Rabenau HF, Kampf G, Cinatl J, et al. Efficacy of various disinfectants against SARS coronavirus. J Hosp Infect 2005;61(2):107–11. https://doi.org/10.1016/j.jhin.2004.12.023.

90. Kampf G, Todt D, Pfaender S, et al. Persistence of coronaviruses on inanimate surfaces and their inactivation with biocidal agents. J Hosp Infect 2020;104(3):246–51. https://doi.org/10.1016/j.jhin.2020.01.022.

91. Ong SWX, Tan YK, Chia PY, et al. Air, surface environmental, and personal protective equipment contamination by severe acute respiratory syndrome coronavirus 2 (SARS-CoV-2) from a symptomatic patient. JAMA 2020;323(16):1610–2. https://doi.org/10.1001/jama.2020.3227.

92. Kitano T, Piche-Renaud PP, Groves HE, et al. Visitor restriction policy on pediatric wards during novel coronavirus (COVID-19) outbreak: a survey study across North America. J Pediatr Infect Dis Soc 2020;9(6):766–8. https://doi.org/10.1093/jpids/piaa126.

93. Darcy Mahoney A, White RD, Velasquez A, et al. Impact of restrictions on parental presence in neonatal intensive care units related to coronavirus disease 2019. J Perinatol 2020;40(Suppl 1):36–46. https://doi.org/10.1038/s41372-020-0753-7.

94. Tworek JA, Khan F, Sekedat MD, et al. The utility of rapid nucleic acid amplification testing to triage symptomatic patients and to screen asymptomatic preprocedure patients for SARS-CoV-2. Open Forum Infect Dis 2021;8(1):ofaa607. https://doi.org/10.1093/ofid/ofaa607.

95. Lin EE, Blumberg TJ, Adler AC, et al. Incidence of COVID-19 in pediatric surgical patients among 3 US Children's Hospitals. JAMA Surg 2020;155(8):775–7. https://doi.org/10.1001/jamasurg.2020.2588.

96. Otto WR, Geoghegan S, Posch LC, et al. The epidemiology of severe acute respiratory syndrome coronavirus 2 in a pediatric healthcare network in the United States. J Pediatr Infect Dis Soc 2020;9(5):523–9. https://doi.org/10.1093/jpids/piaa074.

97. Aslam A, Singh J, Robilotti E, et al. SARS CoV-2 surveillance and exposure in the perioperative setting with universal testing and personal protective equipment (PPE) policies. Clin Infect Dis 2020. https://doi.org/10.1093/cid/ciaa1607.

98. Bence CM, Jarzembowski JA, Belter L, et al. COVID-19 pre-procedural testing strategy and early outcomes at a large tertiary care children's hospital. Pediatr Surg Int 2021;37(7):871–80. https://doi.org/10.1007/s00383-021-04878-2.

99. Haidar G, Ayres A, King WC, et al. Preprocedural SARS-CoV-2 testing to sustain medically needed health care delivery during the COVID-19 pandemic: a prospective observational study. Open Forum Infect Dis 2021;8(2):ofab022. https://doi.org/10.1093/ofid/ofab022.

100. Bowyer B, Thukral C, Patel S, et al. Outcomes of symptom screening and universal COVID-19 reverse transcriptase polymerase chain reaction testing before endoscopy in a community-based ambulatory surgery center. Gastrointest Endosc 2021;93(5):1060–1064 e1. https://doi.org/10.1016/j.gie.2020.10.001.

101. Larsen CG, Bub CD, Schaffler BC, et al. The impact of confirmed coronavirus disease 2019 (COVID-19) infection on ambulatory procedures and associated delays in care for asymptomatic patients. Surgery 2021;169(6):1340–5. https://doi.org/10.1016/j.surg.2021.01.005.

102. Tande AJ, Pollock BD, Shah ND, et al. Impact of the COVID-19 vaccine on asymptomatic infection among patients undergoing pre-procedural COVID-19 molecular screening. Clin Infect Dis 2021. https://doi.org/10.1093/cid/ciab229.

103. Patel A, Jernigan DB, 2019-nCoV CDC Response Team. Initial public health response and interim clinical guidance for the 2019 novel coronavirus outbreak - United States, December 31, 2019-February 4, 2020. MMWR Morb Mortal Wkly Rep 2020;69(5):140–6. https://doi.org/10.15585/mmwr.mm6905e1.

104. Dollard P, Griffin I, Berro A, et al. Risk assessment and management of COVID-19 among travelers arriving at designated U.S. airports, January 17-September 13, 2020. MMWR Morb Mortal Wkly Rep 2020;69(45):1681–5. https://doi.org/10.15585/mmwr.mm6945a4.

105. Haischer MH, Beilfuss R, Hart MR, et al. Who is wearing a mask? Gender-, age-, and location-related differences during the COVID-19 pandemic. PLoS One 2020;15(10):e0240785. https://doi.org/10.1371/journal.pone.0240785.
106. Guy GP Jr, Lee FC, Sunshine G, et al. Association of state-issued mask mandates and allowing on-premises restaurant dining with county-level COVID-19 case and death growth rates - United States, March 1-December 31, 2020. MMWR Morb Mortal Wkly Rep 2021;70(10):350–4. https://doi.org/10.15585/mmwr.mm7010e3.
107. Joo H, Miller GF, Sunshine G, et al. Decline in COVID-19 hospitalization growth rates associated with statewide mask mandates - 10 states, March-October 2020. MMWR Morb Mortal Wkly Rep 2021;70(6):212–6. https://doi.org/10.15585/mmwr.mm7006e2.
108. Kanu FA, Smith EE, Offutt-Powell T, et al. Declines in SARS-CoV-2 transmission, hospitalizations, and mortality after implementation of mitigation measures-Delaware, March-June 2020. MMWR Morb Mortal Wkly Rep 2020;69(45):1691–4. https://doi.org/10.15585/mmwr.mm6945e1.
109. Van Dyke ME, Rogers TM, Pevzner E, et al. Trends in county-level COVID-19 incidence in counties with and without a mask mandate - Kansas, June 1-August 23, 2020. MMWR Morb Mortal Wkly Rep 2020;69(47):1777–81. https://doi.org/10.15585/mmwr.mm6947e2.
110. Barrios LC, Riggs MA, Green RF, et al. Observed face mask use at six universities - United States, September-November 2020. MMWR Morb Mortal Wkly Rep 2021;70(6):208–11. https://doi.org/10.15585/mmwr.mm7006e1.
111. Hutchins HJ, Wolff B, Leeb R, et al. COVID-19 mitigation behaviors by age group - United States, April-June 2020. MMWR Morb Mortal Wkly Rep 2020;69(43):1584–90. https://doi.org/10.15585/mmwr.mm6943e4.
112. Green DN, Blumenkamp CK. Facemasking behaviors, preferences, and attitudes among emerging adults in the united states during the COVID-19 pandemic: an exploratory study. Cloth Text Res J 2021. https://doi.org/10.1177/0887302X211006775.
113. Gallaway MS, Rigler J, Robinson S, et al. Trends in COVID-19 incidence after implementation of mitigation measures - Arizona, January 22-August 7, 2020. MMWR Morb Mortal Wkly Rep 2020;69(40):1460–3. https://doi.org/10.15585/mmwr.mm6940e3.
114. Lyu W, Wehby GL. Comparison of estimated rates of coronavirus disease 2019 (COVID-19) in border counties in Iowa without a stay-at-home order and border counties in Illinois With a Stay-at-Home Order. JAMA Netw Open 2020;3(5):e2011102. https://doi.org/10.1001/jamanetworkopen.2020.11102.
115. Fuller JA, Hakim A, Victory KR, et al. Mitigation policies and COVID-19-associated mortality - 37 European Countries, January 23-June 30, 2020. MMWR Morb Mortal Wkly Rep 2021;70(2):58–62. https://doi.org/10.15585/mmwr.mm7002e4.
116. Lash RR, Donovan CV, Fleischauer AT, et al. COVID-19 contact tracing in two counties - North Carolina, June-July 2020. MMWR Morb Mortal Wkly Rep 2020;69(38):1360–3. https://doi.org/10.15585/mmwr.mm6938e3.
117. Spencer KD, Chung CL, Stargel A, et al. COVID-19 case investigation and contact tracing efforts from health departments - United States, June 25-July 24, 2020. MMWR Morb Mortal Wkly Rep 2021;70(3):83–7. https://doi.org/10.15585/mmwr.mm7003a3.
118. Honein MA, Christie A, Rose DA, et al. Summary of guidance for public health strategies to address high levels of community transmission of SARS-CoV-2 and related deaths, December 2020. MMWR Morb Mortal Wkly Rep 2020;69(49):1860–7. https://doi.org/10.15585/mmwr.mm6949e2.

Updates in the Epidemiology, Approaches to Vaccine Coverage and Current Outbreaks of Measles

Nadine Peart Akindele, MD[a,b,*]

KEYWORDS

- Measles • Measles virus • Vaccines

KEY POINTS

- Measles, caused by measles virus continues to be a disease associated with significant morbidity and mortality in areas whereby vaccine access and health care resources are limited.
- The epidemic of measles in 2019 speaks to the need for continued vaccination efforts to limit the spread of disease.
- Research is ongoing regarding the management of measles, as well as the improved surveillance and monitoring of the disease in efforts to continue to reduce measles cases and associated morbidity and mortality.

INTRODUCTION

Measles is a viral exanthem that occurs in childhood after infection with measles virus (MeV). The origins of measles have been traced back to that of Rinderpest virus, a cattle pathogen that is now eradicated. Based on recent selection-aware molecular clock modeling of a 1912 MeV strain, it is believed that MeV diverged from Rinderpest as a spill-over event from cattle as early as the 6th century BCE, likely at the time the population growth was substantial enough to support the transmission of the virus.[1]

Before the time of vaccination, measles deaths contributed significantly to childhood mortality, particularly for children less than age 5. This high mortality was substantially reduced with the introduction of measles vaccines in the 1960s[2] and with the aid of global vaccine programs the numbers of cases and mortality continued to decrease. Still despite the numerous global efforts behind vaccine administration

Funding sources: NIH T32-AI052071-18, NIH R01-AI131226, The Bauernschmidt Committee of the Eudowood Board at Johns Hopkins School of Medicine.
[a] Department of Pediatrics, Division of Pediatric Infectious Diseases, Johns Hopkins University, School of Medicine, 200 N Wolfe Street, Room 3150, Baltimore, MD 21287, USA; [b] United States Food and Drug Administration, Silver Spring, MD 20993, USA
* 200 N Wolfe Street, Room 3150, Baltimore, MD 21287.
E-mail address: npeart1@jhmi.edu

Infect Dis Clin N Am 36 (2022) 39–48
https://doi.org/10.1016/j.idc.2021.11.010
0891-5520/22/© 2021 Elsevier Inc. All rights reserved.

id.theclinics.com

and access, as well as efforts to improve nutrition and access to medical care, in 2018, measles was the cause of more than 140,000 deaths, primarily in children less than 5 years of age. In the United States, the outbreaks of measles in 2019 increased awareness of this vaccine-preventable disease associated with high morbidity and mortality. Additionally, the suspensions of vaccine campaigns due to the COVID-19 pandemic have highlighted concerns with vaccine access and ongoing transmission of this disease. This Clinics review of measles will discuss the latest information on the epidemiology, pathophysiology, immune response, clinical manifestations, diagnosis, management, and prevention of measles.

DISCUSSION
What Is the Current Epidemiology of Measles?

Cases of measles have drastically declined over the years due to the introduction of safe and effective measles-containing vaccines (MCVs). Elimination was first documented in the United States in 2000, and the continued maintenance of herd immunity had provided substantial protection against the resurgence of infection. In addition to vaccination, improved nutrition and health care have been contributing factors to the decrease in measles deaths and complications. Still, despite the low number of cases in the Americas, measles continues to be a disease that heavily burdens low-resource nations in Asia and Africa.[3] Access to vaccination may be limited and nutrition in some communities remains poor, with vitamin A deficiency being a major factor in measles-associated mortality.[4] This along with the movement toward vaccine hesitancy, which has primarily been fueled by misinformation surrounding vaccines and which has been a detriment to immunization programs in several countries, contributed to the sudden increase in cases seen around the world, including in the United States (**Fig. 1**). In 2019, the World Health Organization (WHO) reported more than 869,770 cases and an estimated 207,500 deaths worldwide.[3]

Measles is transmitted by the respiratory route (**Fig. 2**.). The incubation period is about 10 days from the time of infection to the development of fever and 14 days to the development of the hallmark maculopapular rash. The virus is highly contagious as defined by the reproductive number (R0), or the average number of secondary cases in a susceptible population that an infected individual can cause. The R0 of

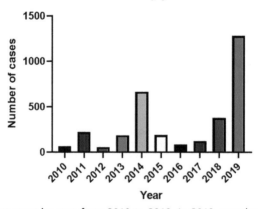

Fig. 1. Measles virus cases by year from 2010 to 2019. In 2019, measles virus cases surged, with cases at the highest levels in the US since 1992 (*Data from* CDC, https://www.cdc.gov/measles/cases-outbreaks.html).

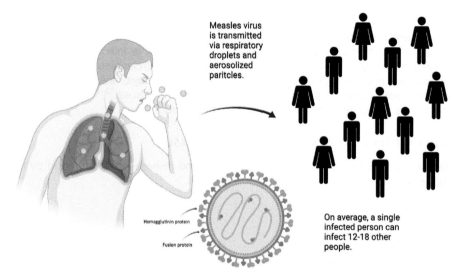

Measles virus is transmitted via respiratory droplets and aerosolized paritcles.

Hemagglutinin protein

Fusion protein

On average, a single infected person can infect 12-18 other people.

Fig. 2. Transmission and Reproductive number (R0) of measles virus. Transmission is via the respiratory route, through respiratory droplets and aerosols. Measles virus is highly contagious with an R0 of 12 to 18, meaning on average, one infected person will spread the virus to 12 to 18 others.

measles is one of the highest at 12 to 18[5] (see **Fig. 2.**) when compared with SARS-CoV-2 (R0 2.4–3.4)[5] and influenza (R0 1.2–1.4).[6] Because of this high reproductive number, a high level of population immunity (>94%) is required to interrupt transmission and eliminate measles, meaning the absence of continuous disease transmission for greater than 12 months. There is no animal reservoir although nonhuman primates (NHPs) can be infected and share immunologic responses and clinical manifestations similar to humans after infection.

Transmission in temperate climates tends to reflect a seasonal distribution with transmission occurring in the late winter and early spring. In tropical climates, the transmission tends to peak during the rainy seasons.

What Causes Measles?

Measles is a highly contagious childhood exanthem caused by MeV, which belongs to the family *Paramyxoviridae*. Other well-known viruses in this family include mumps virus (MuV), the parainfluenza viruses, and the zoonotic Nipah virus (NiV), and like these other viruses, MeV is an enveloped, negative sense, single-stranded, RNA virus.[7] The family *Paramyxoviridae* is divided into two subfamilies, *Paramyxovirinae* and *Pneumovirinae*. The genus *Morbillivirus*, which includes MeV, is within the subfamily *Pneumovirinae*.[8] The MeV genome is 16kb long and contains 6 genes that encode 8 proteins, including nucleocapsid (N), phosphoprotein (P), 2 nonstructural proteins, C and V, which are also encoded by the P gene, matrix (M), fusion (F), hemagglutinin (H), and large polymerase (L). H and F are surface glycoproteins responsible for attachment to a host cell membrane, fusion, and cell entry.[8] The remainder of the proteins are responsible for the packaging of the virion RNA (N), viral RNA transcription, and translation (P and L, subunits of the RNA-dependent RNA polymerase),[9] virus assembly (M) and evading the host immune response (C and V).[10]

Pathogenesis of Measles

After respiratory infection with wild-type (WT) MeV, the virus spreads from the respiratory tract to the lymphoid tissue. Infected peripheral blood mononuclear cells (B and

T cells and monocytes) then spread the virus to epithelial cells of nonlymphoid organs.[11,12] The hallmark rash that occurs 10 to 14 days after infection is due to the MeV-specific cellular immune response associated with virus clearance. Although infectious virus is not typically detected in lymphocytes after 21 days, viral RNA clearance is slower, taking weeks to months to clear from cells and tissues.[13–15] Recovery from infection is associated with life-long protective immunity.

WHAT ARE THE CLINICAL MANIFESTATIONS OF MEASLES?

Measles is transmitted by the respiratory route and disease is characterized by the following:

- Cough
- Coryza/runny nose
- Conjunctivitis
- Koplik spots
- Maculopapular rash
- Fever

Measles was responsible for more than 2 million deaths each year before the introduction of the vaccines in 1963, making it a leading cause of child morbidity and mortality at that time.[16] Complications of measles are the major reason for morbidity and mortality associated with the disease and usually manifest as pneumonia, but blindness and neurologic manifestations also occur.[17]

Complications

Measles mortality is primarily due to the secondary immunodeficiency that accompanies primary infection.[18] Because life-long immunity is also established, the immune suppression is typically described as paradoxic. Lymphopenia is common during acute disease[19] followed by reductions in both T cell function[20] and humoral immunity over time.[21] This paradoxic immune suppression is believed to lead to the increased susceptibility of a person infected with measles to secondary infections. Pneumonia, as well as gastrointestinal and upper respiratory tract infections, can occur after measles infection and both viral and bacterial pathogens can be found as culprits.[22] Increased vitamin A utilization and subsequent deficiency occurs and can exacerbate the complications of primary infection with MeV.[23] Prior deficiency of vitamin A can be associated with more severe measles cases.[4] Acute neurologic complications of measles include autoimmune demyelinating disease and acute disseminated encephalomyelitis. Subacute sclerosing panencephalitis (SSPE) is a neurologic complication associated with persistent infection that occurs several years (average of 7 years) after primary infection. Although rare and reported to occur in only 5 to 10 cases per million reported measles cases,[23] this serious complication of measles leads to cognitive decline, myoclonus, gait abnormalities, vision loss, and death.[17]

What Are the Treatment Options for Measles?

Several treatment options for measles have been explored; however, only Vitamin A has been shown to decrease the mortality associated with disease and is recommended.[24] Ribavirin has in vitro activity against MeV and has been used successfully in select case reports[25] but has significant toxicity that limits its widespread adoption and the use in clinical trials. Interferon alpha has primarily been studied in animal models;[26] however, for similar reasons as with ribavirin, clinical data are limited. Vitamin A, however, has been studied in clinical trials and has been shown in meta-analyses to reduce mortality in children aged less than 2 years (risk ratio (RR): 0.21; 95% confidence interval (CI): 0.07–0.66) as well as pneumonia-specific mortality (RR: 0.57; 95% CI: 0.24–1.37)[24] when given in 2 doses over the course of 2 days. The mechanism of action is not fully understood; however, measles may increase the body's utilization of vitamin A due to the rapid destruction of epithelial surfaces.[24] Additionally, the ability of vitamin A to support the proliferation of lymphocytes may play a role, as its immunologic properties have been studied with other infectious diseases, including HIV, malaria, and diarrheal infections.[27] Currently, the WHO recommends a 2-day treatment with 200,000 international units (IU) per day for children greater than 1 year of age, 100,000 IU per day for infants 6 to 12 months of age and 50,000 IU per day for infants less than 6 months of age. Additionally, it is recommended that children with clinical evidence of vitamin A deficiency be given a third dose approximately 2 to 4 weeks later.[4,24,27] Although prophylactic antibiotics are not indicated, severe complications of measles including secondary bacterial pneumonia and gastrointestinal disease, may warrant the use of antibiotics.

How to Prevent Measles?

Primary prevention

Since 1963, there has been a highly effective and safe live attenuated virus vaccine for measles. The vaccine was developed in the mid-20th century by the passage of WT MeV isolated from the blood of a boy in Boston, through renal and amnion cells and then through chicken embryo fibroblast (CEF) cells.[28] The first live attenuated vaccine strain licensed in 1963 frequently produced a rash and fever after administration. Continued passage of this virus strain through various cell types led to further attenuation and has produced the most common vaccine strains used today.[29,30] The Moraten (Attenuvax) vaccine strain which was passed further in CEF cells is the only strain used in the United States today. The Edmonston–Zagreb (EZ) vaccine strain was passed through human WI-38 cells and is used widely internationally. MCVs are often combined with other live attenuated virus vaccines, such as mumps and rubella. The measles–mumps–rubella (MMR) vaccine, for example, is a combined vaccine that is widely used today. The vaccine is administered subcutaneously, though other modes of delivery have been explored. Aerosolized MCVs were found to be inferior to subcutaneous injection with a lower proportion of those who seroconverted in the aerosolized group (85.4%, 95% CI: 82.5–88.0) when compared with the subcutaneous group (94.6%, 95% CI: 92.7–96.1).[31] Microarray patches[32] have also been studied and were shown to induce protective antibody levels in a higher proportion of monkeys when compared with those who received the subcutaneous injection,[33] though it has not yet been studied in humans. If found to be effective, the latter could be a useful means to increase access of the vaccination to areas of low resource with high transmission, as it is a needle-free, heat-stable option, that requires minimal medical expertise to administer. While stabilizers (such as sorbitol and gelatin) and antibiotics (such as neomycin) are possible components of the current subcutaneous MCVs, they do not contain adjuvants such as thiomersal.[34]

The measles vaccine series is given in the US in 2 doses, as recommended by the Advisory Committee on Immunization Practices (ACIP), the American Academy of Pediatrics (AAP), and the American Academy of Family Physicians (AAFP) in the 1980s due to an increase in outbreaks despite the introduction of the single dose in the 1960s. The immune response to the vaccine is similar as to what occurs after primary infection, with immunoglobulin G first appearing 12 to 15 days after vaccination and reaching its peak at 21 to 28 days after vaccination.[34] Measles antibodies develop in approximately 95% of children vaccinated at 12 months of age and 98% of children vaccinated at 15 months of age. This decreases to 85% to 90% for those vaccinated at 9 months of age, hence the U.S. Centers for Diseases Control and Prevention (US CDC) immunization schedule recommendation to have the first MMR dose at 1 year of age. Notably, several countries do initiate the first dose as early as 9 months of age, due to higher levels of transmission of the virus. It is also reasonable in some settings to administer the vaccine as early as 6 months of age. The WHO recommends the administration of MCVs as early as 6 months of age in the following scenarios:

- During ongoing measles outbreaks
- During vaccination campaigns, when the risk of measles in younger infants is high
- For internally displaced populations and refugees and populations in conflict zones
- For infants known to be HIV-infected or exposed (ie, born to an HIV-infected mother)
- For individual infants at high risk of contracting measles; and
- For infants traveling to countries experiencing measles outbreaks[35]

Children that receive a dose of an MCV at 6 months of age, should still, however, receive their standard routine MMR schedule once they are of age.

Approximately 2%–5% of children who receive only one dose of MMR vaccine fail to respond to it, which is also known as primary vaccine failure. A portion of this vaccine failure is related to the presence of inhibitory maternal antibodies as well as immunologic immaturity of the vaccine recipient.[34] MMR primary vaccine failure can also be related to damaged vaccine or loss of vaccine potency. Suspected but not confirmed vaccine failure could be related to incorrect records and possibly other reasons. Second doses of MMR, which are recommended to be administered at 4 to 6 years of age in the US, are not indicated as a "booster" as is the case with other vaccine types, rather, it was implemented to capture those who did not respond to or did not receive the initial MMR vaccine. Most persons who fail to respond to the first dose will respond to a second dose. It has been shown that more than 97% of those who receive 2 doses of measles vaccine (with the first dose administered no earlier than 1 year of age) develop protective measles immunity[36] especially when given at an older age.[34] Immunity to measles vaccine is less durable than the immunity generated by primary WT MeV infection, though protection typically does last for several years. Secondary vaccine failure has been reported, though is rare.[36] The vaccine is generally well tolerated, with most adverse reactions occurring with the 1st dose. Typical vaccine-related reactions include:

- Injection site redness and pain
- Fever
- Rash
- Thrombocytopenia

Studies have since disproved the earlier false allegations that the MMR vaccine causes autism. One of the largest studies that evaluated this was a retrospective cohort study of more than 500,000 children who received the vaccine, and in this study, there was no association that was found between the vaccine and autism spectrum disorder (relative risk: 0.92, 95% CI: 0.68–1.24).[37]

Measles is an antigenically monotypic virus and so the measles vaccines that were derived over 6 decades ago from common strains of the virus, continue to provide protection against WT strains that have arisen worldwide. The neutralizing epitopes in the surface proteins that induce protection are highly conserved. Because the evolution of the receptor binding sites of H remain restricted, new measles vaccines do not need to be developed to counter new strains.[38] Measles vaccination is estimated to have prevented 25.5 million deaths globally.[3]

In 2001, the Measles & Rubella Initiative (M&R Initiative) was formed by the American Red Cross, the United Nations Foundation, the US CDC, the United Nations Children's Fund (UNICEF), and the WHO to support and fund measures to prevent deaths from measles.[39] These organizations together identify issues that lead to undervaccination in high-risk communities and focus on implementing strategies to overcome low vaccine rates. Examples of such strategies include developing novel methods to increase the dissemination of information and limit vaccine misinformation with current technologies, including social media. They also work to improve monitoring and surveillance of measles and vaccination rates.

Secondary prevention

Secondary protection for unimmunized or high-risk individuals exposed to measles can be achieved with one of the 2 methods: MMR or immunoglobulin (IG) administration. MMR is preferred if it can be administered within 3 days of exposure. Some hosts who are immunocompromised cannot receive the live vaccine, however. In those settings, it is appropriate to give IG within 6 days from the time of exposure. A study on unimmunized children in New York during a 2013 outbreak demonstrated that both MMR and intramuscular (IM) IG were effective in preventing clinical measles with a measured effectiveness of 83.4% (CI: 34.4, 95.8) for MMR and 100% (CI: 56.2, 99.8) for IMIG.[40] It should be noted that if IG is administered, if not contraindicated and the patient is greater than 12 months of age, individuals should also receive MMR or MMRV 6 months after intramuscularly administered IG or 8 months after intravenously administered IG.[41,42]

Current Measles Outbreaks

Although several advances have been made toward decreasing measles outbreaks, globally, there is still a struggle to achieve the 3 milestones established by The World Health Assembly (WHA) in 2010. The milestones, which were created with efforts to achieve measles control by 2015 were as follows: (1) increase routine vaccination coverage with 1 dose of a measles containing vaccine (MCV1) to at least 90% nationally and at least 80% in every district, (2) reduce global annual measles incidence to less than 5 cases per million population, and (3) reduce global measles mortality by 95% from the 2000 estimate.[43] Globally, MCV1 coverage in 2018 was estimated to be 86%, according to WHO and UNICEF (WUENIC) (Table 1).[43]

Table 1 Regional MCV1 coverage by WHO region	
Region	Percentage MCV1 Coverage
African (AFR)	74
Americas (AMR)	90
Eastern Mediterranean (EMR)	82
European (EUR)	95
South-East Asia (SEAR)	89
Western Pacific (WPR)	95

Data from Moss WJ, Shendale S, Lindstrand A, et al. Feasibility assessment of measles and rubella eradication. Vaccine. 2021;39(27):3544-3559. https://doi.org/10.1016/j.vaccine.2021.04.027

In 2019, 9 countries accounted for 73% of all reported measles cases: Central African Republic, Democratic Republic of Congo, Georgia, Kazakhstan, Madagascar, North Macedonia, Samoa, Tonga, and Ukraine.[3] After 2019, due to the COVID-19 pandemic, almost 41 countries put off their measles vaccine campaigns for 2020 and 2021. Due to this, there is concern that this may fuel more and bigger outbreaks than what was experienced in 2019, as previous experiences with Ebola outbreaks in Liberia, Guinea, and Sierra Leone revealed that the suspension of vaccine activity led to increased incidences of measles cases.[44] As of 2021, the top 3 countries with measles outbreaks are Nigeria, Pakistan and India.[45] The WHO has recently published updated recommendations for measles management to reduce the morbidity and mortality associated with recent measles outbreaks.[23]

CLINICS CARE POINTS

- Measles is a highly contagious respiratory virus, associated with significant morbidity and mortality, especially for children less than 5 years of age.
- Measles continues to be a major threat to public health despite the presence of a highly safe and effective vaccine, due to ongoing issues with vaccine access and delivery as well as recent suspensions in vaccine programs due to the COVID-19 pandemic.
- Ongoing efforts to increase vaccine coverage have continued, though globally, the set goals have not yet been achieved.

DISCLAIMER

Dr. N. PeartAkindele contributed to this article in her personal capacity. The views expressed in this article are her own and do not necessarily represent the views of the Food and Drug Administration or the United States Government.

ACKNOWLEDGMENTS

I am grateful to my mentors, Diane E Griffin, MD, PhD and William Moss, MD, MPH, who provided support in the editing and review of this article. Images and figures were created with the help of BioRender.com and Graphpad Prism.

DISCLOSURE

The author has nothing to disclose.

REFERENCES

1. Düx A, Lequime S, Patrono LV, et al. Measles virus and rinderpest virus divergence dated to the sixth century BCE. Science (New York, NY) 2020; 368(6497):1367–70.
2. Gastanaduy PA, Redd SB, S. CN, et al. Manual for the surveillance of vaccine-preventable diseases, Chapter 7: Measles. 2019. Page last reviewed: May 13, 2019
3. Patel MK, Goodson JL, Alexander JP Jr, et al. Progress Toward Regional Measles Elimination — Worldwide, 2000–2019. MMWR Morb Mortal Wkly Rep 2020; 69(45):1700–5.
4. Hussey GD, Klein M. A Randomized, Controlled Trial of Vitamin A in Children with Severe Measles. N Engl J Med 1990;323(3):160–4.

5. Guerra FM, Bolotin S, Lim G, et al. The basic reproduction number (R(0)) of measles: a systematic review. Lancet Infect Dis 2017;17(12):e420–8.

6. Chowell G, Miller MA, Viboud C. Seasonal influenza in the United States, France, and Australia: transmission and prospects for control. Epidemiol Infect 2008; 136(6):852–64.

7. Cox RM, Plemper RK. Structure and organization of paramyxovirus particles. Curr Opin Virol 2017;24:105–14.

8. Plattet P, Alves L, Herren M, et al. Measles Virus Fusion Protein: Structure, Function and Inhibition. Viruses 2016;8(4):112.

9. Bankamp B, Horikami SM, Thompson PD, et al. Domains of the Measles Virus N Protein Required for Binding to P Protein and Self-Assembly. Virology 1996; 216(1):272–7.

10. Iwasaki M, Takeda M, Shirogane Y, et al. The matrix protein of measles virus regulates viral RNA synthesis and assembly by interacting with the nucleocapsid protein. J Virol 2009;83(20):10374–83.

11. de Swart RL, Ludlow M, de Witte L, et al. Predominant infection of CD150+ lymphocytes and dendritic cells during measles virus infection of macaques. Plos Pathog 2007;3(11):e178.

12. de Vries RD, Lemon K, Ludlow M, et al. In vivo tropism of attenuated and pathogenic measles virus expressing green fluorescent protein in macaques. J Virol 2010;84(9):4714–24.

13. Nelson AN, Putnam N, Hauer D, et al. Evolution of T Cell Responses during Measles Virus Infection and RNA Clearance. Scientific Rep 2017;7(1):11474.

14. Nelson AN, Lin W-HW, Shivakoti R, et al. Association of persistent wild-type measles virus RNA with long-term humoral immunity in rhesus macaques. JCI Insight 2020;5(3).

15. Lin W-HW, Kouyos RD, Adams RJ, et al. Prolonged persistence of measles virus RNA is characteristic of primary infection dynamics. Proc Natl Acad Sci 2012; 109(37):14989–94.

16. Moss WJ. Measles. Lancet 2017;390(10111):2490–502.

17. Garg RK, Mahadevan A, Malhotra HS, et al. Subacute sclerosing panencephalitis. Rev Med Virol 2019;29(5):e2058.

18. Griffin DE. Immune responses during measles virus infection. Curr Top Microbiol Immunol 1995;191:117–34.

19. Griffin DE. Measles virus-induced suppression of immune responses. Immunol Rev 2010;236(1):176–89.

20. Tamashiro VG, Perez HH, Griffin DE. Prospective study of the magnitude and duration of changes in tuberculin reactivity during uncomplicated and complicated measles. Pediatr Infect Dis J 1987;6(5):451–4.

21. Mina MJ, Kula T, Leng Y, et al. Measles virus infection diminishes preexisting antibodies that offer protection from other pathogens. Science 2019;366(6465): 599–606.

22. Beckford AP, Kaschula RO, Stephen C. Factors associated with fatal cases of measles. A retrospective autopsy study. S Afr Med J 1985;68(12):858–63.

23. WHO. Guide for clinical case management and infection prevention and control during a measles outbreak. Geneva2020.

24. Huiming Y, Chaomin W, Meng M. Vitamin A for treating measles in children. Cochrane Database Syst Rev 2005;2005(4):Cd001479.

25. Gururangan S, Stevens RF, Morris DJ. Ribavirin response in measles pneumonia. J Infect 1990;20(3):219–21.

26. Takahashi T, Hosoya M, Kimura K, et al. The cooperative effect of interferon-α and ribavirin on subacute sclerosing panencephalitis (SSPE) virus infections, in vitro and in vivo. Antiviral Res 1998;37(1):29–35.

27. Villamor E, Fawzi WW. Effects of Vitamin A Supplementation on Immune Responses and Correlation with Clinical Outcomes. Clin Microbiol Rev 2005;18(3):446–64.

28. Enders JF, Peebles TC. Propagation in tissue cultures of cytopathogenic agents from patients with measles. Proc Soc Exp Biol Med 1954;86(2):277–86.

29. Krugman S, Muriel G, Fontana VJ. Combined live measles-rubella vaccine. Am J Dis Child 1972;123(5):518.

30. Katz SL, Enders JF, Holloway A. Studies on an attenuated measles-virus vaccine. II. Clinical, virologic and immunologic effects of vaccine in institutionalized children. N Engl J Med 1960;263:159–61.

31. Low N, Bavdekar A, Jeyaseelan L, et al. A randomized, controlled trial of an aerosolized vaccine against measles. N Engl J Med 2015;372(16):1519–29.

32. Badizadegan K, Goodson JL, Rota PA, et al. The potential role of using vaccine patches to induce immunity: platform and pathways to innovation and commercialization. Expert Rev Vaccin 2020;19(2):175–94.

33. Joyce JC, Carroll TD, Collins ML, et al. A Microneedle Patch for Measles and Rubella Vaccination Is Immunogenic and Protective in Infant Rhesus Macaques. J Infect Dis 2018;218(1):124–32.

34. WHO, De Swart RL, Moss WJ. The immunological Basis for immunization series. Geneva; 2020.

35. WHO. Measles vaccines: WHO position paper – April 2017. Wkly Epidemiol Rec 2017;92(17):205–27.

36. Mathias RG, Meekison WG, Arcand TA, et al. The role of secondary vaccine failures in measles outbreaks. Am J Public Health 1989;79(4):475–8.

37. Madsen KM, Hviid A, Vestergaard M, et al. A population-based study of measles, mumps, and rubella vaccination and autism. N Engl J Med 2002;347(19):1477–82.

38. Muñoz-Alía M, Nace RA, Zhang L, et al. Serotypic evolution of measles virus is constrained by multiple co-dominant B cell epitopes on its surface glycoproteins. Cell Rep Med 2021;2(4):100225.

39. Initiative MaR. Measles Rubella Strateg Framework 2021;1–48.

40. Arciuolo RJ, Jablonski RR, Zucker JR, et al. Effectiveness of Measles Vaccination and Immune Globulin Post-Exposure Prophylaxis in an Outbreak Setting—New York City, 2013. Clin Infect Dis 2017;65(11):1843–7.

41. Gastañaduy PA, Goodson JL. Measles (Rubeola). CDC; 2019.

42. General CDC. Recommendations on Immunization. Morbidity Mortality Weekly Rep 2011;60(2).

43. Moss WJ, Shendale S, Lindstrand A, et al. Feasibility assessment of measles and rubella eradication. Vaccine 2021;39(27):3544–59.

44. Masresha BG, Luce R Jr, Weldegebriel G, et al. The impact of a prolonged ebola outbreak on measles elimination activities in Guinea, Liberia and Sierra Leone, 2014-2015. Pan Afr Med J 2020;35(Suppl 1):8.

45. CDC. Global Measles Outbreaks. 2021. Available at: https://www.cdc.gov/globalhealth/measles/data/global-measles-outbreaks.html?CDC_AA_refVal=https%3A%2F%2Fwww.cdc.gov%2Fglobalhealth%2Fmeasles%2Fglobalmeaslesoutbreaks.htm. Accessed June 8, 2021.

Tuberculosis in Children

Devan Jaganath, MD, MPH[a], Jeanette Beaudry, MD, PhD[b],
Nicole Salazar-Austin, MD, ScM[c],*

KEYWORDS

- Tuberculosis • TB • Child • Treatment • Diagnosis • Prevention

KEY POINTS

- LTBI diagnosis requires assessment of risk factors, immunologic evidence of infection, and exclusion of symptomatic TB disease.
- LTBI treatments have moved away from the traditional 9 months of isoniazid toward shorter rifamycin-containing regimens.
- The integration of clinical, radiographic, and microbiologic data is needed to support a diagnosis of TB disease.
- Multidrug therapy for at least 6 months is currently used to treat TB disease, with additional considerations in formulation and administration required for children.
- New diagnostics for more accurate and faster detection, and shorter treatment courses for LTBI and TB disease seek to improve TB outcomes in children.

NATURE OF THE PROBLEM

Tuberculosis (TB) is an infectious disease caused by *Mycobacterium tuberculosis* complex (Mtb).[1] Each year, 7.5 million children are infected with TB and 1.1 million children develop TB disease worldwide, representing 12% of the global TB burden.[2] At the same time, children have a disproportionately higher mortality, with 230,000 deaths annually.[2] The high mortality rate is a reflection of the challenges in diagnosing and treating TB in children, especially the most vulnerable including children younger than 5 years old and children with HIV coinfection.[3–6] The incidence of TB disease further increases when they enter adolescence and begin to develop adult-type disease.[5,7]

In the United States, TB cases have shifted toward foreign-born adults,[8,9] but 4% of the national TB disease prevalence is still in children less than 15 years old and 10% are adolescents and young adults 15 to 24 years old.[8] Disparities exist with disproportionately higher rates among non-White ethnic groups and in the US-affiliated islands.[9] Treatment

[a] Division of Pediatric Infectious Diseases, University of California, San Francisco, 1001 Potrero Avenue, Building 3, Room 635A, Box 1234, San Francisco, CA 94110, USA; [b] Division of Pediatric Infectious Diseases, Johns Hopkins University School of Medicine, 200 N. Wolfe Street, Room 3150, Baltimore, MD 21287, USA; [c] Division of Pediatric Infectious Diseases, Johns Hopkins University School of Medicine, 200 N Wolfe Street, Room 3147, Baltimore, MD 21287, USA
* Corresponding author.
E-mail address: nsalaza1@jhmi.edu

Infect Dis Clin N Am 36 (2022) 49–71
https://doi.org/10.1016/j.idc.2021.11.008
0891-5520/22/© 2021 Elsevier Inc. All rights reserved.

of TB infection in children and adolescents is critical to prevent progression to TB disease and to prevent them from becoming the future reservoir for TB transmission.[10]

In this review, we outline the current approach to diagnosis and treatment of TB infection and disease in children, focusing on the main issues that arise during clinical care and concluding with emerging diagnostic and therapeutic options.

TUBERCULOSIS INFECTION
Diagnosis

Latent TB infection (LTBI) represents a state where the child has evidence of an immune response to Mtb, but does not have signs and symptoms of TB disease. In this stage, the mycobacteria are thought to be controlled but not eliminated by the immune system.[11] As a consequence, children with LTBI are not infectious.[1] LTBI evaluation requires a combination of risk factor assessment and immunologic evidence of infection, while ensuring there is no clinical or radiographic evidence of TB disease.

The American Academy of Pediatrics (AAP) recommends screening for TB risk factors at the first well-child visit, every 6 months for the first year of life, and then annually.[12] Schools may require TB screening as a requirement for entry and juvenile detention centers may perform initial screening as a congregate setting. Multiple screening tools are available, and the suggested questions are outlined in **Table 1**. The risk factors for infection or progression to TB disease fall into three categories: (1) birth or significant time spent in a TB-endemic setting; (2) known or suspected TB exposure, or a high risk of TB exposure; and (3) immunosuppression. Immunosuppression is caused by HIV infection, cancer, organ transplantation, biologic response modifiers (including anti–tumor necrosis factor-α inhibitors), and prolonged steroid use. Children with HIV are at an increased risk of TB disease, and should be tested annually if previously negative.[12] Additional risk factors, such as renal failure requiring hemodialysis, homelessness, or ingestion of unpasteurized milk products, should be included as relevant to the local demographics of TB disease in the community.

Tuberculosis Infection Testing

Testing for TB infection in low-incidence settings, such as the United States, should be performed only for those with risk factors because testing the general population has a low positive predictive value and increases the likelihood of false positivity.[13] Testing options for TB infection include the tuberculin skin test (TST), also referred to as purified protein derivative, and interferon-γ release assays (IGRAs). For children that have been recently exposed to TB, negative testing is repeated 8 to 10 weeks after the last exposure to Mtb to allow for the development of an adaptive immune response.[14] Because LTBI testing reflects an immune response after exposure to TB, there is low utility in serial or future testing after a positive result.

Tuberculin skin testing

TST involves intradermal injection of a tuberculin protein mixture, with measurement of the induration caused by a delayed hypersensitivity reaction after 2 to 3 days.[1] The cutoff for induration is 5 mm for children with a TB contact, symptoms concerning for TB, or are immunocompromised (including HIV), and 10 mm for children younger than 5 years old or who have lived in a TB-endemic setting.[12] A 15-mm cutoff is for children 5 years and older without risk factors. The advantages of TST are that it is performed in the community without a laboratory and is affordable, making it attractive for large-scale screening activities. However, tuberculin needs to be refrigerated, testing requires two visits, technical placement is difficult, and interreader reliability is variable.[15]

Table 1
Summary and comparison of TB screening questions for children with LTBI

Category	AAP Red Book[12]	California Pediatric TB Risk Assessment[85]	Pediatric Tuberculosis Collaborative Group[13]
Birth or significant time spent in TB-endemic setting	Was your child born in a high-risk country?[a]	Birth, travel, or residence in a country with an elevated TB rate for at least 1 mo	Was your child born outside the United States?
	Has your child traveled to a high-risk country?[a] How much contact did your child have with the resident population?		Has your child traveled outside the United States?
Immunosuppression[b]	Immunosuppressed populations	Immunosuppression, current or planned	
Known or suspected TB contact or high-risk of exposure	Has a family member had a positive tuberculin skin test result?	Close contact to someone with infectious TB disease during lifetime	Has your child been exposed to anyone with TB disease?
	Has a family member or contact had tuberculosis disease?		Does your child have close contact with a person who has a positive TB skin test?

[a] Countries other than the United States, Canada, Australia, New Zealand, or Western and North European countries.
[b] HIV, organ transplant recipient, steroids (prednisone ≥2 mg/kg/d, or ≥15 mg/d for ≥2 wk), anti–tumor necrosis factor-α inhibitor, or other immunosuppressive medication.

The overall performance of TST is moderate in children, with sensitivity ranging from 67% to 85%,[15–18] and specificity ranging from 70% to 92%.[15,18] TST can cross-react with other non-TB mycobacteria (NTM), including *Mycobacterium avium* complex, and the bacille Calmette-Guérin (BCG) vaccine, leading to false-positive results.[14] BCG vaccine is often given at birth, and the cross-reaction wanes over time,[19] but is more likely to persist if the individual received the vaccine or a booster when older (local guidelines are available at http://www.bcgatlas.org/). False-negative results can occur in children who are less than 6 months old, immunosuppressed, have severe TB disease, recent TB infection, other concomitant bacterial infections, and if recently given a live virus vaccine including measles.[17] In addition, technical challenges in storing, administering, and reading TSTs can lead to false-negative results.

Interferon-γ release assays
IGRAs are blood-based assays that measure T-cell release of interferon-γ after exposure to TB-specific antigens ESAT-6 and CFP-10.[1] The two most common assays are QuantiFERON Gold Plus (Qiagen, Germantown, MD) and T-SPOT.TB test (Oxford-Immunotec, Abingdon, United Kingdom), with cutoffs determined by the amount of interferon-γ detected relative to the background from a negative control. If the positive

and/or negative controls fail, the assays result as indeterminate or invalid. T-SPOT.TB also has a borderline category that is between a negative and positive result.

Compared with TST, IGRAs have similar sensitivity (57%–85%),[16–18] but improved specificity (85%–100%).[16–18] The higher specificity is because IGRAs do not cross-react with the BCG vaccine and are less likely to interact with other NTMs. In addition, only a single visit is needed, unlike the TST.[14] Consequently, IGRAs are preferred over TST for LTBI testing in the United States,[1,14] and is required for all immigrants 2 years and older as part of the civil surgeon medical evaluation.[20] Although TST has been preferred for children younger than 2 years old, growing evidence suggests that IGRAs perform similarly to TST in young children and discordant results have not resulted in missed TB cases,[21] although both have reduced sensitivity in younger children.[12,18] The AAP still recommends that a TST be used for children younger than 2 years old, but they do allow IGRA testing.[12]

Several limitations of IGRAs can impact their implementation. IGRAs use blood samples that are invasive and difficult to obtain in children, and requires laboratory infrastructure.[15,22,23] IGRAs are more expensive than the TST, although a family may have reduced costs by not requiring an additional visit.[18] Indeterminate, invalid, or borderline results can complicate interpretation and negates the benefits of a single visit if repeat testing is needed. Also, false negatives can still occur with IGRAs in individuals who are immunosuppressed, young children, early TB infection, or advanced TB disease.[17]

Interpretation of tuberculin skin test or interferon-γ release assay results

Interpretation of either a TST or IGRA should take into account the risk factors that initiated LTBI testing. A positive result from either a TST or IGRA in a child with TB risk factors should be considered a true positive unless there is a clear alternative diagnosis. We generally do not obtain a TST and IGRA, unless we are concerned about a false negative and want to repeat testing. In children less than 2 years old with BCG vaccination, a positive TST should account for the child's TB risk factors, but if concerned for a false positive an IGRA is performed. If TST and IGRA results are discordant, we would consider the likelihood of a false positive by TST, whether any technical factors may have led to a false negative by one of them, or the possibility of alternative diagnoses including NTM infection if TST positive and IGRA negative. However, we would again consider the risk factors of the child for TB progression and complications, and would have a low threshold for classifying them as positive if no clear alternative explanation exists. Indeterminate, invalid, or borderline IGRA results should be repeated, either with the same or different IGRA, or with a TST.

Excluding tuberculosis disease

Neither TST nor IGRA can differentiate TB infection from disease, and it is critical to rule out symptomatic disease before initiating LTBI treatment.[12] Symptom screening should include fever, cough, weight loss, or failure to thrive, with a complete clinical examination including growth assessment and evaluation of extrapulmonary manifestations including lymphadenopathy. Two-view anteroposterior and lateral chest radiographs (CXR) are recommended in the United States, especially because children can have subtle or absent symptoms. If abnormal, we would consider further evaluation of TB disease including sputum-based testing before initiating LTBI treatment.

Treatment of Latent Tuberculosis Infection

Isoniazid monotherapy has been the mainstay of LTBI treatment presumed to be susceptible to isoniazid and rifampin for decades. Meta-analyses of isoniazid prophylaxis in adults and children showed isoniazid preventive therapy reduces the risk of TB disease by 60% over the subsequent 2 years.[24,25] Some studies have shown effectiveness of greater than 90% when restricting the analysis to those who were adherent.[26] However, the effectiveness of isoniazid for TB prevention has been limited by low adherence and completion rates because of prolonged treatment durations (6–9 months) and by the risk of hepatotoxicity. Rifamycin-based treatment regimens are now the preferred regimens for LTBI treatment because of higher treatment completion rates and decreased hepatotoxicity.[27,28] These regimens include 3 months of once-weekly isoniazid plus rifapentine (3HP), 4 months of daily rifampin (4R), and 3 months of daily isoniazid plus rifampin (3HR). Drug-drug interactions with rifamycins, particularly with HIV antiretroviral therapy, may limit their use in some populations.

Isoniazid and rifapentine weekly for 3 months

3HP is a preferred regimen among children aged 2 years and older. This regimen is noninferior to 9 months of daily isoniazid in adults, children aged 2 to 17 years, and adults with HIV.[29–31] Although not well studied in children with HIV, this regimen is expected to be as efficacious in this population. Although initial studies were done with directly observed therapy, programmatic data have shown high completion rates with self-administered therapy and directly observed therapy is no longer mandatory.[27,32,33] Children tolerate 3HP well with lower rates of adverse events compared with adults; this includes hepatoxicity, which has not yet been shown in children. Side effects of 3HP include isolated rash and mild, self-resolving influenza-like symptoms including fever, fatigue, headache, dizziness, nausea, myalgia, and rarely hypotension and syncope, which typically occur several hours after ingestion of the third or fourth dose.

Rifapentine is a potent inducer of the cytochrome P-450 enzyme and the P-glycoprotein transport systems and drug-drug interactions are anticipated. 3HP is administered in children taking an efavirenz-based antiretroviral therapy regimen, but not to children on integrase inhibitors, protease inhibitors, and some nonnucleoside reverse transcriptase inhibitors including nevirapine. Planned studies will assess the drug-drug interaction with dolutegravir in children.

Dosing for the 3HP regimen in children is shown in **Table 2**. Currently, rifapentine is only formulated as a 150-mg film-coated tablet. The pharmacokinetics of the crushed tablet have been studied and current dosing recommendations account for an estimated 30% reduction in oral bioavailability associated with crushing the tablet.[34] Crushed tablets are bitter tasting, but tolerable and should be mixed with high-fat foods, such as ice cream or pudding, to enhance absorption. Although some parents prefer daily regimens to enhance adherence, others may prefer intermittent regimens to decrease the total number of doses required. Drawbacks of the 3HP regimen include the lack of dosing for children aged less than 2 years, the lack of a child-friendly formulation, the high cost of the regimen, and drug-drug interactions.

Rifampin daily for 4 months

Four months of daily rifampin is a preferred regimen for adults and children of all ages. Compared with 9 months of isoniazid (9H), 4R has noninferior efficacy, an improved safety profile, and higher rates of treatment completion with self-administered therapy.[33,35,36] Drug-induced hepatitis remains the most common severe adverse event, but is less common than with 9H. There are limited data for efficacy of the 4R regimen in people living with HIV, but no reason to believe it would be less efficacious.

Side effects of rifampin include minor gastrointestinal symptoms (common) and dermatologic reactions (rare).[35] Hepatotoxicity is reported but rare, occurring in 0%

Table 2
Regimens, dosing, formulations, efficacy, adverse reactions, and significant drug-drug interactions for LTBI treatment

Regimen	Dosage	Formulations	Recommended Populations	Efficacy with 9H as a Reference	Hepatotoxicity in Children	Other Adverse Events	Significant Drug-Drug Interactions
Rifapentine plus isoniazid weekly for 3 mo (3HP)	*Children (2–11 years old):* Isoniazid 25 mg/kg Rifapentine 10.0–14.0 kg, 300 mg 14.1–25.0 kg, 450 mg 25.1–32.0 kg, 600 mg 32.1–49.9 kg, 750 mg ≥50.0 kg, 900 mg *Adults and children (≥12 years old):* Isoniazid 15 mg/kg Rifapentine as above, maximum doses Isoniazid 900 mg Rifapentine 900 mg	RPT: 150-mg film-coated tablet; may be taken whole or crushed (should be maintained in blister packs until ready to use) INH tablet: 100-mg (scored) or 300-mg tablet; may be crushed	Adults and children ≥2 years old, people living with HIV	Noninferior to 9H: Cumulative rate difference: −0.74% (UL 95% CI, 0.32%; predefined NI margin, 0.75%)[29]	No hepatotoxicity identified in children during trials[29] or programmatic roll out to date[32,33,86]	Hypersensitivity reactions with influenza-like syndrome, rash, drug-induced liver injury, hypotension, syncope	Protease inhibitors, integrase inhibitors, maraviroc; anticonvulsant agents, azole antifungal agents, macrolides and tetracyclines, hormone-replacement therapy, and warfarin
Rifampin daily for 3–4 mo (4R)	*Children:* 15–20 mg/ kg [a] *Maximum dose:* 600 mg	Oral capsule: 150 mg and 300 mg; may be opened and used as sprinkles Oral suspension (10 mg/mL)[a]	Adults and children of all ages Limited data for people living with HIV (not recommended in the United States)	Similar efficacy to 9H: Rate difference, −0.37 cases per 100 person-years (95% CI, −0.88 to 0.14)[35]	Range, 0%–0.1%[33,35,87–89]	Nausea, decreased appetite, orange discoloration of bodily fluids	Dolutegravir (dose should be increased to twice daily), protease inhibitors, rilpivirine, elvitegravir, maraviroc; oral contraceptives, azole antifungal agents, calcium channel blockers

| Rifampin plus isoniazid daily for 3 mo (3RH) | Children: Isoniazid 10–20 mg/kg Rifampin 15–20 mg/kg Maximum doses: Isoniazid 300 mg Rifampin 600 mg | RIF oral capsule: 150 mg and 300 mg; may be opened and used as sprinkles INH tablet: 100-mg (scored) or 300-mg tablet; may be crushed Worldwide: 75/50 RH dispersible tablet available | Adults and children of all ages, people living with HIV | Similar efficacy to 9H[90] | Hepatitis found in 0%–0.5% of children; transient liver enzymes found in up to 6% of children[90-95] | Nausea, decreased appetite, orange discoloration of bodily fluids, drug-induced liver injury | Dolutegravir (dose should be increased to twice daily), protease inhibitors, rilpivirine, elvitegravir, maraviroc; oral contraceptives, azole antifungal agents, calcium channel blockers |
| Isoniazid daily for 9 mo (9H) | Children: 10–15 mg/kg[b] Maximum dose: 300 mg | INH tablet: 100-mg (scored) or 300-mg tablet; may be crushed | Adults and children of all ages, people living with HIV | — | ~1% | Drug-induced liver injury | Azole antifungal agents, MAO inhibitors, phenytoin, SSRI antidepressants, valproic acid, acetaminophen |

Abbreviations: CI, confidence interval; INH, isoniazid; MAO, monoamine oxidase; NI, non-inferior; RH, rifampin/isoniazid; RIF, rifampin; RPT, rifapentine; SSRI, selective serotonin reuptake inhibitor.

a Some experts use rifampin at 20 to 30 mg/kg for the daily regimen when prescribing for infants and toddlers.
b Centers for Disease Control and Prevention recommends dosage of 10 to 20 mg/kg.

to 2% of children.[35] Rifampin results in temporary orange discoloration of bodily fluids, such as saliva, urine, sweat, and tears.

Dosing for rifampin is shown in **Table 2**. Rifampin is formulated as capsules (150 mg and 300 mg), which can be opened and sprinkled in food and as an extemporaneous solution (10 mg/mL) made at compounding pharmacies.

Rifampin is a potent inducer of the cytochrome P-450 enzyme and the P-glycoprotein transport systems, resulting in multiple clinically significant drug interactions. Concomitant use of certain classes of drugs should be avoided where possible including oral contraceptives, azole antifungal agents, and calcium channel blockers. Other drug classes require close monitoring and/or dosage adjustments including HMG-CoA reductase inhibitors, warfarin, glucocorticoids, methadone, and tacrolimus. Rifampin has significant drug interactions with antiretroviral agents including integrase inhibitors, protease inhibitors, and some nonnucleoside reverse transcriptase inhibitors including nevirapine. Importantly, this limits the use of rifampin not only among children with HIV, but also HIV-exposed, uninfected children who remain on nevirapine prophylaxis.[37] Twice-daily dolutegravir was safe and sufficient to overcome the enzyme-inducing effect of rifampin for children.[38]

Isoniazid and rifampin daily for 3 months

A regimen of 3 months of daily isoniazid and rifampin is recommended for adults and children of all ages including those children with HIV, although use in this population may be limited by drug interactions. Overall, for HIV-negative adults and children, this regimen has been shown to have similar efficacy, hepatotoxicity, and adverse events requiring discontinuation of therapy as those receiving at least 6 months of isoniazid. Other side effects apart from hepatotoxicity include gastrointestinal intolerance and rash.

Dosing for the 3HR regimen is shown in **Table 2**. In the United States, these drugs are formulated separately and result in a high pill burden, limiting the utility of this daily regimen. Globally, the dispersible fixed-dose combination (75/50 mg) makes this regimen attractive while we await a child-friendly formulation of rifapentine. Although this regimen may be used in children with HIV, drug interactions have been shown between rifampin and multiple antiretroviral agents as described previously, limiting its use in some children.

Six or 9 months of isoniazid

Although rifamycin-based therapies are now preferred, 6H and 9H are alternative regimens to treat LTBI in children with or without HIV who are unable to take a preferred regimen because of drug-drug interactions or intolerability.[27] Isoniazid has been well-studied in many populations including adults and children with and without HIV. Drug-induced hepatitis remains the most common severe adverse event, occurring in about 1% of children. Early symptoms include poor appetite, nausea, and abdominal pain. When symptoms are identified early and the drug is stopped, hepatotoxicity is reversible.

Dosing for 6H and 9H are shown in **Table 2**. Isoniazid comes in 100-mg scored tablets that are easily crushed and mixed with formula, breast milk, or food. Isoniazid solution causes significant gastrointestinal disturbance and is not tolerated in more than 50% of children. There are few drug interactions with isoniazid, making it an attractive regimen for children with HIV and children taking medicines known to interact with rifamycins.

Treatment of latent tuberculosis after exposure to drug-resistant tuberculosis

There are no established regimens for LTBI after exposure to isoniazid and rifampin-resistant TB. Observational data suggest monotherapy with a fluoroquinolone may be sufficient for treatment,[39] but some experts recommend dual therapy. Consultation with pediatric disease experts is recommended.

Latent tuberculosis infection treatment and development of drug resistance

Concerns over the development of drug resistance have hindered implementation of LTBI treatment. Resistance can largely be avoided by adequately ruling out TB disease before the initiation of LTBI treatment to avoid monotherapy and the risk of resistance.[40] Early TB disease may be missed with clinical evaluation. Because early disease and most pediatric disease is paucibacillary, the risk of developing resistance with one- or two-drug LTBI treatment, even in the presence of TB disease, is considered rare.

Nitrosamines

In August 2020, the Food and Drug Administration reported that nitrosamines had been identified in rifapentine and rifampicin, including 1-cyclopentyl-4-nitrosopiperazine (CPNP) and 1-methyl-4-nitrosopiperazine (MNP). Although no data show an associated between CPNP or MNP and cancer, this is assumed based on long-term animal studies with similar compounds. The risk of cancer with any of these short-course LTBI treatment regimens is unknown. When weighing the alternatives of withholding LTBI treatment or using isoniazid monotherapy, the risk of developing TB disease, hepatoxicity, or liver failure far outweighed the potential future cancer risk. The Food and Drug Administration has temporarily raised the acceptable nitrosamine threshold in rifamycins while pharmaceutical companies work to lower nitrosamine levels in all rifamycins.

TUBERCULOSIS DISEASE
Diagnosis

Currently, no single test can reliably and accurately diagnose TB disease in children. Instead, we depend on the child's TB risk factors combined with clinical, radiographic, and microbiologic evidence to support a diagnosis,[41,42] recognizing the limitations of each approach. Given the challenges in TB diagnosis, and that 96% of pediatric TB deaths are in children who were not started on treatment,[3] it is critical to have a low threshold to initiate empiric treatment if there is sufficient, albeit incomplete, evidence to suggest TB.

Clinical evaluation

Clinical signs and symptoms for TB disease in children include fever, prolonged cough (>1–2 weeks), weight loss, and failure to thrive. Although pulmonary TB is the most common type, children are more likely than adults to have extrapulmonary manifestations, including lymph node, abdominal, bone, joint, and central nervous system (CNS) disease. Thus, a complete clinical examination is essential, including evaluation of growth. In spinal TB, collapse of the vertebral bodies may create a kyphosis known as a gibbus deformity. CNS disease can manifest with altered mental status, cranial nerve palsies, headache, vomiting, or seizures.[43]

Radiographic findings

Children should receive a two-view (anteroposterior and lateral) CXR. CXR findings reflect the pathophysiology of pediatric pulmonary TB, which is often primary TB disease as opposed to reactivation disease seen in adolescents and adults.[17,44] Primary pulmonary TB disease manifests with mediastinal lymphadenopathy, which may or may not have a granulomatous parenchymal inflammation (Ghon focus), referred together as the Ghon complex.[17,45]

Each component (lymph node and parenchymal inflammation) can then progress to create further complications. The lymphadenopathy can cause airway obstruction that can lead to lung collapse, a postobstructive expansile pneumonia, or create a ball-valve effect to hyperinflate the lungs. Lung consolidation, cavitation, and bronchiectasis can result either from evolution of the parenchymal involvement or from extension of a lymph node into the lung tissue or bronchioles. This can further extend to the pleura, and cause a pleural effusion or empyema. In disseminated disease, a diffuse small nodular "miliary" pattern reflects the hematogenous spread. Adolescents can have adult-type TB, which can present with cavitation, upper lobe consolidations, and fibrosis or scarring, and are more likely to have a pleural effusion than younger children.[46]

The wide range and nonspecific radiographic manifestations in children make it difficult to diagnose TB solely by CXR.[47–49] Chest ultrasound has been evaluated to assess mediastinal lymphadenopathy,[47] but is operator-dependent. There is a limited role for chest computed tomography (CT) given the findings are still nonspecific with additional cost and radiation, but it can better detect lymphadenopathy and may have a benefit if considering other etiologies that would warrant advanced imaging.

For abdominal TB, imaging (ultrasound, CT, MRI) may reveal lymphadenopathy, hepatosplenomegaly with tuberculomas, and thickening of the terminal ileum. CNS TB is evaluated by MRI or CT, and can have several presentations including ring-enhancing tuberculomas, abscess, and leptomeningeal enhancement, especially in the basilar region.[17,50]

Respiratory sample testing

The standard evaluation for TB includes the collection of respiratory specimens for Mtb testing.[1,12] Sample types can include expectorated or induced sputum, or gastric aspirates. Three specimens should be obtained every 8 to 24 hours, with at least one early morning specimen. Children are often admitted for three morning fasting gastric aspirate samples. All samples should be sent for acid-fast bacilli (AFB) smear microscopy (Ziehl-Neelsen or fluorescent staining) and mycobacterial culture, and at least one specimen sent for nucleic acid amplification testing (NAAT). Although positive results are specific for TB, sensitivity is often low in children given their paucibacillary disease (**Table 3**). Most children have smear-negative disease, and the yield of culture can be less than 40%,[16,51] with slightly higher sensitivity and faster results in liquid

Table 3
Accuracy of diagnostics for TB disease in children

	Sensitivity Range, %	Specificity Range, %
AFB smear microscopy[1,17,96]	7–29	≥90
Mycobacterial culture[51]	1.5–65	100
Xpert MTB/RIF or Ultra[a]		
Respiratory specimens[b,52,53]	65–73	97–100
Stool[52,53,63,64]	57–67	98–99
Lymph node[17,52]	80–94	99
Cerebral spinal fluid[17,52]	67–85	94–99
Urine lateral-flow lipoarabinomannan[a,56–60,62,97]	28–73	61–91

[a] Based on a microbiologic reference standard.
[b] Includes expectorated sputum, induced sputum, or gastric aspirate.

mycobacterial growth in tube compared with solid culture media.[1] The NAAT known as Xpert MTB/RIF (Cepheid, Sunnyvale, CA) has a sensitivity of 65% to 73% with sputum or gastric aspirates; the next-generation Xpert MTB/RIF Ultra has a lower limit of detection and new "trace" category that improved sensitivity to 70% to 73% in children.[52,53] The yield of testing is lower in children less than 5 years of age, and is further impacted by the sample quality, type, and number collected.[54,55] Bronchoalveolar lavage may improve the quality of the specimen, but does not significantly increase yield and is invasive.

Nonsputum testing for intrathoracic tuberculosis

An IGRA or TST is performed to evaluate for immunologic evidence of TB infection. Given the moderate sensitivity of TST and IGRAs, especially in vulnerable groups including young and immunosuppressed children, a negative result needs to be interpreted with caution and should not be used alone to rule out TB. Pleural effusions can have lymphocytic predominance, elevated protein, and elevated lactate dehydrogenase. Pleural fluid adenosine deaminase greater than or equal to 40 U/L has been associated with an 89% to 99% sensitivity and 88% to 97% specificity for TB.[1] Pleural TB is difficult to diagnose, and pleural tissue biopsy is valuable for pathologic assessment of acid-fast bacteria, granulomas, and culture. Urine-based testing with lipoarabinomannan (LAM) has had limited performance in children (see **Table 3**), with sensitivity ranging from 28% to 73%[56–60] and specificity 61% to 91%.[56–60] Accuracy improves with HIV coinfection, and currently the World Health Organization (WHO) recommends urine LAM for children with HIV.[60] Next-generation LAM assays are being developed (eg, SILVAMP TB LAM, Fujifilm, Tokyo, Japan) that have improved sensitivity and can detect 42% to 65% of confirmed TB in children,[61,62] and may be considered in future guidelines. Stool-based testing has been suggested in young children because they swallow their sputum. Stool culture has limited performance, but NAATs, including Xpert MTB/RIF, have shown about 57% to 67% sensitivity,[52,53,63,64] and has been included as an option for testing in recent WHO guidelines.[53]

Extrapulmonary tuberculosis specimen testing

Fine-needle aspiration of lymph nodes and bone biopsies are sent for pathology, AFB staining, mycobacterial culture, and NAAT. Similarly, joint fluid aspiration is further assessed with AFB staining, culture, and NAAT. For CNS TB, the cerebrospinal fluid (CSF) profile can have a mild leukocytosis with lymphocytic predominance, and has an elevated protein.[17] CSF culture is low yield and often requires a large volume, but NAAT can be sent on the CSF with sensitivity of 67% to 85% and specificity 94% to 99%.[17,52] CSF testing should also be performed in children younger than 2 years old regardless of neurologic symptoms given the risk of disseminated disease.[12]

Resistance testing

Culture-based methods can evaluate for phenotypic susceptibility to first-line and second-line agents, but is slow and requires technical expertise.[65] Genotypic testing of known resistance-conferring mutations provides a faster approach, and includes evaluation of the rpoB mutation in rifampin resistance with Xpert MTB/RIF, and line probe assays and sequencing approaches that can assess mutations for first-line drugs and second-line options including aminoglycosides and fluoroquinolones. Although faster, genotypic methods can have reduced sensitivity and there are silent mutations that do not predict phenotypic resistance. Thus, when feasible, phenotypic approaches should still be done to further confirm drug resistance.

Treatment of Tuberculosis Disease

Treatment of presumed or drug-susceptible pulmonary tuberculosis in children

The purpose of TB treatment in children is to rapidly kill or inhibit multiplication of Mtb, which when combined with an immune response, prevents rapid dissemination of disease and results in cure. Treatment duration is typically 6 months to ensure eradication of rapidly dividing and slowly metabolizing mycobacteria subpopulations, or persister mycobacteria, believed to cause relapse after treatment cessation.

First-line TB treatment includes three or four drugs: rifampin, isoniazid, and pyrazinamide with or without ethambutol (RHZE). The 2-month initiation phase includes three or four drugs with the purpose of rapidly reducing mycobacterial burden. The subsequent 4-month continuation phase includes rifampin and isoniazid, targeting elimination of persistent mycobacteria. Dosing for first-line drugs is provided in **Table 4**.

Rifampin and pyrazinamide provide sterilizing activity of these slowly metabolizing mycobacterial subpopulations and in combination have allowed for a shorter treatment duration of 6 months. Isoniazid has two purposes: to reduce the burden of rapidly metabolizing mycobacteria during the initiation phase, and to protect against

Table 4
Dosing, formulations, and adverse reactions for first-line treatment of pediatric pulmonary TB disease

Drug	Dose	Formulations[a]	Adverse Reactions
Rifampin	10–20 mg/kg[b] (max 600–900 mg)	Oral capsule (150 mg, 300 mg)[c] Oral suspension (10 mg/mL)[d] IV injection	Hepatotoxicity Hypersensitivity Red/orange-tinged secretions GI upset Rash
Isoniazid	10–15 mg/kg (max 300 mg)	Oral tablet (100 mg, 300 mg) Oral solution (50 mg/5 mL)[e] IM injection (100 mg/mL)	Hepatotoxicity Peripheral neuropathy Hypersensitivity GI upset Rash
Pyrazinamide	30–40 mg/kg (max 2000 mg)	Scored tablet (500 mg) Oral suspension (100 mg/mL)[d]	Hepatotoxicity Hyperuricemia GI upset
Ethambutol	15–25 mg/kg (max 1600 mg)	Oral tablet (100 mg, 400 mg) Oral suspension (50 mg/mL)[d]	Optic neuritis[f] Hypersensitivity

Abbreviations: GI, gastrointestinal; IM, intramuscular; IV, intravenous.
[a] Fixed dose combinations not available in the United States.
[b] Author recommends highest tolerated dose within range, as formulations allow.
[c] Often given as sprinkles by opening the capsule.
[d] Requires compounding pharmacy.
[e] Often poorly tolerated (GI upset); most patients prefer crushed tablet mixed with food, formula, or breast milk.
[f] Ethambutol has been associated with optic neuropathy whose early symptoms cannot be easily reported or detected in young children. The World Health Organization reviewed ethambutol toxicity and found doses of 20 mg/kg (range, 15–25 mg/kg) daily for 2 months was not associated with ocular toxicity and could be given without ophthalmology follow-up.

the development of rifampin resistance during the continuation phase. Ethambutol prevents the development of drug resistance among first-line companion drugs. Ethambutol is used when there is (1) unknown drug susceptibility patterns for the child or source case and either the risk of isoniazid monoresistance or HIV prevalence is significant, (2) extensive "adult-type" or smear-positive pulmonary disease present, or (3) severe form of extrapulmonary TB present. Drugs are not generally interchangeable; any need to modify the standard regimen because of drug resistance, allergy, or intolerance should be discussed with a pediatric TB specialist.

Because children often do not have microbiologic confirmation of TB, the drug regimen is based on the drug susceptibility testing from the likely source case or epidemiology and the risk of drug resistance. Risk factors for drug-resistant TB include prior TB treatment, contacts of patients with known drug-resistant TB or poor initial response to therapy (eg, persistent smear positivity after appropriate treatment), and immigration from or travel to countries with a high prevalence of drug-resistant TB. When risk factors for drug resistance are present, every effort should be made to identify an isolate to guide treatment.

Treatment of tuberculosis meningitis
Childhood tuberculous meningitis is associated with significant morbidity and mortality, and despite treatment only one in three children survive without neurologic sequelae.[66] Treatment with standard doses of RHZE results in low CSF concentrations of rifampin and ethambutol.[67–69] Adult trials have shown early intensified treatment with high-dose rifampicin, either orally or intravenously, and levofloxacin, when isoniazid monoresistance is present, reduces morbidity and mortality.[68,70–72] Modeling studies suggest rifampin doses of at least 30 mg/kg orally or 15 mg/kg intravenous and levofloxacin dosing of at least 20 to 30 mg/kg orally are likely necessary to attain similar exposures in children as were studied in adults.[73] Ongoing studies are evaluating this dosing and outcomes in children with tuberculous meningitis.

In cases where drug-susceptible TB is likely based on source case susceptibilities or epidemiology, rifampin, isoniazid, and pyrazinamide are recommended. There are few randomized controlled trials to guide the selection of the fourth drug. CDC guidelines recommend ethambutol; however, given its poor CNS penetration, the AAP recommends either ethionamide or an aminoglycoside.[12] Ethionamide is a thioamide and prodrug requiring activation by mycobacterial EthA with good CNS penetration.[74] Along with isoniazid, it inhibits mycolic acid synthesis via InhA. Gastrointestinal disturbance and reversible hypothyroidism are common during long-term therapy, but are both often tolerated. Aminoglycosides, most commonly streptomycin, are intravenous and carry the risk of ototoxicity and nephrotoxicity. In cases where drug resistance is identified or suspected or ethionamide is not available, initial treatment with a fluoroquinolone and/or linezolid, which both penetrate the CNS well, may be beneficial.[71,75,76] Accumulating data in adults suggest levofloxacin may improve outcomes in drug-resistant tuberculous meningitis, including isoniazid monoresistant TB.[71]

Adjuvant steroids
Adjuvant corticosteroids reduce mortality from TB meningitis by 25% in people of all ages and pediatric studies have shown improved intellectual outcomes in children randomized to receive corticosteroids.[77,78] Corticosteroids have also been shown to reduce the development of constrictive pericarditis and relieve obstruction most commonly from lymphadenitis.[79] Finally, steroids are sometimes used in severe

miliary disease to mitigate alveolocapillary block or in abdominal TB to reduce the risk of strictures.

Administering tuberculosis treatment to children

Drug doses and formulations of first-line therapy for pulmonary TB in children are shown in **Table 4**. First-line TB medications are crushed and mixed in sugar-free chocolate pudding or grape jelly to enhance acceptability in young children.[80] Although medications in these compounds have been shown to be stable for up to 4 hours, practically any food the child prefers can be used to mask the taste as long as it is taken quickly after crushing and mixing with food. Rifampin and pyrazinamide can be compounded into suspensions, which is often necessary in very young children to obtain the appropriate dose given formulations available in the United States. Crushed isoniazid tablets should be used whenever possible; isoniazid solution causes nearly half of children to have significant gastrointestinal upset. Pyridoxine supplementation often accompanies use of isoniazid to prevent peripheral neuropathy, but in children is limited to exclusively breastfed infants, children with malnutrition, and children living with HIV.

Monitoring tuberculosis treatment

Monthly follow-up to assess for treatment response, drug toxicity, and adherence is typically sufficient. Drug-related hepatotoxicity is rare in children and routine assessment of serum transaminases is not recommended and limited to children with underlying liver disease. Caregivers should be counseled on early symptoms of hepatitis including nausea, vomiting, and abdominal pain, which may prompt assessment of liver function testing. Treatment response is assessed clinically, by following symptoms, weight gain, and development; radiologically, by following CXR and other imaging; and microbiologically, with repeat sputa samples assessing for smear and culture conversion. The microbiologic assessment is often not necessary in young children with paucibacillary disease who have negative smear and culture at diagnosis. Repeat radiographs are not mandatory, but are often helpful when a child has not shown significant clinical improvement and there are concerns about possible drug resistance. Hilar adenopathy can take 1 to 2 years to resolve and should not be considered a poor response to therapy.

Therapeutic drug monitoring is used to determine drug concentrations at timed intervals to determine the appropriateness of drug dosing. This is not routinely recommended in TB care, but is useful in children with malabsorptive conditions, those at risk for drug-drug interactions, renal insufficiency with or without renal-replacement therapy, diabetes mellitus, and those with poor clinical response to first-line therapy with known or assumed susceptibility to first-line agents.[81]

Duration of treatment

Treatment duration for drug-sensitive pulmonary TB disease in children is typically 6 months. This is extended in adult populations when there is cavitation on initial or follow-up chest imaging and culture remains positive after 2 months of treatment. Certain extrapulmonary TB conditions require longer therapy including tuberculous meningitis (6–12 months) and TB of the bone, joint, or spine (6–9 months). Treatment of TB with resistance to either rifampicin, isoniazid, or pyrazinamide is also typically longer, including treatment of *Mycobacterium bovis*, which is inherently resistant to pyrazinamide.

Box 1
Summary of approach to the diagnosis of TB infection

Clinical Care Points 1: Summary of our approach to the diagnosis of TB infection
- We assess risk factors that increase the risk of TB infection or progression to TB disease, in particular birth in, residence to, or travel to a TB-endemic setting; immunosuppression; or contact with an individual with TB disease.
- LTBI testing should be done on all children with risk factors. We perform IGRAs on all children 2 years and older; if the child is younger than 2, we perform a TST, but if it is not available or feasible, or there is concern for false positivity, we use an IGRA.
- We do not perform both TST or IGRA unless one test is invalid/indeterminate, there is concern for false negativity, or to evaluate for other etiologies including NTM infection.
- We consider positive results for a TST or IGRA a true positive in children with TB risk factors unless there is a clear alternative explanation.
- We exclude TB disease by symptom screen, physical examination, and two-view CXR. If there is no evidence of TB disease, we proceed with LTBI treatment. If there are clinical signs of TB or radiographic abnormalities, we would next consider the collection of respiratory specimens for TB disease evaluation.

Treatment of drug-resistant tuberculosis in children

Treatment of drug-resistant TB is often longer and requires at least four or five anti-TB drugs. Drug choice should consider the drug resistance pattern of the child or source case isolate and drug penetration to the site of disease. Dosing and availability of child-friendly formulations of second-line drugs are improving but still lacking. Up-to-date information on dosing and formulations is found at the sentinel-project.org. Regimens to treat drug-resistant TB should be designed with a pediatric TB specialist.

Emerging advances for childhood tuberculosis diagnosis and treatment

Several new diagnostics for LTBI and TB disease are under evaluation.[82] For LTBI, skin-based testing has been developed that incorporates ESAT-6 and CFP-10 rather than the nonspecific tuberculin mixture, and new platforms could allow IGRA testing closer to the point-of-care. For TB disease, pathogen-based tests include the measurement of cell-free DNA or other TB-specific antigens, such as ESAT-6 and CFP-10 in plasma or urine. Host-based assays are also being assessed, including

---

Box 2
Approach to LTBI treatment in children

Clinical Care Points 2. How we approach LTBI treatment in children
- Regimen choice should consider age, formulation, likely adherence, and possible drug-drug interactions with rifamycins.
- Vitamin B_6 is indicated for exclusively breastfed infants, children with malnutrition, and children living with HIV.
- None of the newly recommended short-course regimens require directly observed therapy, including 3HP.
- Parents should be counseled about the early symptoms of hepatoxicity (nausea, poor appetite, emesis, and abdominal pain) and should immediately return to care should they develop.
- Children should be followed by their pediatrician monthly to evaluate for drug toxicity and adherence. All medications should be weight-adjusted monthly.
- In most situations, liver function testing is only indicated when the child is symptomatic of hepatitis.
- Children exposed to drug-resistant TB should be referred to a pediatric TB expert.

Box 3
Approach to TB diagnosis in children

Clinical Care Points 3: How we approach TB diagnosis in children
- We screen for TB risk factors and symptoms, and perform a complete physical examination, including growth assessment.
- We obtain an IGRA or TST, two-view CXR, and three respiratory specimens for AFB smear and culture, and at least one for Mtb NAAT.
- For TB lymphadenitis, we obtain fine-needle aspirations on an enlarged lymph node for pathology, AFB staining, mycobacterial culture, and NAAT.
- A CT or MRI should be obtained for concerns for CNS TB, and CSF sent for NAAT in addition to a standard CSF profile.
- Without microbiologic confirmation, we still diagnose a child with TB if they have risk factors, signs, and symptoms of TB without a clear alternative cause.

---

gene- and protein-based signatures or the measurement of T-cell markers. In addition, there are efforts to optimize LAM and stool testing, and the use of oral swabs to make respiratory specimen collection less invasive. Image analysis with artificial intelligence has led to large advancements in computer-aided detection of TB in CXRs; further work is needed to extend it to children. For resistance testing, new molecular tests are being evaluated and next-generation sequencing may provide a broader assessment of all the possible mutations that can confer drug resistance. Lastly, there is a growing appreciation of the wider spectrum of TB, including incipient and subclinical TB,[83] and there are ongoing efforts to characterize and diagnose these different states to inform earlier and specific treatment regimens.

Continued advances in LTBI treatment are also anticipated. Worldwide, children 12 years and older have access to 1HP or 1 month of daily rifapentine and isoniazid for TB treatment. Ongoing studies in adults and children will clarify efficacy in different populations and the dosing, safety, and tolerability of this regimen in children. A child-friendly formulation of rifapentine is not expected for at least 5 to 10 years. Ongoing studies of injectable bedaquiline in mice may prove useful in humans and could allow

---

Box 4
Approach to TB treatment in children

Clinical Care Points 4. How we approach TB treatment in children
- First we assess the child's risk for drug-resistant TB.
- Assuming no risk factors for drug resistance, three- or four-drug therapy with rifampin, isoniazid, and pyrazinamide with or without ethambutol is started as empiric therapy.
- During the 2-month initiation phase, all three or four drugs are used to rapidly decrease the mycobacterial burden. During the continuation phase, rifampin and isoniazid are used to eradicate persisting mycobacteria.
- Vitamin B_6 is indicated for exclusively breastfed infants, children with malnutrition, and children living with HIV.
- Children should be followed monthly to evaluate for treatment response, drug toxicity, and adherence. All medications should be weight-adjusted monthly.
- Directly observed therapy is the standard of care in all settings.
- In most situations, liver function testing is only indicated when the child is symptomatic of hepatitis.
- Therapy is extended beyond 6 months with certain forms of TB, poor response to therapy, with cavitation, and persistently positive smears at Month 2, or if there is poor adherence.

for a single injection to treat LTBI in drug-sensitive and drug-resistant exposure. Finally, advances in TB vaccine research may also aid treatment and prevention of TB infection and TB disease.

Shortened treatment regimens in adults and children signify a major advance for TB treatment not seen for decades. For children, the SHINE trial found 4 months of RHZE (2 months of intensive phase and 2 months of continuation phase) was noninferior to the standard 6-month RHZE regimen in children with minimal TB disease. Similarly, in adolescents and adults, a 4-month regimen of rifapentine, isoniazid, pyrazinamide, and moxifloxacin (RHZM) was noninferior to the standard 6-month regimen of RHZE in all efficacy analyses and is already recommended by WHO.[84] Although some work needs to be done before these regimens are ready for implementation, there is great hope for shortened regimens, improved adherence, and better treatment outcomes in the near future.

Beyond the development of new diagnostics and therapeutic regimens, we need to improve the care cascade for LTBI and TB disease to increase the proportion of children and adolescents who are screened, tested, and treated. This requires greater engagement with providers and families to understand the individual, community, and structural barriers to TB care. It is also important to improve early recognition of TB disease and encourage use of algorithms for clinical diagnosis.

SUMMARY

The successful care of children and adolescents with TB requires a recognition of the risk factors and clinical and radiographic signs of TB, especially when microbiologic testing is negative, and partnership with caregivers to safely complete the minimum 3 months of treatment of LTBI and 6 months for TB disease. Our approach to diagnosing and treating LTBI and TB disease is outlined in **Boxes 1–4**. Ongoing efforts seek to improve the performance and ease of TB diagnostics for children, with shorter treatment regimens and better formulations for LTBI and TB disease.

DISCLOSURE

The authors have nothing to disclose. D. Jaganath, J. Beaudry, and N. Salazar-Austin are funded by the National Institutes of Health. N. Salazar-Austin also receives research support from UNITAID.

REFERENCES

1. Lewinsohn DM, Leonard MK, LoBue PA, et al. Official American Thoracic Society/ Infectious Diseases Society of America/Centers for Disease Control and Prevention Clinical Practice Guidelines: diagnosis of tuberculosis in adults and children. Clin Infect Dis 2017;64(2):111–5.

2. World Health Organization. Global Tuberculosis Report 2020. Geneva: World Health Organization. 2019. Available at. https://www.who.int/publications/i/item/ 9789240013131. Accessed June 2 2021.

3. World Health Organization. Roadmap towards ending TB in children and adolescents. Geneva: World Health Organization. 2018. Available at. https://www.who. int/tb/publications/2018/tb-childhoodroadmap/en/. Accessed January 18 2020.

4. Swaminathan S, Rekha B. Pediatric tuberculosis: global overview and challenges. Clin Infect Dis 2010;50(Suppl 3):S184–94.

5. Marais BJ, Gie RP, Schaaf HS, et al. The natural history of childhood intra-thoracic tuberculosis: a critical review of literature from the pre-chemotherapy era. Int J Tuberc Lung Dis 2004;8(4):392–402.

6. Martinez L, Cords O, Hoursburgh CR, et al. Pediatric TB Contact Studies Consortium. The risk of tuberculosis in children after close exposure: a systematic review and individual-participant meta-analysis. Lancet 2020;395:973–84.

7. Dodd PJ, Prendergast AJ, Beecroft C, et al. The impact of HIV and antiretroviral therapy on TB risk in children: a systematic review and meta-analysis. Thorax 2017;72(6):559–75.

8. Deutsch-Feldman M, Pratt RH, Price SF, et al. Tuberculosis—United States, 2020. MMWR Morb Mortal Wkly Rep 2021;70(12):409–14.

9. Cowger TL, Wortham JM, Burton DC. Epidemiology of tuberculosis among children and adolescents in the USA, 2007–17: an analysis of national surveillance data. Lancet Public Health 2019;4(10):e506–16.

10. Rangaka MX, Cavalcante SC, Marais BJ, et al. Controlling the seedbeds of tuberculosis: diagnosis and treatment of tuberculosis infection. The Lancet 2015; 386(10010):2344–53.

11. Pai M, Behr MA, Dowdy D, et al. Tuberculosis Nat Rev Dis Primers 2016;2(1): 16076.

12. American Academy of Pediatrics. Tuberculosis. In: Kimberlin DW, Jackson MA BM, Long SS, editors. Red Book: 2018 Rep Committee Infect Dis. American Academy of pediatrics. 2018. p. 829–53.

13. Targeted tuberculin skin testing and treatment of latent tuberculosis infection in children and adolescents. Pediatrics 2004;114(Supplement 4):1175–201.

14. National Society of Tuberculosis Clinicians and National Tuberculosis Controllers Association. Testing and Treatment of Latent Tuberculosis Infection in the United States: Clinical Recommendations. Available at: http://www.tbcontrollers.org/resources/tb-infection/clinical-recommendations/#.YD5DHq-P6hd.   Accessed July 2021.

15. Holmberg PJ, Temesgen Z, Banerjee R. Tuberculosis in children. Pediatr Rev 2019;40(4):168–78.

16. Dunn JJ, Starke JR, Revell PA. Laboratory diagnosis of *Mycobacterium* tuberculosis infection and disease in children. J Clin Microbiol 2016;54(6):1434–41.

17. Starke JR, Donald PR. Handbook of child and adolescent tuberculosis. Oxford University Press; 2016.

18. Cruz AT, Reichman LB. The case for retiring the tuberculin skin test. Pediatrics 2019;143(6):e20183327.

19. Farhat M, Greenaway C, Pai M, et al. False-positive tuberculin skin tests: what is the absolute effect of BCG and non-tuberculous mycobacteria? Int J Tuberc Lung Dis 2006;10(11):1192–204.

20. Centers for Disease Control and Prevention. Tuberculosis Technical Instructions for Civil Surgeons. Available at. https://www.cdc.gov/immigrantrefugeehealth/civil-surgeons/tuberculosis.html. Accessed July 2021.

21. Kay AW, Islam SM, Wendorf K, et al. Interferon-γ release assay performance for tuberculosis in childhood. Pediatrics 2018;141(6):e20173918.

22. Mazurek GH, Jereb J, Vernon A, et al. Updated guidelines for using interferon gamma release assays to detect *Mycobacterium tuberculosis* infection—United States, 2010. MMWR Recomm Rep 2010;59(Rr-5):1–25.

23. World Health Organization. Latent tuberculosis infection: updated and consolidated guidelines for programmatic management. Available at. Available at:

https://apps.who.int/iris/bitstream/handle/10665/260233/9789241550239-eng.
pdf. Accessed July 2021.

24. Ayieko J, Abuogi L, Simchowitz B, et al. Efficacy of isoniazid prophylactic therapy
in prevention of tuberculosis in children: a meta-analysis. BMC Infect Dis 2014;
14:91.

25. Smieja MJ, Marchetti CA, Cook DJ, et al. Isoniazid for preventing tuberculosis in
non-HIV infected persons. Cochrane Database Syst Rev 2000;2:CD001363.

26. Ferebee SH. Controlled chemoprophylaxis trials in tuberculosis. A general review.
Bibl Tuberc 1970;26:28–106.

27. Sterling TR, Njie G, Zenner D. Guidelines for the treatment of latent tuberculosis
infection: recommendations from the National Tuberculosis Controllers Association and CDC. MMWR 2020;69(NO. RR-1):1–11. https://doi.org/10.15585/mmwr.
rr6901a1.

28. WHO consolidated guidelines on tuberculosis: tuberculosis preventive treatment.
Geneva: World Health Organization; 2020. Licence: CC BY-NC-SA 3.0 IGO.

29. Villarino ME, Scott NA, Weis SE, et al. Treatment for preventing tuberculosis in
children and adolescents: a randomized clinical trial of a 3-month, 12-dose
regimen of a combination of rifapentine and isoniazid. JAMA Pediatr 2015;
169(3):247–55.

30. Sterling TR, Villarino ME, Borisov AS, et al. Three months of rifapentine and isoniazid for latent tuberculosis infection. *N Engl J Med* 2011;365(23):2155–66.

31. Sterling TR, Scott NA, Miro JM, et al. Three months of weekly rifapentine and
isoniazid for treatment of *Mycobacterium tuberculosis* infection in HIV-
coinfected persons. AIDS 2016;30(10):1607–15.

32. Sandul AL, Nwana N, Holcombe JM, et al. High rate of treatment completion in
program settings with 12-dose weekly isoniazid and rifapentine for latent *Mycobacterium tuberculosis* infection. Clin Infect Dis 2017;65(7):1085–93.

33. Cruz AT, Starke JR. Completion rate and safety of tuberculosis infection treatment
with shorter regimens. Pediatrics 2018;141(2). https://doi.org/10.1542/peds.
2017-2838.

34. Weiner M, Savic RM, Kenzie WR, et al. Rifapentine pharmacokinetics and tolerability in children and adults treated once weekly with rifapentine and isoniazid for
latent tuberculosis infection. J Pediatr Infect Dis Soc. 2014;3(2):132–45.

35. Diallo T, Adjobimey M, Ruslami R, et al. Safety and side effects of rifampin versus
isoniazid in children. N Engl J Med 2018;379(5):454–63.

36. Menzies D, Adjobimey M, Ruslami R, et al. Four months of rifampin or nine
months of isoniazid for latent tuberculosis in adults. N Engl J Med 2018;379(5):
440–53.

37. McIlleron H, Denti P, Cohn S, et al. Prevention of TB using rifampicin plus isoniazid reduces nevirapine concentrations in HIV-exposed infants. J Antimicrob
Chemother 2017. Epub ahead of printdoi:10.1093/jac/dkx112.

38. Waalewijn H, Mujuru H, Amuge P, et al. Adequate dolutegravir exposure dosed
BID with rifampicin in children 6 to <18 years. Paper presented at: CROI 2020 Vir-
tual Conference on Retroviruses and Opportunistic Infections; March 8–11, 2020;
Boston, Massachusetts Abstract Number 847

39. Bamrah S, Brostrom R, Dorina F, et al. Treatment for LTBI in contacts of MDR-TB
patients, Federated States of Micronesia, 2009-2012. Int J Tuberc Lung Dis 2014;
18(8):912–8.

40. Balcells ME, Thomas SL, Godfrey-Faussett P, et al. Isoniazid preventive therapy
and risk for resistant tuberculosis. Emerg Infect Dis 2006;12(5):744–51.

41. World Health Organization. Guidance for national tuberculosis programmes on the management of tuberculosis in children. 2nd edition. Geneva: World Health Organization; 2014.

42. The Union's desk guide for diagnosis and management of TB in children. Paris: International Union Against Tuberculosis and Lung Disease; 2016.

43. Shah I, Pereira NMD. Tuberculous meningitis in children: a review article. Curr Infect Dis Rep 2020;22(4):11. https://doi.org/10.1007/s11908-020-0720-7.

44. Marais BJ, Gie RP, Schaaf HS, et al. A proposed radiological classification of childhood intra-thoracic tuberculosis. Pediatr Radiol 2004;34(11):886–94.

45. Pillay T, Andronikou S, Zar HJ. Chest imaging in paediatric pulmonary TB. Paediatric Respir Rev 2020;36:65–72. https://doi.org/10.1016/j.prrv.2020.10.002.

46. Snow KJ, Cruz AT, Seddon JA, et al. Adolescent tuberculosis. Lancet Child Adolesc Health 2020;4(1):68–79.

47. Heuvelings CC, Bélard S, Andronikou S, et al. Chest ultrasound compared to chest X-ray for pediatric pulmonary tuberculosis. Pediatr Pulmonol 2019;54(12): 1914–20.

48. Andronikou S, Grier D, Minhas K. Reliability of chest radiograph interpretation for pulmonary tuberculosis in the screening of childhood TB contacts and migrant children in the UK. Clin Radiol 2021;76(2):122–8.

49. Kaguthi G, Nduba V, Nyokabi J, et al. Chest radiographs for pediatric TB diagnosis: interrater agreement and utility. Interdiscip Perspect Infect Dis 2014;291841.

50. Schaller MA, Wicke F, Foerch C, et al. Central nervous system tuberculosis: etiology, clinical manifestations and neuroradiological features. Clin Neuroradiol 2019;29(1):3–18.

51. DiNardo AR, Detjen A, Ustero P, et al. Culture is an imperfect and heterogeneous reference standard in pediatric tuberculosis. Tuberculosis (Edinb) 2016;101S: S105–8.

52. Kay AW, González Fernández L, Takwoingi Y, et al. Xpert MTB/RIF and Xpert MTB/RIF Ultra assays for active tuberculosis and rifampicin resistance in children. Cochrane Database Syst Rev 2020;(8). https://doi.org/10.1002/14651858. CD013359.pub2.

53. World Health Organization. WHO consolidated guidelines on tuberculosis. Module 3: diagnosis - Rapid diagnostics for tuberculosis detection 2021 update. Geneva: World Health Organization; 2021.

54. Zar HJ, Workman LJ, Prins M, et al. Tuberculosis diagnosis in children using Xpert Ultra on different respiratory specimens. Am J Respir Crit Care Med 2019;200(12):1531–8.

55. Song R, Click ES, McCarthy KD, et al. Sensitive and feasible specimen collection and testing strategies for diagnosing tuberculosis in young children. JAMA Pediatr 2021;175(5):e206069.

56. Kroidl I, Clowes P, Reither K, et al. Performance of urine lipoarabinomannan assays for paediatric tuberculosis in Tanzania. Eur Respir J 2015;46(3):761–70.

57. LaCourse SM, Pavlinac PB, Cranmer LM, et al. Stool Xpert MTB/RIF and urine lipoarabinomannan for the diagnosis of tuberculosis in hospitalized HIV-infected children. Aids 2018;32(1):69–78.

58. Nicol MP, Allen V, Workman L, et al. Urine lipoarabinomannan testing for diagnosis of pulmonary tuberculosis in children: a prospective study. Lancet Glob Health 2014;2(5):e278–84.

59. Gautam H, Singla M, Jain R, et al. Point-of-care urine lipoarabinomannan antigen detection for diagnosis of tuberculosis in children. Int J Tuberc Lung Dis 2019; 23(6):714–9.
60. World Health Organization. Lateral flow urine lipoarabinomannan assay (LF-LAM) for the diagnosis of active tuberculosis in people living with HIV: Policy update. 2019. Available at: https://www.who.int/tb/publications/2019/LAMPolicyUpdate 2019/en/. Accessed July 28 2020.
61. Nicol MP, Schumacher SG, Workman L, et al. Accuracy of a novel urine test, Fujifilm SILVAMP tuberculosis lipoarabinomannan, for the diagnosis of pulmonary tuberculosis in children. Clin Infect Dis 2021;72(9):e280–8.
62. Nkereuwem E, Togun T, Gomez MP, et al. Comparing accuracy of lipoarabinomannan urine tests for diagnosis of pulmonary tuberculosis in children from four African countries: a cross-sectional study. Lancet Infect Dis 2021;21(3): 376–84.
63. Mesman AW, Rodriguez C, Ager E, et al. Diagnostic accuracy of molecular detection of *Mycobacterium tuberculosis* in pediatric stool samples: a systematic review and meta-analysis. Tuberculosis (Edinb) 2019;119:101878.
64. MacLean E, Sulis G, Denkinger CM, et al. Diagnostic accuracy of Stool Xpert MTB/RIF for detection of pulmonary tuberculosis in children: a systematic review and meta-analysis. J Clin Microbiol 2019;57(6). https://doi.org/10.1128/jcm. 02057-18.
65. Curry International Tuberculosis Center. Drug-resistant tuberculosis: a survival guide for clinicians, 3rd edition. Available at: https://www.currytbcenter.ucsf.edu/ products/view/drug-resistant-tuberculosis-survival-guide-clinicians-3rd-edition. Accessed July 2021.
66. Swindells S, Ramchandani R, Gupta A, et al. One month of rifapentine plus isoniazid to prevent HIV-related tuberculosis. N Engl J Med 2019;380(11):1001–11.
67. Cresswell FV, Te Brake L, Atherton R, et al. Intensified antibiotic treatment of tuberculosis meningitis. Expert Rev Clin Pharmacol 2019;12(3):267–88.
68. Ruslami R, Ganiem AR, Dian S, et al. Intensified regimen containing rifampicin and moxifloxacin for tuberculous meningitis: an open-label, randomised controlled phase 2 trial. Lancet Infect Dis 2013;13(1):27–35.
69. Pilheu JA, Maglio F, Cetrangolo R, et al. Concentrations of ethambutol in the cerebrospinal fluid after oral administration. Tubercle 1971;52(2):117–22.
70. Cresswell FV, Meya DB, Kagimu E, et al. High-dose oral and intravenous rifampicin for the treatment of tuberculous meningitis in predominantly HIV-positive Ugandan adults: a phase II open-label randomised controlled trial. Clin Infect Dis 2021. https://doi.org/10.1093/cid/ciab162.
71. Heemskerk AD, Nguyen MTH, Dang HTM, et al. Clinical outcomes of patients with drug-resistant tuberculous meningitis treated with an intensified antituberculosis regimen. Clin Infect Dis 2017;65(1):20–8.
72. Heemskerk AD, Bang ND, Mai NT, et al. Intensified antituberculosis therapy in adults with tuberculous meningitis. N Engl J Med 2016;374(2):124–34.
73. Savic RM, Ruslami R, Hibma JE, et al. Pediatric tuberculous meningitis: model-based approach to determining optimal doses of the anti-tuberculosis drugs rifampin and levofloxacin for children. Clin Pharmacol Ther 2015;98(6):622–9.
74. Thee S, Garcia-Prats AJ, Donald PR, et al. A review of the use of ethionamide and prothionamide in childhood tuberculosis. Tuberculosis 2016;97:126–36.
75. Sun F, Ruan Q, Wang J, et al. Linezolid manifests a rapid and dramatic therapeutic effect for patients with life-threatening tuberculous meningitis. Antimicrob Agents Chemother 2014;58(10):6297–301.

76. Li HM, Lu J, Liu JR, et al. Linezolid is associated with improved early outcomes of childhood tuberculous meningitis. Pediatr Infect Dis J 2016;35(6):607–10.

77. Schoeman JF, Van Zyl LE, Laubscher JA, et al. Effect of corticosteroids on intracranial pressure, computed tomographic findings, and clinical outcome in young children with tuberculous meningitis. Pediatrics 1997;99(2):226–31.

78. Prasad K, Singh MB, Ryan H. Corticosteroids for managing tuberculous meningitis. Cochrane Database Syst Rev 2016;4(4):CD002244.

79. Wiysonge C, Ntsekhe M, Thabane L, et al. Interventions for treating tuberculous pericarditis. Cochrane Database Syst Rev 2017;13(9):CD000526.

80. Peloquin CA, Durbin D, Childs J, et al. Stability of antituberculosis drugs mixed in food. Clin Infect Dis 2007;45(4):521.

81. Alsultan A, Peloquin CA. Therapeutic drug monitoring in the treatment of tuberculosis: an update. Drugs 2014;74(8):839–54.

82. Treatment Action Group. The Tuberculosis Diagnostics Pipeline Report: Advancing the Next Generation of Tools. Available at: https://www.treatmentactiongroup.org/wp-content/uploads/2020/10/pipeline_TB_Diagnostics_2020_final.pdf. accessed July 2021.

83. Drain PK, Bajema KL, Dowdy D, et al. Incipient and subclinical tuberculosis: a clinical review of early stages and progression of infection. Clin Microbiol Rev 2018;31(4). https://doi.org/10.1128/cmr.00021-18.

84. Dorman SE, Nahid P, Kurbatova EV, et al. Four-month rifapentine regimens with or without moxifloxacin for tuberculosis. New England Journal of Medicine 2021;384(18):1705–18.

85. California Tuberculosis Controllers Association. Latent tuberculosis infection guidance for the prevention of tuberculosis in California. Available at. Available at: https://ctca.org/guidelines/guidelines-latent-tuberculosis-infection-guideline/. Accessed July 2021.

86. Hatzenbuehler LA, Starke JR, Graviss EA, et al. School-based study to identify and treat adolescent students at risk for tuberculosis infection. Pediatr Infect Dis J 2016;35(7):733–8.

87. Villarino ME, Ridzon R, Weismuller PC, et al. Rifampin preventive therapy for tuberculosis infection: experience with 157 adolescents. Am J Respir Crit Care Med 1997;155(5):1735–8.

88. Page KR, Sifakis F, Montes de Oca R, et al. Improved adherence and less toxicity with rifampin vs isoniazid for treatment of latent tuberculosis: a retrospective study. Arch Intern Med 2006;166(17):1863–70.

89. Lardizabal A, Passannante M, Kojakali F, et al. Enhancement of treatment completion for latent tuberculosis infection with 4 months of rifampin. Chest 2006;130(6):1712–7.

90. Spyridis NP, Spyridis PG, Gelesme A, et al. The effectiveness of a 9-month regimen of isoniazid alone versus 3- and 4-month regimens of isoniazid plus rifampin for treatment of latent tuberculosis infection in children: results of an 11-year randomized study. Clin Infect Dis 2007;45(6):715–22.

91. Bright-Thomas R, Nandwani S, Smith J, et al. Effectiveness of 3 months of rifampicin and isoniazid chemoprophylaxis for the treatment of latent tuberculosis infection in children. Arch Dis Child 2010;95(8):600–2.

92. Ormerod LP. Rifampicin and isoniazid prophylactic chemotherapy for tuberculosis. Arch Dis Child 1998;78(2):169–71.

93. Ormerod LP. Reduced incidence of tuberculosis by prophylactic chemotherapy in subjects showing strong reactions to tuberculin testing. Arch Dis Child 1987;62(10):1005–8.

94. Jasmer RM, Snyder DC, Chin DP, et al. Twelve months of isoniazid compared with four months of isoniazid and rifampin for persons with radiographic evidence of previous tuberculosis: an outcome and cost-effectiveness analysis. Am J Respir Crit Care Med 2000;162(5):1648–52.
95. Ena J, Valls V. Short-course therapy with rifampin plus isoniazid, compared with standard therapy with isoniazid, for latent tuberculosis infection: a meta-analysis. Clin Infect Dis 2005;40(5):670–6.
96. Kunkel A. Abel Zur Wiesch P, Nathavitharana RR, Marx FM, Jenkins HE, Cohen T. Smear positivity in paediatric and adult tuberculosis: systematic review and meta-analysis. BMC Infect Dis 2016;16:282.

Management and Prevention of *Staphylococcus aureus* Infections in Children

Ibukunoluwa C. Kalu, MD[a,1], Carol M. Kao, MD[b,1],
Stephanie A. Fritz, MD, MSCI[b,*]

KEYWORDS

- *Staphylococcus aureus* • Colonization • Decolonization • Skin infection
- Bacteremia • Osteomyelitis • Pneumonia • Meningitis

KEY POINTS

- *S aureus* is a common and challenging cause of infection in children, ranging in severity from asymptomatic colonization, to skin and soft tissue infection, to bacteremia, osteomyelitis, necrotizing pneumonia, and endocarditis.
- *S aureus* is the leading cause of skin and soft tissue infections, for which systemic antibiotics should be administered in addition to drainage to optimize cure and prevent recurrence.
- Management of *S aureus* infection entails prompt assessment of the source of infection and initiation of appropriate antibiotics based on local antibiotic susceptibility patterns.
- In outpatient settings, preventive strategies include optimization of hygiene measures and decolonization regimens performed by all household members with a history of SSTI in the prior year.
- In hospitals, preventive strategies, including active surveillance and decolonization of both MRSA-colonized and MSSA-colonized critically ill infants with expected prolonged hospitalizations, can reduce morbidity and mortality.

INTRODUCTION

Staphylococcus aureus is a gram-positive pathobiont, a common skin commensal with the potential to cause a broad spectrum of infections including toxin-mediated disease, skin and soft tissue infections (SSTIs), and invasive, life-threatening infections

[a] Department of Pediatrics, Division of Pediatric Infectious Diseases, Pediatric Infection Prevention, Duke University Medical Center, 315 Trent Drive, Hanes House #365, DUMC 3499, Durham, NC 27710, USA; [b] Department of Pediatrics, Division of Pediatric Infectious Diseases, Washington University School of Medicine, 660 South Euclid Avenue, MSC 8116-43-10, St Louis, MO 63110, USA
[1] These authors contributed equally to this article
* Corresponding author.
E-mail address: fritz.s@wustl.edu
Twitter: @IbukunMD((I.C.K.); @StephaureusLab (S.A.F.)

Infect Dis Clin N Am 36 (2022) 73–100
https://doi.org/10.1016/j.idc.2021.11.006
0891-5520/22/© 2021 Elsevier Inc. All rights reserved.

id.theclinics.com

including bacteremia, endocarditis, pneumonia, and osteomyelitis.[1] S aureus remains one of the most common pathogens responsible for pediatric health care–associated infections, particularly central line–associated bloodstream infections (CLABSIs) and surgical site infections (SSIs).[2,3]

S aureus is continually evolving, developing mechanisms to evade antibiotic treatment. Soon after the introduction of penicillin for widespread use in the 1940s, S aureus strains resistant to penicillin emerged, causing an epidemic of infections among individuals in health care and community settings. To combat these penicillin-resistant S aureus strains, the semisynthetic penicillin, methicillin, was introduced. Unfortunately, only several years after the introduction of methicillin, strains resistant to this new "silver bullet" also emerged, and continue to pose challenges for clinicians, particularly as these strains confer resistance not only to methicillin, but to the entire class of β-lactam antibiotics.[4] From the time of their emergence in the 1960s until the 1990s, these methicillin-resistant S aureus (MRSA) strains predominantly caused nosocomial infections. In the late 1990s, clinically and genetically distinct strains of MRSA emerged, infecting otherwise healthy hosts without the traditional health care–associated risk factors for MRSA infections. These strains were coined "Community-Associated (CA)" MRSA; the most frequent circulating strain in the United States, determined by pulse-field gel electrophoresis, is the USA300 clone.[5,6] The emergence of these strains has resulted in an epidemic of SSTIs as well as invasive, necrotizing infections.[6,7]

SSTI is the most frequent entity caused by S aureus and includes impetigo, folliculitis, cellulitis, and cutaneous abscesses (furuncles and carbuncles). The incidence of SSTIs rose significantly in the early 2000s driven by the emergence of the CA-MRSA USA300 clone. From 1997 to 2005, visits to ambulatory centers (outpatient physician offices and emergency departments) by patients with purulent SSTI rose from 4.6 million to 9.6 million annually.[8,9] Although the incidence of these infections has recently plateaued, and decreased in some populations, the overall burden of these infections remains high (8.4 million ambulatory visits annually).[10,11] Recently, there has been an increase in methicillin-susceptible S aureus (MSSA) strains possessing the USA300 genetic background, though with increased resistance to non–β-lactam antibiotics.[12,13]

S aureus is one of the most frequent causes of bloodstream infections (BSIs) and musculoskeletal infections in children. The estimated rate of S aureus bacteremia is 1.5 to 3.5 per 1000 pediatric hospital admissions.[14–16] An investigation of pediatric BSIs using the Premier Healthcare Database revealed that, among children beyond the neonatal period, 25% of BSIs were caused by S aureus (16% MSSA and 9% MRSA).[17] The mortality associated with S aureus bacteremia in children is as high as 6%.[18,19] Owing to great strides in health care infection-prevention practices, the incidence of nosocomial MRSA BSIs in the United States has decreased. Approximately half of all S aureus infections in health care settings are caused by MSSA, and the incidence of MSSA BSIs has remained steady. In hospitalized patients, the rate of CA-MRSA bacteremia has not changed, whereas CA-MSSA infections have significantly increased.[20]

Approximately 30% of healthy people are colonized with S aureus, and 2% to 10% with MRSA. Colonization poses risk for subsequent infection in both healthy and hospitalized individuals.[21–25] The anterior nares have traditionally been described as the most common site of S aureus colonization. In children, however, non-nasal sites (eg, inguinal folds, axillae, umbilicus, oropharynx) may be more common reservoirs for S aureus.[23,26] Thus, among high-risk populations, many hospital infection-prevention programs perform active surveillance (nasal screening) to detect S aureus colonization among vulnerable populations, to inform targeted decolonization using topical antimicrobials or antiseptics.[27] Importantly, understanding the burden of *S aureus* colonization among hospitalized patients promotes antimicrobial stewardship. For example, among adult patients, absence of nasal *S aureus* colonization has a high (>96%) negative predictive value for *S aureus* infections at other anatomic sites.[28]

CLINICAL ENTITIES AND TREATMENT
Antibiotic Overview

Management of *S aureus* infections includes prompt initiation of appropriate antibiotics, rapid assessment for the source of infection, and possible sites of metastatic infection, with urgent eradication of infectious sources or metastatic foci, when feasible. As geographic variation in antimicrobial susceptibilities exists, empiric therapy should be selected based on local antibiotic susceptibility patterns. Definitive antibiotic choice and length of therapy depend on the site and severity of infections and the antibiotic susceptibility of the infecting isolate. Intravenous antibiotics provide optimal initial therapy for invasive *S aureus* infections, and transition to oral options are appropriate for some infections. Classes of antibiotics used for pediatrics include semisynthetic penicillins (oxacillin, nafcillin), cephalosporins (cefazolin, ceftriaxone, ceftaroline), tetracyclines (doxycycline), oxazolidinone (linezolid), lincosamides (clindamycin), sulfonamides (trimethoprim-sulfamethoxazole [TMP-SMX]), and cyclic lipopeptides (daptomycin) **(Table 1)**. Adjunctive therapy may be indicated for relapsed or prolonged *S aureus* infections, although the impact on mortality and clinical outcomes remains unclear.[29]

Bloodstream Infection

S aureus is a common cause of BSI in children, resulting in significant morbidity and mortality **(Table 2)**.[15] *S aureus* BSI can be secondary to, or result in, infectious foci at another site, including a central venous catheter (CVC), bone, lung, or skin and soft tissue. However, BSI without an obvious source occurs in 5% to 30% of cases and is associated with higher mortality.[14,30] Risk factors for BSI include *S aureus* colonization, congenital heart disease, underlying immunosuppression (leukemia/lymphoma, hemoglobinopathy, primary immunodeficiency, solid-organ transplantation), and prematurity.[29,31] Of note, an increase in rates of *S aureus* BSI occurred concurrently with the emergence of USA300 CA-MRSA and subsequent increase in SSTIs.[32]

Prolonged *S aureus* bacteremia is associated with an increased risk of complications such as septic emboli, thrombi, and metastatic foci of infection.[16] Each additional day of bacteremia has been associated with a 50% (95% confidence interval, 26%–79%) increased odds of bacteremia-related complications.[33] Risk factors for prolonged *S aureus* bacteremia include methicillin-resistance, musculoskeletal infection, endovascular infection, and delayed intervention for source control.[14,16] Children with risk factors for infective endocarditis (IE; eg, congenital heart disease and fever), clinical features suggestive of IE, or persistent bacteremia for greater than 72 hours should be thoroughly assessed for complications using echocardiogram, as well as imaging of other anatomic sites as indicated by swelling, inflammation, or pain.[29,34]

Presence of a CVC may increase the risk of prolonged bacteremia. CVC removal is recommended for patients with *S aureus* bacteremia given the ability of *S aureus* to adhere to foreign material, making eradication difficult.[35] Efforts have been made to optimize bacteremia prevention strategies among hospitalized patients, including bathing with topical antiseptics to decrease bacterial bioburden on the skin. In a multicenter trial of children in pediatric intensive care units (ICUs), daily chlorhexidine

Table 1
Systemic antibiotics for *S aureus* infections and associated adverse effects.

Antibiotic Class	Specific Medications	Activity Against MRSA	Activity Against MSSA	Reported Adverse Effects	Special Considerations
β-Lactam antibiotics (penicillins, cephalosporins, β-lactam inhibitors, carbapenems)	Oxacillin/Nafcillin		X	• Bone marrow suppression with prolonged use • Transaminase elevation • Thrombophlebitis • Diarrhea • *Clostridioides difficile* infection	• Class of choice for MSSA infections • Inactive against MRSA except ceftaroline
	Cefazolin/Cephalexin		X		
	Cefepime		X		
	Ceftriaxone		X		
	Ceftaroline	X	X		
	Amoxicillin-clavulanate		X		
	Ampicillin-sulbactam		X		
	Piperacillin-tazobactam		X		
	Meropenem		X		
	Ertapenem		X		
Glycopeptide	Vancomycin	X	X	• Tissue penetration variable depending on degree of inflammation • Nephrotoxicity	• Therapeutic monitoring necessary • Higher MICs (>1) have been associated with treatment failure
Lipopeptide	Daptomycin	X	X	• Elevation in creatinine phosphokinase (CPK)	• Inactivated by pulmonary surfactant; should not be used for the treatment of pneumonia or left-sided endocarditis • Approved for use in children ≥12 mo of age
Lincosamides	Clindamycin[a]	X	X	• Diarrhea • *Clostridioides difficile* infection	• Poor taste of oral suspension • Excellent oral bioavailability and tissue/bone penetration, poor CNS penetration

Class	Drug(s)	Adverse effects	Comments
(continued from previous page)			• *S aureus* may exhibit either constitutive or inducible resistance • Most HA-MRSA isolates resistant to clindamycin
Oxazolidinones	Linezolid Tedizolid	• Bone marrow suppression (more likely to occur beyond 3 wk of treatment) • Peripheral and optic neuropathy (more likely to occur beyond 3 wk of treatment) • Lactic acidosis • Diarrhea, emesis	• Activity against VISA and VRSA • Excellent oral bioavailability • Use with caution in patients taking serotonergic or adrenergic agents
Tetracycline	Doxycycline[a] Minocycline[a] Tigecycline Omadacycline	• Use caution in children <8 y of age due to tooth enamel discoloration and decreased bone growth; short courses (<3 wk) are unlikely to result in harm • Photosensitivity	• Excellent oral bioavailability • Tigecycline has low serum concentration
Lipoglycopeptides	Telavancin Dalbavancin Oritavancin	• Gastrointestinal symptoms (nausea, vomiting)	• Limited data available in children • Dalbavancin and oritavancin are administered once weekly
Quinolones	Delafloxacin Levofloxacin[a] Moxifloxacin[a]	• Tendinopathies • QT interval prolongation	• Excellent oral bioavailability

(continued on next page)

Table 1
(continued)

Antibiotic Class	Specific Medications	Activity Against MRSA	Activity Against MSSA	Reported Adverse Effects	Special Considerations
Others	Trimethoprim-Sulfamethoxazole (TMP-SMX)	X	X	• TMP-SMX not recommended in infants younger than 2 mo of age due to risk of bilirubin displacement	• Rifampin should not be used as monotherapy due to the rapid development of resistance
	Rifampin	X			• Rifampin may be combined with another agent for hardware-associated infections

Notes: Antibiotics included are those available for use in the United States. Choice of antibiotic to treat *Staphylococcus aureus* infection is dependent upon susceptibility of infecting organism; empiric therapy should be selected based on local antibiotic susceptibility patterns.

Abbreviations: MIC, minimum inhibitory concentration; MRSA, methicillin-resistant *Staphylococcus aureus*; MSSA, methicillin-susceptible *S aureus*; HA-MRSA, health care–associated methicillin-resistant *S aureus*; VISA, vancomycin-intermediate *S aureus*; VRSA, vancomycin-resistant *S aureus*.

a Susceptibility is variable.

Adapted from Refs.[34,48]

Table 2
Staphylococcus aureus infection entities

Infection Site	Epidemiology	Clinical Presentation	Duration of Antibiotic Therapy
Bloodstream (Bacteremia)	*S aureus* accounts for 5%–30% of BSIs without localizing source and CLABSIs.[30,31,33] Increased risk of persistent bacteremia and treatment failure with retained foreign body, >2 infected sites, and endovascular infection.[14,16]	Fever Lethargy	2–6 wk depending on the source of bacteremia
Central Nervous System (Meningitis, Epidural abscess)[a]	Uncommon (<1% of all pediatric meningitis), <5% of *S aureus* invasive infections.[65] Mortality in children is low. Associated with device placement, trauma, prematurity, intraventricular hemorrhage, or CNS malformation.	Fever Altered mental status Back pain	Meningitis: 2 wk Brain, spinal epidural abscess, subdural empyema: 4–6 wk
Lungs (Pneumonia, empyema)	Rare (<1% of all pediatric pneumonias). Bullous lung disease more common among infants. Common cause of necrotizing pneumonia.[57] Increased risk of complications: pleural space involvement and lung abscesses.	Fever Cough Chest pain	7–21 d depending on the severity of infection and clinical improvement
Endovascular (endocarditis, thrombophlebitis, septic embolism)[a]	Common cause of endocarditis with high mortality and morbidity.	Fever Chest pain	4–6 wk

(continued on next page)

Table 2
(continued)

Infection Site	Epidemiology	Clinical Presentation	Duration of Antibiotic Therapy
	Typical signs of endocarditis may not be present in children.[42]		
Bone, Muscle, Joint (osteomyelitis, pyomyositis, osteoarthritis)	Most common cause of musculoskeletal infections in children.[45,47]	Fever Focal joint or extremity pain Arthralgia	Septic arthritis: 3–4 wk Osteomyelitis: 3–6 wk
Skin and Soft Tissue Infection	Represents >60% of *S aureus* infections.	Pain Rash Erythema Swelling Purulence	7–10 d

Abbreviations: BSI, bloodstream infection; CLABSI, central line–associated bloodstream infection; CNS, central nervous system; MRSA, methicillin-resistant *Staphylococcus aureus*.

bathing yielded a 34% reduction in risk of bacteremia compared with daily bathing with soap and water.[36]

Vancomycin combined with a beta-lactam is recommended as empiric treatment for *S aureus* bacteremia until antimicrobial susceptibility is available.[29] Treatment duration depends on the source of the bacteremia and the presence of complications such as endovascular infection or metastatic foci of infection. In pediatrics, 7 to 14 days of IV antibiotic therapy is generally recommended for uncomplicated bacteremia, though more research is needed to derive the optimal length of IV therapy.[29] Endovascular infection, musculoskeletal infection, critical illness, and initial subtherapeutic vancomycin levels have been associated with MRSA BSI treatment failure.[33,37]

To assess response to antibiotic therapy, it is essential to document clearance of bacteremia. Thus, it is recommended to obtain daily blood cultures until blood cultures are negative for 2 days.[38] As the yield of positivity is low, additional blood cultures to document sterility following 2 days of negative cultures are not typically indicated unless the patient's clinical condition deteriorates. Infectious disease consultation for *S aureus* BSI has been demonstrated to improve patient management and outcomes, including decreased mortality and recurrence of bacteremia.[29,39]

Endocarditis/Endovascular Infection

S aureus is the most common cause of IE. The overall mortality for *S aureus* IE is as high as 66% (see **Table 2**).[40] In the International Collaboration on Endocarditis Prospective Cohort Study conducted from 2000 to 2003, *S aureus* caused 32% of all IE cases, of which 27% were MRSA. MSSA IE cases tended to result in a higher incidence of systemic embolization compared with MRSA (26% vs 18%, $P = .06$), but MRSA IE was associated with a longer duration of bacteremia (43% vs 9%, $P < .001$) and a trend toward increased mortality.[41]

The clinical presentation of IE can be nonspecific and indolent with symptoms such as malaise, weight loss, or myalgias. The typical signs of IE, including new-onset heart murmur, congestive heart failure, and embolic phenomenon, are often not present in children.[42] When endocarditis is suspected in a child, it is recommended to obtain 3 sets of blood cultures, ideally through separate venipunctures, before initiation of antibiotics. Unlike adults, transthoracic echocardiography (TTE) can be sufficient in children.[43] However, transesophageal echocardiography should be obtained in children who have had prior cardiac surgeries, have congenital anomalies, are at high risk for aortic root abscesses, or in whom TTE does not provide sufficient information.[44] Negative echocardiography does not exclude IE.

Bactericidal, rather than bacteriostatic, antibiotics should be used to treat endovascular infection (endocarditis, septic thrombophlebitis, mycotic aneurysms) for the duration of therapy. *S aureus* bacteremia commonly persists after initiation of appropriate therapy, particularly if the source of infection has not been removed (eg, CVC). For MRSA endocarditis, vancomycin or daptomycin are recommended for a minimum of 6 weeks. For MSSA IE, oxacillin/nafcillin or cefazolin should be used for at least 4 to 6 weeks and vancomycin can be used as an alternative in those highly allergic to beta-lactam antibiotics. Given the difficulty of eradicating *S aureus* from foreign material, if prosthetic material is present, the addition of rifampin for 6 weeks and gentamicin for the initial 2 weeks of treatment is recommended; patients receiving this regimen should be closely monitored for adverse side effects.[44]

Acute Hematogenous Osteomyelitis, Septic Arthritis, Pyomyositis

S aureus is the most common cause of musculoskeletal infections (see **Table 2**).[45–47] In children, infections in the bone, joint, and muscle most commonly arise from

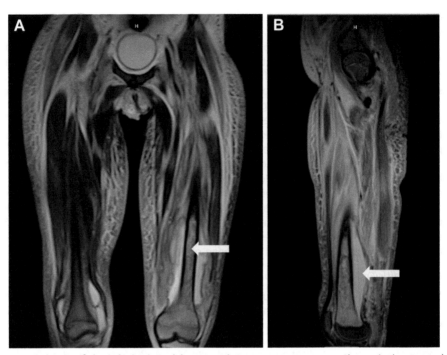

Fig. 1. *A)* MRI of the left thigh and femur with intravenous contrast. Shown is the coronal view demonstrating a T2 hyperintense signal in the left distal femoral metaphysis (*arrow*), which extends 19 cm proximal to the distal femoral physis consistent with acute MRSA hematogenous osteomyelitis. (*B*) Shown is the sagittal view demonstrating a T2 hyperintense, rim-enhancing subperiosteal abscess measuring 2.8 x 4.5 × 13.0 cm (*arrow*) and hyperintensity in the vastus intermedius, medialis, lateralis, and semitendinosus muscles, and diffuse subcutaneous edema throughout the left thigh.

hematogenous seeding, and more rarely from a contiguous focus of infection, such as a decubitus ulcer, or through direct inoculation from trauma or a surgical procedure. *S aureus* accounts for up to 60% of pyomyositis cases in children and commonly affects the pelvic and lower extremity muscles.[46] *S aureus* accounts for up to 78% of acute hematogenous osteomyelitis (AHO) in children; 33% of these cases are caused by MRSA.[48] AHO most frequently occurs in the long bones of the lower extremities and the pelvis, followed by the long bones of the upper extremities.[49,50] Multifocal osteomyelitis has been reported in 5% to 10% of patients with AHO and up to 35% of patients have contiguous septic arthritis.[49,51] AHO may be complicated by the formation of an intraosseous or subperiosteal abscess (**Fig. 1**) and has also been associated with thrombotic complications including deep venous thrombosis adjacent to the site of infection and septic pulmonary emboli.[52,53]

The clinical presentation of *S aureus* musculoskeletal infection in children includes fever, pain, erythema, warmth, point tenderness, and limited range of motion. For children with lower extremity osteomyelitis, patients frequently present with limp or inability to bear weight.[47] Detailed clinical evaluation should be prioritized in children with osteomyelitis. Although procalcitonin, a common inflammatory biomarker, is not recommended, the initial diagnostic investigation should include serum C-reactive protein (CRP). The baseline CRP value can be followed during the clinical course to assess response to therapy.[48] Blood cultures should be obtained before antimicrobial therapy. Although the sensitivity of early plain radiographs for suspected AHO infection is low, it is reasonable to start with plain radiography of the affected limbs. However, further imaging such as MRI to confirm the diagnosis is often needed.[54] End of treatment imaging studies should not be routinely obtained in uncomplicated AHO unless there is involvement of physis; end of therapy imaging is recommended for patients with complicated AHO.[48]

When feasible, a bone biopsy or aspirate of purulent material obtained via surgical procedure or interventional radiology should be performed to obtain microbiological studies that can guide targeted antimicrobial therapy. Although blood cultures may reveal the causative organism in ~50% of patients with *S aureus* musculoskeletal infection, aspirate or biopsy increases the yield and may be the only specimen revealing the organism.[48,51,54] Surgical debridement and drainage of a joint space or subperiosteal or intraosseous abscess should be performed to prevent long-term morbidity. If patients are clinically stable and an upcoming surgical procedure is planned, waiting to start antibiotics until after the procedure is reasonable. For rapidly deteriorating patients, prompt administration of antibiotics reduces the risk of mortality;the yield of cultures obtained within 24 to 48 hours of antibiotic initiation is similar to those obtained before the onset of antibiotic therapy.[48]

Empiric antimicrobial therapy should include coverage against *S aureus* and CA-MRSA based on patient risk factors and local susceptibility data.[48] Definitive treatment should be based on microbiologic study results. Early transition from IV to oral antibiotics with good bioavailability and bone concentration has been demonstrated to be effective in children with uncomplicated musculoskeletal infections who are clinically stable.[45,48] However, a paucity of data exist to guide the optimal length of hospitalization and IV antibiotic therapy before transitioning to oral antibiotic therapy. In one retrospective study, patients who were discharged home and successfully treated with oral antibiotics received a median of 7 days (interquartile range, 5–10 days) of IV antibiotic therapy before hospital discharge. Ultimately, the optimal duration and route of antibiotic therapy should be individualized based on the patient's clinical response; some patients with a complicated course, including multifocal or deep-seated infection, prolonged bacteremia, immunocompromised state, and very young age may require a longer course of IV antibiotics.[53] Recently published clinical practice guidelines for pediatric AHO state that 3 to 4 weeks of total antibiotic therapy may be adequate for children with uncomplicated AHO who have shown clinical response to initial therapy, whereas longer courses of antibiotics may be needed with more virulent pathogens, extensive infection, or complicated cases.[48] Three to 4 weeks of antibiotics are generally recommended for the treatment of septic arthritis, although concomitant osteomyelitis is not uncommon and may warrant longer treatment.

Up to 10% of children with *S aureus* AHO will experience acute complications (eg, treatment failure within 6 weeks of antibiotic therapy initiation, prolonged hospitalization) as well as long-term morbidity (eg, growth arrest of the affected limb or limb length discrepancy, pathologic fractures, avascular necrosis, chronic dislocation, chronic osteomyelitis).[51,53] The development of orthopedic complications after AHO has been associated with prolonged fever, delayed source control, need for multiple surgical procedures, bacteremia, and AHO with concomitant septic arthritis (**Box 1**).[45,51,53] In 2 large pediatric retrospective studies, methicillin resistance was not associated with adverse outcomes; however, methicillin resistance was associated with decreased range of motion at end of therapy in one pediatric study compared with individuals with non-*S aureus* musculoskeletal infection.[45,51,53] The *S aureus* strain type may be more important than antibiotic susceptibility (ie,

---

Box 1
Factors associated with complications in pediatric patients with acute hematogenous osteomyelitis

Factors Associated with Acute Complications[53]
  Fever (body temperature >100.4°F) for more than 48 hours after starting antibiotics
  Bone abscess
  Associated suppurative arthritis
  Disseminated disease
  Delayed source control (surgical intervention more than 3 days after hospital admission)

Factors Associated with Chronic Complications[51,53]
  Prolonged fever (body temperature >100.4°F) for more than 4 days following hospital admission
  Disseminated disease
  Delayed source control (surgical intervention more than 3 days after hospital admission)
  Requirement for bone debridement
  CRP ≥100 mg/L 2 to 4 days after antibiotic initiation
  Staphylococcus aureus strain type (agr group III)

Abbreviation: agr, accessory gene regulator.

---

methicillin-resistant vs susceptible).[51] A multidisciplinary approach to S aureus musculoskeletal infections and the development of clinical practice guidelines can decrease time to diagnostic MRI, increase the proportion of patients with tissue culture and identification of the infecting organism, increase prescription of targeted antibiotic therapy, and decrease hospital length of stay and hospital readmission rates.[54] Severity of illness scores have been devised to predict patients at high risk of developing AHO complications, which may inform treatment and follow-up plans.[53]

Pneumonia

S aureus is an important cause of community-acquired pneumonia (CAP) and can be rapidly progressive, resulting in severe, fulminant respiratory failure (see **Table 2**).[55] S aureus pneumonia is associated with increased disease severity and worse outcomes, with increased length of hospital stay, need for ICU admission, and use of mechanical ventilation.[56,57] S aureus is also an important contributor to hospital-acquired pneumonia, ventilator-associated pneumonia, and healthcare-associated pneumonia. Risk factors for S aureus pneumonia in children include underlying cystic fibrosis and mechanical ventilation.

Children typically present with severe pneumonia with or without effusion, necrotizing or cavitary infiltrates, or empyema (**Fig. 2**).[57] Viral codetection is common, and children may present with preceding or concurrent upper respiratory tract infection. In particular, necrotizing pneumonia caused by S aureus strains producing Panton-Valentine leucocidin has been associated with preceding flu-like illness.[58] Influenza-S aureus codetection has high morbidity and mortality rates. MRSA coinfection of the lungs during the 2009 influenza A (H1N1) outbreak resulted in an 8-fold increased relative risk of mortality among previously healthy children.[59]

Blood cultures should be obtained in children requiring hospitalization for CAP, those with severe or complicated CAP, or those who fail to improve after initial antibiotic therapy. Of the children enrolled in the prospective Etiology of Pneumonia in the Community surveillance study diagnosed with S aureus CAP, 26% also had bacteremia, 52% had a positive pleural fluid culture, and 39% had positive culture from bronchoalveolar lavage fluid or endotracheal aspirate.[60] Sputum sample or

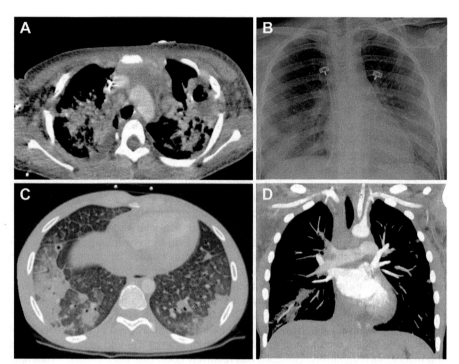

Fig. 2. *A*) Chest CT with contrast. Shown is a patient with extensive MRSA multifocal necrotizing pneumonia throughout both lungs with a lung abscess in the left upper lobe measuring 4.0 x 2.6 × 3.9 cm and additional cavitary lesions in the right middle lobe. There is also moderate global cardiomegaly with a possible vegetation measuring 12 mm along the lateral leaflet of the mitral valve, and moderate pericardial effusion with pericardial enhancement. (*B*) Chest radiograph with scattered bilateral infiltrates from a patient with MSSA bacteremia. (*C, D*) Chest CT angiography with contrast showing bilateral opacities with areas of early cavitation, multiple septic pulmonary emboli including nonocclusive thrombi within the pulmonary arteries.

tracheal aspirate for Gram stain and culture should also be obtained in children with severe CAP. Drainage of pleural effusion or empyema, if present, should be considered based on the size of the effusion and the degree of respiratory compromise.[61]

Empiric coverage for *S aureus* is recommended in cases of severe pneumonia defined as requirement for ICU admission, necrotizing or cavitary infiltrates, or presence of empyema.[62] For initial treatment of MRSA or MSSA pneumonia, vancomycin or clindamycin (based on local susceptibility data) in addition to a beta-lactam is recommended, although linezolid and ceftaroline fosamil are alternative antibiotics with MRSA coverage.[61] Daptomycin should not be administered for pneumonia given inactivation by pulmonary surfactant.

Central Nervous System Infection (Meningitis, Epidural Abscess, Ventricular Shunt Infection)

S aureus central nervous system (CNS) infection is uncommon and typically occurs as a complication of neurosurgical procedures, CNS instrumentation (eg, ventricular shunt), bacteremia, or extension from a parameningeal focus. *S aureus* has been implicated in 13% to 25% of ventricular shunt infections and is the most common cause of spinal epidural abscesses (see **Table 2**).[63,64] In a prospective surveillance study of *S aureus* at a large children's hospital, CNS infections accounted for 5% of all invasive *S aureus* infections.[65] The majority (70%) of these cases were associated with a CNS device, typically a ventriculoperitoneal shunt, 13% were associated with hematogenous meningitis, and 10% were associated with spinal epidural abscess. MSSA accounted for 67% of infections in the case series. Overall mortality and morbidity in children was low.[65]

S aureus CNS infections typically present with fever, headaches, neck or back pain, nausea, vomiting, and neurologic symptoms. Epidural abscesses classically present with back pain, fever, and neurologic symptoms (**Fig. 3**). CNS shunt infections present with fever and signs of increased intracranial pressure.[66,67] Given the severity of *S aureus* CNS infections, a high degree of clinical suspicion is needed. Imaging studies should be considered, particularly if a child presents with neurologic signs and symptoms accompanied by *S aureus* bacteremia.

Management of *S aureus* CNS infection typically requires surgical intervention. Due to potential spinal cord compression, emergent surgical intervention is critical in management of spinal epidural abscesses to prevent long-term neurologic sequelae. For treatment of CNS shunt infections, it is essential to remove all components of an infected device, place an external CSF drain, and initiate antibiotic treatment.[62] Antibiotic choice in treatment of CNS infection should take into account cerebrospinal fluid (CSF) penetration. An anti-staphylococcal beta-lactam antibiotic such as nafcillin or oxacillin is recommended for MSSA CNS infections and vancomycin for MRSA.[68] However, vancomycin has relatively poor CSF penetration even in the presence of inflamed meninges, with a median CSF to serum ratio of 3% and high inter-subject pharmacokinetic variability. Linezolid has relatively good CSF penetration.[69] Rifampin has similar penetration for inflamed and non-inflamed meninges and achieves

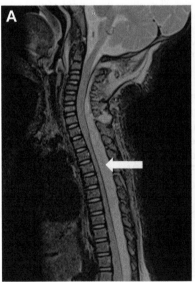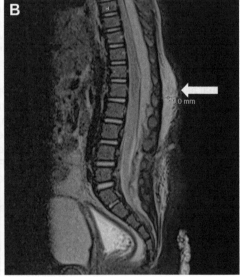

Fig. 3. *A*) MRI brainstem and spine with contrast. Shown is the sagittal view of an extensive MRSA spinal epidural abscess with T2 hyperintense fluid collection and peripheral enhancement extending from the level of C3 to the distal sacrum/coccyx, measuring up to 8 mm in thickness in the mid-thoracic spine in maximum diameter (*arrow*). (*B*) Shown is a T2 hyperintense paraspinal abscess extending from the level of C6-T2 along the left side (*arrow*).

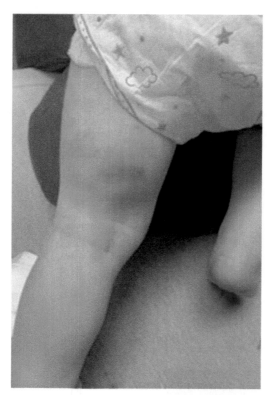

Fig. 4. *Staphylococcus aureus* skin and soft tissue infections. Shown is a toddler with a left posterior thigh abscess with central head and surrounding area of cellulitis.

bactericidal concentrations in the CSF. Given poor CSF penetration of most antibiotics, vancomycin with rifampin is recommended by some experts, although randomized clinical trials have not been performed.[62] Ceftaroline for treatment of MRSA CNS infection has been reported in limited case reports.[70] Phase 1 clinical trials for the use of ceftaroline in pediatric CNS infections are in progress (NCT00633126, NCT02600793).[71]

Skin and Soft Tissue Infection

S aureus is a leading cause of SSTI, manifesting as cellulitis, cutaneous abscesses, folliculitis, and impetigo (see **Table 2, Fig. 4**).[72] SSTIs are a leading cause of pediatric hospitalizations and healthcare utilization, especially given the high likelihood for recurrence, reported to range from 20% to 70%.[15,26,73–76] Risk factors for the development and recurrence of SSTIs include *S aureus* colonization, particularly persistent colonization, colonization of multiple anatomic sites, underlying dermatologic conditions (ie, eczema), personal history of prior SSTI or close contact with someone with SSTIs, participation in contact sports, and certain chronic medical conditions.[21,77,78]

Incision and drainage (I&D) has traditionally been the mainstay for uncomplicated *S aureus* SSTI.[62,79] I&D evacuates infective material, which can be sent for microbiologic culture, and provides pain relief and faster wound healing. Recently, several large, multicenter, placebo-controlled, randomized trials have demonstrated that I&D in conjunction with systemic antibiotic therapy results in a higher likelihood of clinical

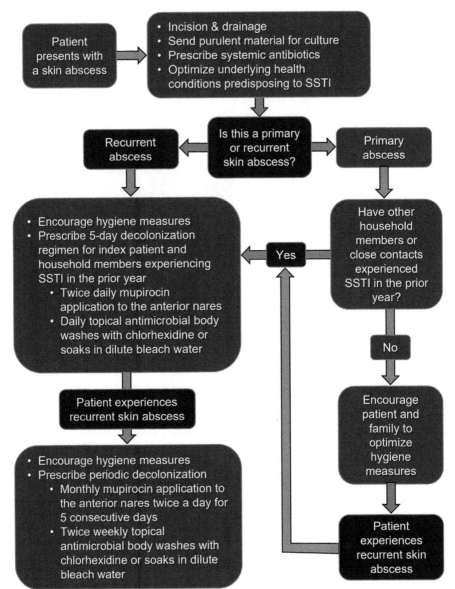

Fig. 5. Recommended approach to the management of patients presenting with skin abscesses based on current evidence. Management of the acute infection includes incision and drainage, culture of the purulent material for organism identification and susceptibility testing, and systemic antibiotic therapy. Decolonization should be recommended for patients who experience recurrent skin abscesses or in settings of ongoing transmission (eg, SSTI in multiple household members) despite optimizing hygiene measures. Specifically, the recommended decolonization regimen is a 5-day protocol consisting of intranasal application of mupirocin (approximately a pea-sized amount to each nostril, applied with a sterile cotton-tipped applicator) twice daily, and daily antimicrobial body washes with either chlorhexidine or dilute bleach water baths. Chlorhexidine should be applied with a clean washcloth to the neck and below (contact with the face and ears should be avoided as ocular and ototoxicity may occur) and should be rinsed off after 1 to 3 minutes. Dilute bleach baths should consist of $\frac{1}{4}$ cup of bleach per $\frac{1}{4}$ filled bathtub for a standard-sized bathtub or 1 teaspoon of bleach per gallon of bathwater for a nonstandard bathtub; individuals should soak in the dilute bleach water for 15 minutes.

cure, regardless of the abscess size. Moreover, administering systemic antibiotics in conjunction with I&D reduces the incidence of recurrent skin infection, likely due to eradication of *S aureus* colonization by systemic antibiotics **(Fig. 5)**.[72,80–83] Despite robust evidence to support the use of systemic antibiotics in conjunction with I&D, antibiotics are prescribed for 69% of ambulatory and ED SSTI visits and only 60% of surveyed pediatric infectious disease providers would recommend antibiotics for treatment of uncomplicated skin abscesses.[10,84]

Cultures from abscesses and purulent SSTIs should be obtained to help guide antibiotic therapy. Empiric choice for treatment of *S aureus* SSTIs should be based on disease severity and local antibiotic susceptibility patterns, which may change over time.[12] In hospitalized children, β-lactams or vancomycin can be started empirically depending on local antimicrobial susceptibility. Clindamycin, linezolid, daptomycin, tetracyclines, or TMP-SMX are alternative options.[62] There is a paucity of data regarding the optimal length of antibiotic therapy for cellulitis and skin abscesses. The optimal duration of treatment should be based on clinical response, and a 7 to 10 day course is generally thought to be sufficient. A randomized-controlled trial comparing 3 versus 10 days of TMP-SMX after drainage for treatment of MRSA skin abscesses found that 3 days of antibiotics resulted in increased treatment failure and subsequent recurrence within 1 month.[85] A subgroup analysis of a randomized trial demonstrated that each additional day of antibiotic therapy (up to 10 days of either clindamycin or TMP-SMX) resulted in an increased likelihood for cure and decreased incidence of SSTI recurrence 6 weeks after the acute infection.[82]

PREVENTION OF *STAPHYLOCOCCUS AUREUS* INFECTIONS
Transmission

To devise effective prevention strategies, it is essential to understand the dynamics of *S aureus* acquisition and transmission. *S aureus* transmission can occur through close personal contact. Households serve as important reservoirs for *S aureus* transmission and indeed, household contacts of individuals with *S aureus* SSTI have a higher prevalence of colonization and SSTI than the general population.[78,86–89] In addition to close personal contact, *S aureus* transmission among household members also occurs through the sharing of personal hygiene items, towels, and beds.[88]

In health care and community settings, environmental surfaces and fomites serve as important reservoirs for *S aureus* acquisition and transmission.[90,91] In a comprehensive investigation of *S aureus* household transmission dynamics among households affected by *S aureus* infections, environmental surfaces, particularly those commonly shared between household members (eg, hand towels, television remote control, video game controller), as well as bed linens, were frequently contaminated with *S aureus*, and specifically, with a strain molecularly concordant with the *S aureus* strain that caused the index patient's infection. Importantly, these surfaces were persistently contaminated over time, perpetuating the cycle of transmission and reacquisition among household members, thus posing risk for recurrent infection.[78,87–89] Thus, integrating environmental hygiene measures may be an important component of *S aureus* eradication and infection prevention; this strategy is currently under study (NCT02572791).

The role of companion animals in *S aureus* transmission dynamics and recurrent SSTIs in owners and veterinary personnel is an important consideration. In the aforementioned household investigation, although *S aureus* colonization of pet dogs and cats was detected (24% of dogs and 13% of cats), and human to pet transmission was observed, these companion animals were rarely a primary source of a transmitted

S aureus strain to their owners.[88,89] Thus, although pet dogs and cats may contribute to overall household transmission dynamics, they likely do not represent natural hosts for S aureus colonization, and their carriage often spontaneously resolves.[92,93] Strategies to reduce transmission between companion animals and their household members include hand washing before and after pet contact, isolating the pet temporarily from a patient undergoing treatment for an active infection, and disinfecting the pet's crate or kennel and washing the pet's bedding.[92,94]

Decolonization

S aureus colonization, and particularly colonization at multiple anatomic sites, is a known risk factor for S aureus infection, though infection typically does not occur without disruption of the skin through inflammatory lesions (eg, eczema), trauma, or microabrasions.[21,75,95] Prevention measures for outpatients will be discussed here (see **Fig. 5**), and specific risk factors and infection prevention strategies for neonates and immunocompromised hosts are described in the following sections. The primary component of S aureus infection prevention is optimization of hygiene measures, including keeping open wounds covered, frequent hand hygiene, regular bathing, using a barrier between bare skin and shared surfaces (eg, athletic or gym equipment), and avoiding sharing personal hygiene items (eg, razors, deodorant, cosmetics) and towels. As bed linens serve as a reservoir of S aureus, they should be laundered weekly. In addition, patients can be encouraged to use lotions in pump or pour bottles to avoid contamination, liquid rather than bar soap, avoiding bath or shower loofas, laundering towels and washcloths after each use, and keeping fingernails trimmed short and clean.[62,73,75] Optimizing the treatment of underlying skin disorders (eg, eczema) is also essential.

Up to 70% of patients with SSTI will experience a recurrence, predominantly with the same molecular strain of S aureus as the primary infection and the strain with which the patient is colonized.[73,76,96] Thus, to prevent recurrent infections, decolonization strategies should be considered for individuals who have optimized hygiene strategies and experience a recurrent SSTI, or in settings in which there is ongoing transmission between household members or other close contacts (eg, infection occurring in multiple household members or athletic team members).[62] These strategies include the application of topical antibiotics or antiseptics to eradicate or decrease the burden of S aureus carriage. Multiple agents and regimens have been investigated for S aureus eradication and have been recently reviewed.[26] A combined decolonization approach of intranasal antibiotic application (eg, mupirocin) and bathing with a topical antiseptic or biocide (eg, chlorhexidine gluconate and dilute bleach water [sodium hypochlorite]) has been most effective for preventing SSTI.[73,75,97]

Mupirocin is a topical antimicrobial agent effective against gram-positive microorganisms. Mupirocin is frequently used in hospital settings to prevent nosocomial infections including SSIs and CLABSIs.[98,99] Chlorhexidine gluconate is a broad-spectrum biocide that is frequently used in health care settings for topical disinfection before invasive procedures and for decolonization among select populations to prevent nosocomial infections.[100] Chlorhexidine comes in several formulations, including a topical liquid, oral rinse, and impregnated cloths. Sodium hypochlorite, or bleach, has broad-spectrum antimicrobial activities. Dermatologists have traditionally recommended bathing in dilute bleach water for patients with eczema, given its effectiveness to improve skin flares, likely due to decreasing the burden of S aureus on the skin.[101]

As S aureus household transmission is an important contributor to persistent colonization or reacquisition and development of recurrent SSTI, several trials have been conducted to evaluate the effectiveness of decolonizing household contacts in addition to the index patient with SSTI. A randomized clinical trial enrolling 183 healthy children with *S aureus* SSTI and colonization and their household contacts compared a household decolonization approach (ie, decolonization regimen performed by all household members) versus decolonization of the index patient alone.[73] The incidence of cumulative SSTI 12 months following the intervention was significantly lower among index patients, as well as household contacts, assigned to the household decolonization arm. A decolonization regimen performed by all household members can be burdensome and costly, especially for large families, and may have the untoward effects of driving antimicrobial resistance and disrupting the commensal skin microbiota. As individuals experiencing SSTI are at increased risk for developing recurrent SSTI, another approach to addressing household transmission and infection prevention is targeting decolonization to household members with a history of SSTI. In a pragmatic, noninferiority trial enrolling 102 healthy children with CA-MRSA skin abscesses and their household contacts, a household decolonization approach, performed by all household members, was compared to a personalized decolonization approach performed by the index patient and household contacts who had experienced an SSTI in the prior year.[102] The incidence of cumulative SSTI 3 months following the decolonization intervention (the primary study outcome) demonstrated noninferiority of the personalized approach to the household approach; these findings persisted over the 12-month longitudinal study period. Adherence to the regimen was higher among participants randomized to the personalized decolonization approach. Given these findings, when prescribing a decolonization regimen for a patient with recurrent SSTI, these measures should also be recommended for household contacts experiencing SSTI in the prior year (see **Fig. 5**). Importantly, in both trials, eradication of *S aureus* carriage and prevention of SSTI waned over time, likely due to ongoing *S aureus* exposure and reacquisition. Thus, a discreet, 5-day decolonization regimen may be inadequate for long-term infection prevention. For patients experiencing ongoing recurrent SSTIs despite optimizing hygiene measures and performing a discreet decolonization regimen, periodic decolonization, performed for 3 months, may provide more sustained protection (NCT02572791). Periodic decolonization includes intranasal application of mupirocin twice daily for 5 consecutive days each month and performing antimicrobial body washes twice weekly (see **Fig. 5**).

Neonates and patients in the neonatal intensive care unit

S aureus colonization and infections are uniquely problematic in neonatal intensive care units (NICUs) because of prolonged hospitalizations of premature infants with friable skin or underlying medical conditions. These infants frequently require invasive procedures and placement of indwelling devices and have immature immune systems. These factors potentially increase the risk of *S aureus* exposure and acquisition. Neonatal *S aureus* infections are frequently preceded by nasal colonization. In recent years, MSSA infection incidence among these vulnerable infants has outpaced the incidence of MRSA infections. Importantly, the rates of morbidity and mortality are similar between infants with MSSA and MRSA infections.[64,98,103]

Among neonates, active *S aureus* surveillance and contact isolation are associated with decreased colonization and infection.[104] In addition to protective isolation to prevent *S aureus* transmission in the NICU, the risk for invasive infection is further reduced through eradicating or decreasing the burden of *S aureus* skin colonization. The most studied agents for neonatal topical decolonization are mupirocin and chlorhexidine gluconate. Given the recent trends in increasing MSSA infections among neonates, one center implemented active surveillance, isolation, and decolonization policy targeting MSSA in addition to MRSA. A review of more than 2700 children before and after policy implementation demonstrated a 73% decrease in MSSA infections immediately after the successful rollout of the intervention, with a sustained 21% quarterly decrease in cultures detecting MSSA.[98] Similar findings have been replicated across multiple studies, further supporting the utility of surveillance and decolonization for *S aureus* prevention in neonatal units.[105] Among these patients, recolonization frequently occurs—up to 39% in one study of decolonized infants—with the same colonizing bacterial strain identified before decolonization.[106] Additive strategies may be necessary for NICUs tackling ongoing *S aureus* outbreaks or in highly endemic settings. These strategies may include antimicrobial stewardship strategies as well as addressing the potential for exposure to caregiver colonization.

As parents may serve as reservoirs for *S aureus* transmission to their infants, particularly in NICUs where skin-to-skin contact is highly encouraged, targeting decolonization directly to parents and/or caregivers may be an effective strategy to prevent neonatal infections. TREAT PARENTS was a double-blind randomized clinical trial assessing the effectiveness of treating *S aureus*-colonized parents with a 5-day regimen of intranasal mupirocin and topical chlorhexidine, compared to placebo, to reduce *S aureus* transmission from parents to their hospitalized infants. Over the 90-day longitudinal study period, 40% of enrolled infants acquired *S aureus* colonization; 57% of infants with *S aureus* acquisition became colonized with an *S aureus* strain concordant with their colonized parents' strains. Importantly, treating parents with topical decolonization significantly reduced the risk of concordant *S aureus* strain acquisition in their infants.[107] Further confirmation of these findings could support widespread utility in the NICU.

Immunocompromised hosts

Children with immunocompromising conditions are at increased risk for *S aureus* infection. Recurrent skin infections are often the first sign of an underlying primary immunodeficiency such as chronic granulomatous disease, leukocyte adhesion defect, or hyperimmunoglobulin E syndrome.[108] Children with malignancy and those who have undergone solid organ or hematopoietic stem cell transplant (HSCT) are at increased risk for *S aureus* infection and complications due to comorbid conditions, presence of CVCs, immunosuppressive medications, and prolonged hospitalizations.[108–110] Despite high risk for complicated infections, mortality directly attributable to *S aureus* bacteremia is low.

General infection prevention principles such as hand hygiene, use of personal protective equipment, and appropriate care of CVCs are essential to prevent *S aureus* infections in immunocompromised children. In contrast to the reduction of *S aureus* infections in critically ill patients through decolonization, chlorhexidine bathing and nasal mupirocin were not effective in preventing *S aureus* infections in children with cancer or undergoing HSCT.[111] Further research is needed in this area given the high morbidity from *S aureus* in immunocompromised individuals.

SUMMARY

S aureus is a unique microorganism, able to infect every organ system or tissue within the human body. Treatment of acute infection, as well as prevention, is complicated by the ability of *S aureus* to exist as a commensal organism while also possessing pathogenic potential. Management of acute infection includes promptly addressing the source of infection and sites of metastatic infection and initiation of effective antibiotics, which should be selected based on anatomic location of infection, severity of infection, and local antibiotic susceptibility patterns. Additional research is needed to determine the optimal route, length, and agent of antimicrobial therapy for *S aureus* infections in children. Topical antimicrobials are frequently used in health care and outpatient settings to eradicate *S aureus* and prevent subsequent infection. Given the role of close contacts in *S aureus* transmission in hospital and community settings, targeting decolonization to these individuals should also be considered. The development of novel prevention and therapeutic strategies, including lytic agents,[112] vaccines,[113] probiotics,[114] microbiota transplants,[115] and phage therapy,[116] are exciting avenues for future research.

CLINICS CARE POINTS

- Optimal management of *S aureus* invasive infection includes addressing the source of infection, such as drainage of purulent collections and removal of infected CVCs or ventricular shunts.

- Antibiotic selection should be based on local susceptibility patterns as well as consideration of antibiotic penetration into the infected space (eg, CNS infection).

- Optimal route and duration of antibiotics should take into consideration severity of infection, complications, and clinical improvement.

- Prolonged *S aureus* bacteremia is associated with an increased risk of complications such as septic emboli, thrombi, and metastatic foci of infection. Daily blood cultures should be obtained until demonstration of 2 days of negative blood cultures to document clearance of bacteremia.

- A multidisciplinary approach to *S aureus* musculoskeletal infections and implementation of institutional clinical practice guidelines results in more efficient and effective care, leading to decreased hospital length of stay and readmission.

- Systemic antibiotics in addition to I&D should be administered to optimize cure and to prevent recurrence of *S aureus* SSTIs.

- For children with recurrent *S aureus* SSTIs, prevention should be aimed at improving hygiene measures and implementing decolonization strategies in all household members with a history of SSTI in the prior year. For those with continued recurrence, periodic decolonization for 3 months is recommended.

DISCLOSURE

This work was supported in part by a grant from the National Institutes of Health (NIH)/ Eunice Kennedy Shriver National Institute of Child Health and Human Development (OT2-HD107559) and the Agency for Healthcare Research and Quality (AHRQ, R01-HS024269). The content is solely the responsibility of the authors and does not necessarily represent the official views of the NIH or AHRQ. ICK reports consulting fees from IPEC Experts, LLC. C.M. Kao reports clinical trials research funding from Pfizer and Merck. S.A. Fritz reports clinical trials research funding from Merck.

REFERENCES

1. Lowy FD. *Staphylococcus aureus* infections. N Engl J Med 1998;339(8):520–32.
2. Weiner-Lastinger LM, Abner S, Benin AL, et al. Antimicrobial-resistant pathogens associated with pediatric healthcare-associated infections: Summary of data reported to the National Healthcare Safety Network, 2015-2017. Infect Control Hosp Epidemiol 2020;41(1):19–30.

3. Akinboyo IC, Young RR, Smith MJ, et al. Burden of healthcare-associated infections among hospitalized children within community hospitals participating in an infection control network. Infect Control Hosp Epidemiol 2021;1–3.

4. Chambers HF, Deleo FR. Waves of resistance: Staphylococcus aureus in the antibiotic era. Nat Rev Microbiol 2009;7(9):629–41.

5. Herold BC, Immergluck LC, Maranan MC, et al. Community-acquired methicillin-resistant Staphylococcus aureus in children with no identified predisposing risk. Jama 1998;279(8):593–8.

6. Kaplan SL, Hulten KG, Gonzalez BE, et al. Three-year surveillance of community-acquired Staphylococcus aureus infections in children. Clin Infect Dis 2005;40(12):1785–91.

7. Naimi TS, LeDell KH, Como-Sabetti K, et al. Comparison of community- and health care-associated methicillin-resistant Staphylococcus aureus infection. JAMA 2003;290(22):2976–84.

8. Edelsberg J, Taneja C, Zervos M, et al. Trends in US hospital admissions for skin and soft tissue infections. Emerg Infect Dis 2009;15(9):1516–8.

9. Hersh AL, Chambers HF, Maselli JH, et al. National trends in ambulatory visits and antibiotic prescribing for skin and soft-tissue infections. Arch Intern Med 2008;168(14):1585–91.

10. Fritz SA, Shapiro DJ, Hersh AL. National Trends in Incidence of Purulent Skin and Soft Tissue Infections in Patients Presenting to Ambulatory and Emergency Department Settings, 2000-2015. Clin Infect Dis 2020;70(12):2715–8.

11. Miller LG, Eisenberg DF, Liu H, et al. Incidence of skin and soft tissue infections in ambulatory and inpatient settings, 2005-2010. BMC Infect Dis 2015;15:362.

12. Sutter DE, Milburn E, Chukwuma U, et al. Changing Susceptibility of Staphylococcus aureus in a US Pediatric Population. Pediatrics 2016;137(4).

13. Orscheln RC, Hunstad DA, Fritz SA, et al. Contribution of genetically restricted, methicillin-susceptible strains to the ongoing epidemic of community-acquired Staphylococcus aureus infections. Clin Infect Dis 2009;49(4):536–42.

14. Cardenas-Comfort C, Kaplan SL, Vallejo JG, et al. Follow-up blood cultures in children with Staphylococcus aureus bacteremia. Pediatrics 2020;146(6).

15. Gerber JS, Coffin SE, Smathers SA, et al. Trends in the incidence of methicillin-resistant Staphylococcus aureus infection in children's hospitals in the United States. Clin Infect Dis 2009;49(1):65–71.

16. Hamdy RF, Dona D, Jacobs MB, et al. Risk Factors for complications in children with Staphylococcus aureus bacteremia. J Pediatr 2019;208:214–220 e2.

17. Spaulding AB, Watson D, Dreyfus J, et al. Epidemiology of bloodstream infections in hospitalized children in the United States, 2009-2016. Clin Infect Dis 2019;69(6):995–1002.

18. Iwamoto M, Mu Y, Lynfield R, et al. Trends in invasive methicillin-resistant Staphylococcus aureus infections. Pediatrics 2013;132(4):e817–24.

19. McMullan BJ, Bowen A, Blyth CC, et al. Epidemiology and mortality of Staphylococcus aureus bacteremia in Australian and New Zealand children. JAMA Pediatr 2016;170(10):979–86.

20. Kourtis AP, Hatfield K, Baggs J, et al. Vital signs: epidemiology and recent trends in methicillin-resistant and in methicillin-susceptible Staphylococcus aureus bloodstream infections - United States. MMWR Morb Mortal Wkly Rep 2019;68(9):214–9.

21. Fritz SA, Epplin EK, Garbutt J, et al. Skin infection in children colonized with community-associated methicillin-resistant Staphylococcus aureus. J Infect 2009;59(6):394–401.

22. Ellis MW, Hospenthal DR, Dooley DP, et al. Natural history of community-acquired methicillin-resistant *Staphylococcus aureus* colonization and infection in soldiers. Clin Infect Dis 2004;39(7):971–9.

23. Kluytmans J, van Belkum A, Verbrugh H. Nasal carriage of *Staphylococcus aureus*: epidemiology, underlying mechanisms, and associated risks. Clin Microbiol Rev 1997;10(3):505–20.

24. Creech CB 2nd, Kernodle DS, Alsentzer A, et al. Increasing rates of nasal carriage of methicillin-resistant *Staphylococcus aureus* in healthy children. Pediatr Infect Dis J 2005;24(7):617–21.

25. Fritz SA, Garbutt J, Elward A, et al. Prevalence of and risk factors for community-acquired methicillin-resistant and methicillin-sensitive *Staphylococcus aureus* colonization in children seen in a practice-based research network. Pediatrics 2008;121(6):1090–8.

26. McNeil JC, Fritz SA. Prevention strategies for recurrent community-associated *Staphylococcus aureus* skin and soft tissue infections. Curr Infect Dis Rep 2019;21(4):12.

27. Akinboyo IC, Zangwill KM, Berg WM, et al. SHEA neonatal intensive care unit (NICU) white paper series: Practical approaches to *Staphylococcus aureus* disease prevention. Infect Control Hosp Epidemiol 2020;41(11):1251–7.

28. Mergenhagen KA, Starr KE, Wattengel BA, et al. Determining the Utility of Methicillin-Resistant *Staphylococcus aureus* Nares Screening in Antimicrobial Stewardship. Clin Infect Dis 2020;71(5):1142–8.

29. McMullan BJ, Campbell AJ, Blyth CC, et al. Clinical Management of *Staphylococcus aureus* Bacteremia in Neonates, Children, and Adolescents. Pediatrics 2020;146(3).

30. Ligon J, Kaplan SL, Hulten KG, et al. *Staphylococcus aureus* bacteremia without a localizing source in pediatric patients. Pediatr Infect Dis J 2014;33(5):e132–4.

31. McNeil JC, Ligon JA, Hulten KG, et al. *Staphylococcus aureus* Infections in Children With Congenital Heart Disease. J Pediatr Infect Dis Soc 2013;2(4):337–44.

32. Tattevin P, Schwartz BS, Graber CJ, et al. Concurrent epidemics of skin and soft tissue infection and bloodstream infection due to community-associated methicillin-resistant *Staphylococcus aureus*. Clin Infect Dis 2012;55(6):781–8.

33. Hamdy RF, Hsu AJ, Stockmann C, et al. Epidemiology of Methicillin-Resistant *Staphylococcus aureus* Bacteremia in Children. Pediatrics 2017;139(6).

34. Liu C, Bayer A, Cosgrove SE, et al. Clinical practice guidelines by the infectious diseases society of america for the treatment of methicillin-resistant *Staphylococcus aureus* infections in adults and children. Clin Infect Dis 2011;52(3): e18–55.

35. Mermel LA, Allon M, Bouza E, et al. Clinical practice guidelines for the diagnosis and management of intravascular catheter-related infection: 2009 Update by the Infectious Diseases Society of America. Clin Infect Dis 2009;49(1):1–45.

36. Milstone AM, Elward A, Song X, et al. Daily chlorhexidine bathing to reduce bacteraemia in critically ill children: a multicentre, cluster-randomised, crossover trial. Lancet 2013;381(9872):1099–106.

37. Hsu AJ, Hamdy RF, Huang Y, et al. Association Between Vancomycin Trough Concentrations and Duration of Methicillin-Resistant *Staphylococcus aureus* Bacteremia in Children. J Pediatr Infect Dis Soc 2018;7(4):338–41.

38. Ten Oever J, Jansen JL, van der Vaart TW, et al. Development of quality indicators for the management of *Staphylococcus aureus* bacteraemia. J Antimicrob Chemother 2019;74(11):3344–51.

39. Duguid RC, Reesi MA, Bartlett AW, et al. Impact of Infectious Diseases Consultation on Management and Outcome of *Staphylococcus aureus* Bacteremia in Children. J Pediatr Infect Dis Soc 2021;10(5):569–75.

40. Tong SY, Davis JS, Eichenberger E, et al. *Staphylococcus aureus* infections: epidemiology, pathophysiology, clinical manifestations, and management. Clin Microbiol Rev 2015;28(3):603–61.

41. Fowler VG Jr, Miro JM, Hoen B, et al. *Staphylococcus aureus* endocarditis: a consequence of medical progress. JAMA 2005;293(24):3012–21.

42. Le Moing V, Alla F, Doco-Lecompte T, et al. *Staphylococcus aureus* Bloodstream Infection and Endocarditis–A Prospective Cohort Study. PLoS One 2015;10(5): e0127385.

43. Humpl T, McCrindle BW, Smallhorn JF. The relative roles of transthoracic compared with transesophageal echocardiography in children with suspected infective endocarditis. J Am Coll Cardiol 2003;41(11):2068–71.

44. Baltimore RS, Gewitz M, Baddour LM, et al. Infective Endocarditis in Childhood: 2015 Update: A Scientific Statement From the American Heart Association. Circulation 2015;132(15):1487–515.

45. Yi J, Wood JB, Creech CB, et al. Clinical Epidemiology and Outcomes of Pediatric Musculoskeletal Infections. J Pediatr 2021;234:236–244 e2.

46. Vij N, Ranade AS, Kang P, et al. Primary Bacterial Pyomyositis in Children: A Systematic Review. J Pediatr Orthop 2021;41(9):e849–54.

47. McNeil JC. Acute Hematogenous Osteomyelitis in Children: Clinical Presentation and Management. Infect Drug Resist 2020;13:4459–73.

48. Woods CR, Bradley JS, Chatterjee A, et al. Clinical Practice Guideline by the Pediatric Infectious Diseases Society and the Infectious Diseases Society of America: 2021 Guideline on Diagnosis and Management of Acute Hematogenous Osteomyelitis in Pediatrics. J Pediatr Infect Dis Soc 2021;10(8):801–44.

49. McNeil JC, Forbes AR, Vallejo JG, et al. Role of Operative or Interventional Radiology-Guided Cultures for Osteomyelitis. Pediatrics 2016;137(5).

50. Keren R, Shah SS, Srivastava R, et al. Comparative effectiveness of intravenous vs oral antibiotics for postdischarge treatment of acute osteomyelitis in children. JAMA Pediatr 2015;169(2):120–8.

51. McNeil JC, Vallejo JG, Kok EY, et al. Clinical and Microbiologic Variables Predictive of Orthopedic Complications Following *Staphylococcus aureus* Acute Hematogenous Osteoarticular Infections in Children. Clin Infect Dis 2019;69(11): 1955–61.

52. Gonzalez BE, Teruya J, Mahoney DH Jr, et al. Venous thrombosis associated with staphylococcal osteomyelitis in children. Pediatrics 2006;117(5):1673–9.

53. Alhinai Z, Elahi M, Park S, et al. Prediction of Adverse Outcomes in Pediatric Acute Hematogenous Osteomyelitis. Clin Infect Dis 2020;71(9):e454–64.

54. Copley LA, Kinsler MA, Gheen T, et al. The impact of evidence-based clinical practice guidelines applied by a multidisciplinary team for the care of children with osteomyelitis. J Bone Joint Surg Am 2013;95(8):686–93.

55. Self WH, Wunderink RG, Williams Dj, et al. *Staphylococcus aureus* Community-acquired Pneumonia: Prevalence, Clinical Characteristics, and Outcomes. Clin Infect Dis 2016;63(3):300–9.

56. Frush JM, Zhu Y, Edwards KM, et al. Prevalence of *Staphylococcus aureus* and Use of Antistaphylococcal Therapy in Children Hospitalized with Pneumonia. J Hosp Med 2018;13(12):848–52.

57. Carrillo-Marquez MA, Hulten KG, Hammerman W, et al. *Staphylococcus aureus* pneumonia in children in the era of community-acquired methicillin-resistance at Texas Children's Hospital. Pediatr Infect Dis J 2011;30(7):545–50.
58. Gillet Y, Issartel B, Vanhems P, et al. Association between *Staphylococcus aureus* strains carrying gene for Panton-Valentine leukocidin and highly lethal necrotising pneumonia in young immunocompetent patients. Lancet 2002; 359(9308):753–9.
59. Randolph AG, Vaughn F, Sullivan R, et al. Critically ill children during the 2009-2010 influenza pandemic in the United States. Pediatrics 2011;128(6):e1450–8.
60. Jain S, Williams DJ, Arnold SR, et al. Community-acquired pneumonia requiring hospitalization among U.S. children. N Engl J Med 2015;372(9):835–45.
61. Bradley JS, Byington CL, Shah SS, et al. The management of community-acquired pneumonia in infants and children older than 3 months of age: clinical practice guidelines by the Pediatric Infectious Diseases Society and the Infectious Diseases Society of America. Clin Infect Dis 2011;53(7):e25–76.
62. Liu C, Bayer A, Cosgrove SE, et al. Clinical practice guidelines by the infectious diseases society of america for the treatment of methicillin-resistant Staphylococcus aureus infections in adults and children: executive summary. Clin Infect Dis 2011;52(3):285–92.
63. Huang PY, Chen SF, Chang WN, et al. Spinal epidural abscess in adults caused by Staphylococcus aureus: clinical characteristics and prognostic factors. Clin Neurol Neurosurg 2012;114(6):572–6.
64. Shane AL, Hansen NI, Stoll BJ, et al. Methicillin-resistant and susceptible *Staphylococcus aureus* bacteremia and meningitis in preterm infants. Pediatrics 2012;129(4):e914–22.
65. Vallejo JG, Cain AN, Mason EO, et al. *Staphylococcus aureus* Central Nervous System Infections in Children. Pediatr Infect Dis J 2017;36(10):947–51.
66. Davis DP, Wold RM, Patel RJ, et al. The clinical presentation and impact of diagnostic delays on emergency department patients with spinal epidural abscess. J Emerg Med 2004;26(3):285–91.
67. Schoenbaum SC, Gardner P, Shillito J. Infections of cerebrospinal fluid shunts: epidemiology, clinical manifestations, and therapy. J Infect Dis 1975;131(5): 543–52.
68. Tunkel AR, Hasbun R, Bhimraj A, et al. 2017 Infectious Diseases Society of America's Clinical Practice Guidelines for Healthcare-Associated Ventriculitis and Meningitis. Clin Infect Dis 2017;64(6):e34–65.
69. Blassmann U, Hope W, Roehr AC, et al. CSF penetration of vancomycin in critical care patients with proven or suspected ventriculitis: a prospective observational study. J Antimicrob Chemother 2019;74(4):991–6.
70. Balouch MA, Bajwa RJ, Hassoun A. Successful use of ceftaroline for the treatment of MRSA meningitis secondary to an infectious complication of lumbar spine surgery. J Antimicrob Chemother 2015;70(2):624–5.
71. Corey A, So TY. Current Clinical Trials on the Use of Ceftaroline in the Pediatric Population. Clin Drug Investig 2017;37(7):625–34.
72. Daum RS, Miller LG, Immergluck L, et al. A Placebo-Controlled Trial of Antibiotics for Smaller Skin Abscesses. N Engl J Med 2017;376(26):2545–55.
73. Fritz SA, Hogan PG, Hayek G, et al. Household versus individual approaches to eradication of community-associated *Staphylococcus aureus* in children: a randomized trial. Clin Infect Dis 2012;54(6):743–51.
74. Fritz SA, Camins BC, Eisenstein KA, et al. Effectiveness of measures to eradicate *Staphylococcus aureus* carriage in patients with community-associated

skin and soft-tissue infections: a randomized trial. Infect Control Hosp Epidemiol 2011;32(9):872–80.

75. Kaplan SL, Forbes A, Hammerman WA, et al. Randomized trial of "bleach baths" plus routine hygienic measures vs. routine hygienic measures alone for prevention of recurrent infections. Clin Infect Dis 2014;58(5):679–82.

76. Bocchini CE, Mason EO, Hulten KG, et al. Recurrent community-associated *Staphylococcus aureus* infections in children presenting to Texas Children's Hospital in Houston, Texas. Pediatr Infect Dis J 2013;32(11):1189–93.

77. Creech CB, Al-Zubeidi DN, Fritz SA. Prevention of Recurrent Staphylococcal Skin Infections. Infect Dis Clin North Am 2015;29(3):429–64.

78. Hogan PG, Mork RL, Thompson RM, et al. Environmental Methicillin-resistant *Staphylococcus aureus* Contamination, Persistent Colonization, and Subsequent Skin and Soft Tissue Infection. JAMA Pediatr 2020;174(6):552–62.

79. Singer AJ, Talan DA. Management of skin abscesses in the era of methicillin-resistant *Staphylococcus aureus*. N Engl J Med 2014;370(11):1039–47.

80. Talan DA, Moran GJ, Krishnadasan A, et al. Subgroup Analysis of Antibiotic Treatment for Skin Abscesses. Ann Emerg Med 2018;71(1):21–30.

81. Talan DA, Mower WR, Krishnadasan A, et al. Trimethoprim-Sulfamethoxazole versus Placebo for Uncomplicated Skin Abscess. N Engl J Med 2016;374(9): 823–32.

82. Lake JG, Miller LG, Fritz SA. Antibiotic Duration, but Not Abscess Size, Impacts Clinical Cure of Limited Skin and Soft Tissue Infection After Incision and Drainage. Clin Infect Dis 2020;71(3):661–3.

83. Hogan PG, Rodriguez M, Spenner AM, et al. Impact of systemic antibiotics on *Staphylococcus aureus* colonization and recurrent skin infection. Clin Infect Dis 2017;66(2):191–7.

84. Parrish KL, Salwan NK, Thompson RM, et al. Skin and Soft Tissue Infection Treatment and Prevention Practices by Pediatric Infectious Diseases Providers. J Pediatr Infect Dis Soc 2020;9(6):760–5.

85. Holmes L, Ma C, Qiao H, et al. Trimethoprim-Sulfamethoxazole Therapy Reduces Failure and Recurrence in Methicillin-Resistant *Staphylococcus aureus* Skin Abscesses after Surgical Drainage. J Pediatr 2016;169:128–134 e1.

86. Fritz SA, Hogan PG, Hayek G, et al. *Staphylococcus aureus* colonization in children with community-associated Staphylococcus aureus skin infections and their household contacts. Arch Pediatr Adolesc Med 2012;166(6):551–7.

87. Mork RL, Hogan PG, Muenks CE, et al. Comprehensive modeling reveals proximity, seasonality, and hygiene practices as key determinants of MRSA colonization in exposed households. Pediatr Res 2018;84(5):668–76.

88. Mork RL, Hogan PG, Muenks CE, et al. Longitudinal, strain-specific *Staphylococcus aureus* introduction and transmission events in households of children with community-associated meticillin-resistant S aureus skin and soft tissue infection: a prospective cohort study. Lancet Infect Dis 2020;20:188–98.

89. Hogan PG, Mork RL, Boyle MG, et al. Interplay of personal, pet, and environmental colonization in households affected by community-associated methicillin-resistant *Staphylococcus aureus*. J Infect 2019;78(3):200–7.

90. Knox J, Uhlemann AC, Miller M, et al. Environmental contamination as a risk factor for intra-household *Staphylococcus aureus* transmission. PLoS ONE 2012; 7(11):e49900.

91. Price JR, Cole K, Bexley A, et al. Transmission of *Staphylococcus aureus* between health-care workers, the environment, and patients in an intensive care

unit: a longitudinal cohort study based on whole-genome sequencing. Lancet Infect Dis 2017;17(2):207–14.

92. Davis MF, Iverson SA, Baron P, et al. Household transmission of meticillin-resistant *Staphylococcus aureus* and other staphylococci. Lancet Infect Dis 2012; 12(9):703–16.

93. Davis MF, Misic AM, Morris DO, et al. Genome sequencing reveals strain dynamics of methicillin-resistant *Staphylococcus aureus* in the same household in the context of clinical disease in a person and a dog. Vet Microbiol 2015; 180(3–4):304–7.

94. Morris DO, Loeffler A, Davis MF, et al. Recommendations for approaches to meticillin-resistant staphylococcal infections of small animals: diagnosis, therapeutic considerations and preventative measures.: Clinical Consensus Guidelines of the World Association for Veterinary Dermatology. Vet Dermatol 2017;28(3): 304–e69.

95. Wertheim HF, Vos MC, Ott A, et al. Risk and outcome of nosocomial *Staphylococcus aureus* bacteraemia in nasal carriers versus non-carriers. Lancet 2004;364(9435):703–5.

96. Al-Zubeidi D, Burnham CD, Hogan PG, et al. Molecular epidemiology of recurrent cutaneous methicillin-resistant *Staphylococcus aureus* infections in children. J Pediatr Infect Dis Soc 2014;3(3):261–4.

97. Ellis MW, Schlett CD, Millar EV, et al. Hygiene strategies to prevent methicillin-resistant *Staphylococcus aureus* skin and soft tissue infections: a cluster-randomized controlled trial among high-risk military trainees. Clin Infect Dis 2014; 58(11):1540–8.

98. Popoola VO, Colantuoni E, Suwantarat N, et al. Active Surveillance Cultures and Decolonization to Reduce *Staphylococcus aureus* Infections in the Neonatal Intensive Care Unit. Infect Control Hosp Epidemiol 2016;37(4):381–7.

99. Kohler P, Sommerstein R, Schonrath F, et al. Effect of perioperative mupirocin and antiseptic body wash on infection rate and causative pathogens in patients undergoing cardiac surgery. Am J Infect Control 2015;43(7):e33–8.

100. Huang SS, Septimus E, Kleinman K, et al. Targeted versus universal decolonization to prevent ICU infection. N Engl J Med 2013;368(24):2255–65.

101. Huang JT, Abrams M, Tlougan B, et al. Treatment of *Staphylococcus aureus* colonization in atopic dermatitis decreases disease severity. Pediatrics 2009; 123(5):e808–14.

102. Hogan PG, Parrish KL, Mork RL, et al. HOME2: Household vs. Personalized Decolonization in Households of Children with Methicillin-Resistant *Staphylococcus aureus* Skin and Soft Tissue Infection - A Randomized Clinical Trial. Clin Infect Dis 2020;73(11):e4568–77. https://doi.org/10.1093/cid/ciaa752.

103. Schuetz CR, Hogan PG, Reich PJ, et al. Factors associated with progression to infection in methicillin-resistant *Staphylococcus aureus*-colonized, critically ill neonates. J Perinatol 2021;41(6):1285–92.

104. Pierce R, Lessler J, Popoola VO, et al. Meticillin-resistant *Staphylococcus aureus* (MRSA) acquisition risk in an endemic neonatal intensive care unit with an active surveillance culture and decolonization programme. J Hosp Infect 2017;95(1):91–7.

105. Wisgrill L, Zizka J, Unterasinger L, et al. Active Surveillance Cultures and Targeted Decolonization Are Associated with Reduced Methicillin-Susceptible *Staphylococcus aureus* Infections in VLBW Infants. Neonatology 2017;112(3): 267–73.

106. Akinboyo IC, Voskertchian A, Gorfu G, et al. Epidemiology and risk factors for recurrent *Staphylococcus aureus* colonization following active surveillance and decolonization in the NICU. Infect Control Hosp Epidemiol 2018;39(11): 1334–9.
107. Milstone AM, Voskertchian A, Koontz DW, et al. Effect of Treating Parents Colonized With *Staphylococcus aureus* on Transmission to Neonates in the Intensive Care Unit A Randomized Clinical Trial. Jama-Journal Am Med Assoc 2020; 323(4):319–28.
108. McNeil JC. *Staphylococcus aureus* - antimicrobial resistance and the immunocompromised child. Infect Drug Resist 2014;7:117–27.
109. McNeil JC, Hulten KG, Kaplan SL, et al. *Staphylococcus aureus* infections in pediatric oncology patients: high rates of antimicrobial resistance, antiseptic tolerance and complications. Pediatr Infect Dis J 2013;32(2):124–8.
110. McNeil JC, Munoz FM, Hulten KG, et al. *Staphylococcus aureus* infections among children receiving a solid organ transplant: clinical features, epidemiology, and antimicrobial susceptibility. Transpl Infect Dis 2015;17(1):39–47.
111. Zerr DM, Milstone AM, Dvorak CC, et al. Chlorhexidine gluconate bathing in children with cancer or those undergoing hematopoietic stem cell transplantation: A double-blinded randomized controlled trial from the Children's Oncology Group. Cancer 2020;127(1):56–66.
112. Fowler VG Jr, Das AF, Lipka-Diamond J, et al. Exebacase for patients with *Staphylococcus aureus* bloodstream infection and endocarditis. J Clin Invest 2020;130(7):3750–60.
113. Clegg J, Soldaini E, McLoughlin RM, et al. *Staphylococcus aureus* Vaccine Research and Development: The Past, Present and Future, Including Novel Therapeutic Strategies. Front Immunol 2021;12:705360.
114. Gluck U, Gebbers JO. Ingested probiotics reduce nasal colonization with pathogenic bacteria (*Staphylococcus aureus*, Streptococcus pneumoniae, and beta-hemolytic streptococci). Am J Clin Nutr 2003;77(2):517–20.
115. Nakatsuji T, Hata TR, Tong Y, et al. Development of a human skin commensal microbe for bacteriotherapy of atopic dermatitis and use in a phase 1 randomized clinical trial. Nat Med 2021;27(4):700–9.
116. Petrovic Fabijan A, Lin RCY, Ho J, et al. Safety of bacteriophage therapy in severe *Staphylococcus aureus* infection. Nat Microbiol 2020;5(3):465–72.

Implant-Associated Spinal Infections in Children

How Can We Improve Diagnosis and Management?

Jason Lake, MD, MPH[a],*, Oren Gordon, MD, PhD[b]

KEYWORDS

- Scoliosis • Spine surgery • Implant • Surgical site infection • Biofilm

KEY POINTS

- Implant-associated spinal infections (IASI) are a regularly encountered complication of pediatric instrumented spinal fixation.
- Biofilms play an important role in the pathophysiology of IASI.
- Virulent pathogens (eg, *Staphylococcus aureus*) tend to cause early infections (≤90 days from index surgery) compared with more indolent pathogens (eg, *Cutibacterium acnes*) that cause late infections (>90 days from index surgery).
- Early infections can be treated with debridement and implant retention, whereas late infections usually require implant removal.
- Advances in therapeutics, such as antibiofilm antibiotics, and imaging may improve IASI treatment outcomes in the future.

INTRODUCTION

Despite advances in implant materials, surgical techniques, and infection prevention practices, implant-associated spinal infection (IASI) remains a serious complication of pediatric instrumented spinal fixation, affecting 1% to 10% of surgeries.[1–3] IASI results in significant patient morbidity, multiple surgeries and hospitalizations, prolonged antibiotic exposure, and health care expenditure.[4]

The infection rate is lowest for adolescent idiopathic scoliosis (AIS), 0.5% to 3%, and highest for neuromuscular scoliosis (eg, cerebral palsy and myelomeningocele), averaging approximately 4% to 13% across underlying diagnoses.[1,3,5,6] Although

[a] Division of Infectious Diseases, Department of Pediatrics, University of Utah School of Medicine, 295 Chipeta Way, Salt Lake City, UT 84132, USA; [b] Division of Infectious Diseases, Department of Pediatrics, Johns Hopkins University School of Medicine, 200 N. Wolfe Street, Baltimore, MD 21287, USA
* Corresponding author.
E-mail address: jason.lake@hsc.utah.edu

Infect Dis Clin N Am 36 (2022) 101–123
https://doi.org/10.1016/j.idc.2021.11.005
0891-5520/22/© 2021 Elsevier Inc. All rights reserved.

infection risk correlates closely with underlying conditions, the preoperative, intraoperative, and postoperative phases each have unique factors that can affect IASI risk, and various prevention efforts have been implemented to mitigate their risk.[7–10]

IASI management depends on factors such as depth and extent of infection, time to onset from index procedure and microbiology.[7,11] Although infection confined to the soft tissue structures superficial to the fascia can be managed with local wound care and limited antibiotics, deeper (subfascial) infection warrants other considerations and will be the focus of this review. Emphasis will be given to early infections (≤90 days from index surgery) versus delayed infections (>90 days from index surgery), detailing best practices based on current knowledge. Controversial issues including early debridement with implant retention and optimal antibiotic duration will be discussed.[11–13] Finally, special attention is given to antibiofilm agents and pathogen-specific imaging, which hold promise to improve patient care.

PATHOPHYSIOLOGY AND MICROBIOLOGY
Microbiology of Early-Onset Versus Late-Onset Infections

Early postoperative IASI occurs ≤90 days after fusion surgery and is most frequently due to relatively virulent pathogens such as *Staphylococcus aureus* and aerobic gram-negative bacilli.[7] *S aureus* accounts for approximately half of infections (**Fig. 1**).[5,7,14] Gram-negative bacteria, mainly Enterobacterales (eg, *Escherichia coli, Proteus mirabilis, Klebsiella pneumonia)* and *Pseudomonas* spp, are found in about 40% of infections, occurring more commonly at the lumbosacral junction due to proximity to the perianal area and are more frequent in patients with neuromuscular conditions.[8,15] These infections may also involve other gut-derived bacteria such as enterococci and anaerobes. The latter may not grow as well in cultures (eg, *Bacteroides* spp and *Peptostreptococcus* spp).[16] Rare cases of candida infections have been reported.[15] Polymicrobial infections account for approximately 30% of early-onset infections (see **Fig. 1**).

Late-onset infections, occurring more than 90 days from surgery, account for 20% of all IASI.[5,17,18] These are more often caused by less virulent pathogens, such as *Cutibacterium acnes* (formerly *Propionibacterium acnes*) and coagulase-negative staphylococci.[7,19] *C acnes* is a slow-growing organism that requires extended incubation time. In one study, the median time to *C acnes* culture positivity was 6 days, whereas 1 day for all other organisms ($P < .001$).[20] Therefore, appropriate handling in the microbiology laboratory is essential to identify this pathogen. *Staphylococcus epidermidis* (coagulase-negative staphylococci) is associated with the use of spinal

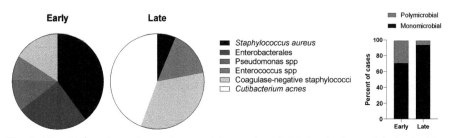

Fig. 1. Microbiology in early-onset versus late-onset pediatric implant-associated spinal infections. (*Data from* 14 studies describing early (N = 114),[1,15,16,18,110] late (N = 139),[15,20,95,103,111] or both early and late infection (N = 496).[5,17,49,112,113])

instrumentation and is recovered in about 30% of infections. Polymicrobial infection is rare in late-onset infections (6%) (see **Fig. 1**).

Antibiotic resistance should be considered with the emergence of antimicrobial-resistant pathogens, such as methicillin-resistant *S aureus* (MRSA), methicillin-resistant *S epidermidis* (MRSE), vancomycin-resistant enterococci, and resistant gram-negative bacteria.[14] Whenever possible, directed therapy should be given based on recovered bacteria and antibiotic susceptibility testing. If bacteria are not recovered, it is imperative that local epidemiology and resistance patterns guide empiric antibiotic therapy.

Biofilm Formation and Infection Persistence

Postsurgical spine infection usually occurs through direct bacterial entry during the surgical procedure. The most common source of this contamination is from the patient's endogenous skin flora. Other causes of infection include operating room personnel, hematogenous seeding, or early postoperative contamination.[14] Certain bacteria (eg, *S aureus*, *Pseudomonas aeruginosa*) can adhere to the surface of implants to form a biofilm. A biofilm is a microbial sessile community characterized by cells that are embedded in a matrix of extracellular polymeric substances that they produce. These cells exhibit an altered phenotype with regard to growth, gene expression, and protein production.[21] Biofilm-forming bacteria grow more slowly than in their planktonic form.[22]

In vitro laboratory investigations document that biofilms may develop within 5 to 6 hours after bacterial inoculation, and the age of the biofilm has major clinical implications related to its tenaciousness and antimicrobial susceptibility. This reduced susceptibility may be intrinsic (as a natural outcome of growth in the biofilm) or acquired (due to transfer of extrachromosomal elements to susceptible organisms in the biofilm).[23,24] The susceptibility of biofilms to antimicrobial agents cannot be determined using standard microdilution testing, as these tests rely upon the response of planktonic rather than biofilm organisms. Instead, susceptibility must be determined directly against biofilm-associated organisms, preferably under conditions that simulate conditions *in vivo*.[24,25] Most often, however, this is not attainable in the clinical microbiology laboratory.

Animal models simulating postsurgical spine infection provide an *in vivo* approach to study the pathophysiology and to evaluate preventative measures, diagnostic tools, and treatment strategies.[26] Recently, novel imaging techniques have demonstrated how biofilm-forming bacteria persist in infected animals and can be traced longitudinally for months using noninvasive bioluminescence imaging and PET.[27–29]

RISK FACTORS

Children and adults have different risk factors for postsurgical spinal infection (SI). For adults, diabetes, obesity, smoking, prior surgical site infection (SSI), longer operative times, posterior approach to spine, and the number of levels fused were all found to increase the risk for infection.[14,30] It has yet to be determined whether minimally invasive spine surgery (even with instrumentation) is associated with lower infection rates versus open surgery.[7]

In children, risk factors differ: In a systemic review of 57 studies, comorbid medical conditions, particularly cerebral palsy or myelodysplasia, urinary or bowel incontinence, and increased implant prominence increased the risk of infection.[8] This review found insufficient evidence for additional risk factors and therefore could make conclusions regarding malnutrition, obesity, number of levels fused, fusion extended to the sacrum/pelvis, blood loss, and use of allograft.[8] Urinary or bowel incontinence was associated with higher infection rates because of gastrointestinal tract flora.[16,31] Evidence regarding an association between UTI and postsurgical infection is conflicting and no convincing relationship has been proven in adults or children.[6,30]

The underlying condition leading to spine surgery is the single most important factor associated with the risk of postsurgical infection in children. This was exemplified in several retrospective studies that included 3588 children who underwent spine surgery and found that patients with neuromuscular etiologies had the highest cumulative incidence of infection (9.2%–14.3%).[1,5,15,32,33] This included cerebral palsy, spina bifida, muscle disease, spinal cord injuries, traumatic brain injuries, paralytic deformities, and chromosome anomalies, but myelomeningocele was associated with the highest risk of infection (17.9%). Even after successful implementation of an infection prevention program, infection rate for this high-risk group was 6.52% compared with 2.73% in other patient populations.[32] Within this high-risk population, the degree of cognitive impairment was found to be associated with infection.[11]

In contrast, patients with AIS had the lowest incidence of infection (0.5%-2.4%).[1,5,15,32] This is consistent with findings from the Scoliosis Research Society database, reporting a low infection rate in AIS, depending on the surgical approach: 0.17%, 1.35%, and 1.37%, for anterior, posterior, and combined instrumentation, respectively.[34]

PREVENTION

Close attention to infection prevention measures is necessary to reduce IASI risk, as failure to provide adequate presurgical and postsurgical mitigation measures has been associated with infection.[19,35,36] Prevention strategies often use a multidisciplinary approach with care bundles or pathways in the preoperative, intraoperative, and postoperative phases.[32,37,38] Standard SSI prevention practices should be observed in all perioperative phases. Recommendations for general SSI prevention practices (eg, bathing, glycemic control, normothermia, etc) are available elsewhere.[9,39] **Table 1** lists practices with particular application in IASI prevention.

CLINICAL MANIFESTATIONS AND DIAGNOSIS
Signs and Symptoms

A high index of suspicion for deep infection is necessary to make the diagnosis and ensure prompt treatment. For both early and delayed infections, clinical manifestations are variable, with fever, pain, and wound changes (eg, discharge and/or dehiscence) often reported.[1,40–42] For late infections, a sinus tract with localized drainage or an abscess may be contiguous with the fusion mass and implant.[13,42,43]

In some cases, infection may not be suspected at all.[44] In several series, when patients underwent surgery for pseudarthrosis (false union), adjacent segment disease, hardware failure, or other noninfectious processes, 38% to 45% of patients were found to be culture positive[45,46]; whether this represents clinically relevant infection or colonization is uncertain. Conversely, when patients have undergone debridement for IASI, pseudarthrosis has been identified in 5% to 62% of cases,[5,47,48] with number of levels fused and body mass index both predictive of pseudarthrosis.[48] Many factors (both infectious and otherwise) are associated with pseudarthrosis and so the relationship between pseudarthrosis and infection remains unclear.

For both early and late infections, laboratory parameters, such as elevated white blood cell (WBC) count, C-reactive protein (CRP), or erythrocyte sedimentation rate (ESR), may be suggestive of infection but are often normal.[1,42,45,49] CRP is a more

Table 1
Implant-associated spinal infection prevention practices

Intervention	Comments
Preoperative	
Staphylococcus aureus screening and decolonization[14,114–116]	Decreases IASI risk • Nasal culture/PCR screening followed by 2% mupirocin and 2% CHG decolonization may decrease SSI risk by 50% or more (R[114]) • Possibly greater effect for deep vs superficial SSI (R[114]) • Mupirocin alone may not decrease risk (R[115]) • May not decrease MSSA infection risk, only MRSA (M[116])
Showering or bathing with soap or antiseptic agent[9,117,118]	May decrease IASI risk • Accepted as standard SSI prevention practice (G[9]) • Evidence for preoperative CHG bathing may be inconclusive (S[118]) • Recommended for patients at high risk of IASI (G[117])
Urinary tract infection screening[3,6,117,119]	Unclear role in IASI prevention • 66% with IASI and UTI had same organism cultured (O[119]) • Urinalysis and urine culture recommended for patients at high risk of IASI (G[117])
Intraoperative	
Parenteral antimicrobial prophylaxis[9,35,39,117,120–123]	Decreases IASI risk • May decrease odds of IASI by up to 63% (M[120]) • First-generation cephalosporin (cefazolin) appropriate in most cases; clindamycin and vancomycin for β-lactam allergy (G[9,39]) • Clindamycin may increase IASI risk by up to 3.5-fold (O[36]) • Broader gram-negative coverage based on local surveillance data (G[39]) • Suboptimal delivery (eg, timing) is a risk-factor for IASI (O[35,121]) • Prolonged surgical antimicrobial prophylaxis (>24 h) is unnecessary even with subfascial drains in place (G,[9] R[122,123])
Skin antisepsis[9,124–127]	Decreases IASI risk • Alcohol-based solutions appear superior to aqueous solutions and are preferred if no contraindications exist (G,[9] S[126]) • CHG and iodophor alcohol-based products likely equivalent (G,[9] O,[127] R,[124,125] S[126])
Topical vancomycin[117,128–132]	May decrease IASI risk • Achieves high concentrations locally with limited systemic absorption (O[128])

(*continued on next page*)

Table 1 (continued)	
Intervention	**Comments**
	• May decrease IASI risk though randomized trials have failed to identify a difference (M,[129] R[130]) • Consider for high-risk patients (G[117]) • May affect epidemiology of infecting pathogens (S[131]) • Potential adverse events have been reported (S[132])
Antibacterial wound irrigation[9,133–135]	May decrease IASI risk • Antibacterial vs non-antibacterial wound irrigations may reduce SSI (S[135]) • Povidone-iodine irrigation may reduce deep IASI (R[133,134]) • Consider use unless contraindications exist (G[9])
Postoperative	
Negative pressure wound therapy[136,137]	May decrease IASI risk • May prevent seroma formation after spinal surgery and reduce SSI risk (M,[136] R[137])
Drains[8,10,19]	Unclear role in IASI prevention • Possible risk factor for late IASI when not used (O[19]) • Limited data do not suggest IASI reduction (S[8,10])

Abbreviations: Evidence type: G, professional or consensus guidelines; M, meta-analysis; N, narrative review; O, observational study; R, randomized controlled trial; S, systematic review.

reliable predictor of infection than ESR or WBC because of more predictable kinetics, and a normal value makes infection unlikely.[7,50,51] CRP trend is more important than a single value both in terms of suggesting infection and in monitoring response to treatment.[52] Given CRP plasma half-life of 19 hours, trending CRP every 3 days is reasonable for monitoring.[53] There is insufficient evidence to evaluate procalcitonin as a tool for diagnosing IASI. Blood cultures are variably positive with reports ranging from 7.7% to 40%, and possibly more likely with early infection.[1,40,42,54]

Imaging

The role of imaging in diagnosing IASI continues to evolve with advantages and disadvantages for each modality. Plain x-rays are often negative in the early course of infection, but pedicle screw or implant loosening, soft tissue swelling, hardware failure, and adjacent segment disease may indicate infection; however, these may also be due to noninfectious causes such as biomechanical stress.[49,55] Ultrasound can identify fluid collections but, similarly, cannot differentiate between infectious and noninfectious etiologies.[56] CT may demonstrate fluid collections and bony changes better than plain x-ray but is less sensitive than MRI.[7] MRI is typically superior to other modalities for detecting fluid collections, bone marrow edema, and soft tissue changes and enhancement.[57] For both contrast-enhanced CT and MRI, implant artifact impairs the ability to differentiate a sterile fluid collection (eg, seroma) from an abscess,[55] though techniques to reduce artifact exist.[58] For MRI, newer, nonferromagnetic implant materials, such as titanium, produce less artifact, though infection abutting hardware can be difficult to distinguish from seroma.[57]

Multiple radionuclide options, including scintigraphy with technetium-99m (^{99m}Tc)-labeled diphosphonate or gallium-67 citrate (^{67}Ga), labeled leukocyte imaging, and fluorine-18 fluorodeoxyglucose-positron emission tomography (^{18}F-FDG-PET), are being used clinically. Both ^{99m}Tc and ^{67}Ga scintigraphy are useful for osteomyelitis (spondylodiscitis) but have decreased specificity in the presence of implants.[59] ^{67}Ga has further practical limitations as multiple imaging sessions are required.[7] Labeled leukocyte imaging is of limited value for diagnosing SI because, for reasons that are poorly understood, at least 50% of the time there is decreased (photopenia) instead of increased uptake at sites of infection; this finding is not sufficiently specific to these infections to make it useful in diagnosis.[60] Modified versions are available but beyond the scope of this review.[59]

^{18}F-FDG-PET is not affected by metallic implant artifact and, compared with other radionuclide studies, has better spatial resolution, sensitivity, and specificity.[61] It can help define the anatomic site of infection and facilitate surgical planning,[62] which may be improved by combining with CT imaging (PET/CT).[63] MRI may be more sensitive for detecting small epidural abscesses, but ^{18}F-FDG-PET/CT appears to be more sensitive and specific for vertebral osteomyelitis.[63] One drawback of ^{18}F-FDG-PET is that implants can result in increased uptake in the first year of implantation,[61] which may make it more appropriate for detecting late infections. ^{18}F-FDG-PET can also be used over time with repeated measurements to evaluate response to treatment, and has already been applied clinically for pulmonary tuberculosis patients.[64] Potential applications of PET to clinical medicine continue to evolve with the development of novel tracers being evaluated for clinical use, including the use of radiolabeled antibiotic to evaluate pharmacokinetics and drug distribution (eg, bone penetration) as well as pathogen-specific tracers to visualize infection *in vivo*.[64,65]

Intraoperative Cultures and Histopathology

Imaging-guided or surgical sampling of tissue for culture and histopathology should be performed. Data from prosthetic joint infections (PJIs) suggest ≥3 specimens be obtained[66]; for PJI and IASI, some recommend 3 to 5 (up to 6) cultures be obtained.[51,67,68] To avoid isolation of skin colonizers, swabs and sinus tract cultures are discouraged.[68] To isolate the causative pathogens, deep cultures should be obtained.[68] When hardware is removed, vortexing and sonication improve culture sensitivity.[69] Cultures may need to be held for 14 days for more indolent pathogens such as C acnes.[68] When there is diagnostic uncertainty and/or if open biopsy is deferred, CT-guided biopsy is a well-tolerated method for identifying SI; however, yield can be variable.[70] Ultrasound-guided biopsy is another option if a fluid collection is present.[56] These invasive procedures are subject to sampling bias. Novel pathogen-specific PET tracers may in the future offer a noninvasive approach to identify the causative pathogen (eg, Enterobacterales) and monitor response to therapy.[71]

TREATMENT AND OUTCOMES
General Principles

IASI treatment requires a combined surgical and medical approach, based on the best available data and tailored to each patient. Though recent literature may support an early transition to oral antibiotics and an overall shorter duration than has historically been used, antibiotic selection, route, and duration will be patient-specific and pathogen-specific.[1,40,54,72–77] Suppressive antibiotics may be considered. Surgical management must also be modified for each patient, though this depends heavily on the time between index procedure and infection.[1,4,40,41,54,72]

Use of Biofilm-Active Antibiotics

Specific therapies for biofilm-related infection are scarce. In many settings, antibiotics (eg, beta-lactams) that target dividing, planktonic bacteria have been favored; however, as biofilms play an important role in IASI, some have suggested antibiofilm agents (eg, fluoroquinolones, rifamycins, oxazolidinones) may improve outcomes.[40,49] Fluoroquinolones can be used as monotherapy for gram-negative infections with good oral bioavailability and bone penetration.[49] Rifampin is the model antibiofilm agent as it has excellent bactericidal activity against susceptible gram-positive bacteria, including S aureus, and inhibits bacterial DNA-dependent RNA polymerase independently of bacterial division, resulting in activity against slowly dividing "dormant" organisms.[78] It is active within acidic environments as well as anaerobic conditions[79] and accumulates within neutrophils[80] and osteoblasts.[81] These properties render rifampin particularly attractive for use in biofilm-related infections. However, the high risk of emergence of resistant mutants requires the concomitant administration of another antibiotic.[78]

Adjuvant rifampin therapy seems promising; however prior studies done in vitro, in animal models, and in few human trials had conflicting results. This is probably due to differences in methodologies used in regard to antibiotic combination, dosing, type and extent of infections treated, and outcome measurements.[78] Rifampin, however, did enhance microbiological clearance when evaluated in clinical studies,[82–84] and in particular populations (eg, PJI), clinical cure was achieved in more than 80% of cases only when rifampin was added.[73,84,85] A small prospective double-blind, randomized control trial that examined the use of adjunctive rifampin for orthopedic implant-associated infection demonstrated cure without removal of the implant only when rifampin was used.[86] Thus, combination therapy with rifampin is currently recommended by the Infectious Diseases Society of America (IDSA) guidelines for the treatment of staphylococcal implant-associated infections.[67] Moreover, some experts recommend the adjunctive use of rifampin for the treatment of MRSA infection even without hardware, particularly for osteomyelitis, though studies evaluating this practice have yielded mixed results.[87]

Despite the extensive clinical use of rifampin, the optimal daily dose and dosage frequency are not well defined. Dosage recommendations for children were extrapolated from the adult dosage based on the assumption that the same dose per kg is appropriate across all ages. The limited pharmacokinetic information in children suggests that young children receiving adult-derived dosages have drug exposures significantly lower than adults.[88,89] In fact, children receiving recommended standard dosages of 10 mg/kg demonstrated very low serum rifampin concentrations, about half of adult levels.[90] Rifampin dosing in children with biofilm-associated S aureus infection, such as IASI, is currently recommended to be 10 to 20 mg/kg/d, given in 1 to 3 doses, with a maximum of 600 mg per dose and 900 mg/d.[67] Given the pharmacokinetic properties of rifampin in children and the probable lower risk of toxicity, the higher dose of at least 20 mg/kg/d would probably be preferred.

Antibiotic Selection

Empiric antibiotic selection will depend on infection timing (eg, early vs late) and the characteristic pathogens (see **Fig. 1**). For both early and late infections, a reasonable initial choice may be an extended-spectrum cephalosporin, such as cefepime, to cover skin flora (eg, gram-positive cocci, such as S aureus), aerobic enteric gram-negatives, including Enterobacterales, and health care–associated gram-negatives, such as *P aeruginosa*. Vancomycin for enterococci and/or resistant gram-positive cocci (eg, MRSA, MRSE) coverage and metronidazole to cover for obligate anaerobes are additional considerations. Modifications can be made based on Gram stain and/or early culture results. Local epidemiology and institutional antibiograms should be taken into consideration. Infectious disease consultation is recommended. Definitive antibiotic selection will depend upon final culture results.

Antibiotic Route

With limited data to support the practice, osteoarticular infections have historically been delivered entirely intravenously.[74–77] There is a growing body of evidence that after a short intravenous (IV) course, antibiotics can be transitioned to an oral/enteral route, assuming high bioavailability, adequate enteral absorption, and appropriate microbiologic susceptibility (**Table 2**). The appropriate time to transition to oral antibiotics is unclear; emerging IASI treatment outcomes suggest that initial IV courses ≤14 days and perhaps even shorter may be possible in most cases.[40,54,72,73] In particular, a recent pragmatic trial demonstrated that with infectious disease consultation, transition to oral antibiotics may be possible within several days of the start of antibiotic treatment for implant-associated infections.[73] It remains unknown whether, when oral antibiotics are an option, IV antibiotics are needed at all.[77]

Antibiotic Duration for IASI

The optimal antibiotic duration is uncertain and depends upon timing of infection onset, clinical course, and goals of treatment (ie, eradication vs suppression). Prolonged courses of treatment were standard of care in the past, but shorter courses of treatment were attempted to avoid adverse events associated with prolonged antibiotic use, including catheter-related complications.[75,76,91,92] More recently, several retrospective series and 2 prospective, noncomparative studies, reported successful treatment of early infection with 12, 8, or 6 weeks of antibiotics (see **Table 2**).[1,40,41,54,72,73] This is consistent with some data for other implant-associated infections[93]; however, in a recent open-label, randomized, controlled trial for PJI, 6 weeks of therapy failed to achieve noninferiority to 12 weeks of therapy, with respective failure rates of 9.4% and 18.1% within 2 years after treatment.[94] Careful evaluation of patient-specific and pathogen-specific considerations should be made, but prolonging therapy for at least 8 to 12 weeks may reduce the risk of treatment failure.

Even shorter durations may be possible for late infections after implant removal. Some authors have suggested that late-onset infections are due to infection of the hardware and surrounding soft tissues without osteomyelitis, even demonstrating hardware removal followed by short-course antibiotic therapy (days to weeks) to be sufficient.[12,95] In one series, patients were successfully treated with 2 days of IV followed by 7 days of PO antibiotics.[95] In another, 21 of 23 patients were cured with 2 to 5 days IV and 7 to 14 days PO (2 patients received IV only).[12] In a series of 23 delayed infections among AIS patients, after implant removal all patients were treated with 2 to 14 days of IV antibiotics followed by 1 to 9 weeks of PO antibiotics. Results were similar for shorter and longer durations.[12]

In our experience, when hardware is removed, by the time of hospital discharge most patients typically receive *1 to 2 weeks* of IV antibiotics from hardware removal. In the absence of a complicated course (eg, concomitant bacteremia, positive surgical cultures after hardware removal, etc), transition to oral antibiotics, when a suitable option exists, is reasonable at or before hospital discharge for an additional 2 to 4 weeks,

Table 2
Studies assessing medical and surgical management for early and late implant-associated spinal infections

Author (Year)	N	Time-To-Onset, Days	Primary Surgical Intervention	Antibiotic Duration	Notes
Early infections (≤90 d from index surgery to onset infectious symptoms)					
Bosch-Nicolau et al,[40] 2019	76	Median: 13.5	DAIR	2 wk IV followed by PO for 6 or 10 wk (8- or 12-wk total)	• At 1-y follow-up (n = 71), 81% (21/26) who received 8 wk vs 87% (39/45) who received 12 wk were infection-free at 1-y after antibiotic discontinuation (P = .51) • >70% received antibiofilm agent (fluoroquinolone, rifampin, linezolid)
Fernandez-Gerlinger[b] et al,[72] 2019	85	Median: 16	DAIR	10 d IV followed by PO (6-wk total)	• 87% (74) with instrumentation: 67 (86%) of those successfully treated had hardware vs 7 (100%) of treatment failures • 93% (79) switched from IV to PO antibiotics • Spinopelvic arthrodesis (OR: 15.3, 95% CI: 1.7–134.3), number of operated vertebrae (OR: 1.26 per vertebrae, 95% CI: 1.1–1.5), and infection with Enterobacterales and enterococci (OR: 16.3, 95% CI: 1.85–143.4) associated with treatment failure in univariate analysis; multivariate not performed due to lack of power

Study	N	Median	Treatment	Antibiotic Duration	Outcomes
Lamberet[a] et al,[1] 2018	26	Median: 13	DAIR	Median total: 19 wk (IQR: 12–26) Median time-to-PO: 17 wk (IQR: 8–39)	• 20% treated with a total of 6 wk • 17 (71%) received fluoroquinolone + rifampin • No treatment failures reported at ≥24 mo though 2 required second procedure and an additional 12 wk antibiotics
Glotzbecker[a] et al,[41] 2016	82	Median: 15 (IQR: 10–25)	DAIR or removal	6 wk total IV (IQR: 4–6)	• Median of 2 procedures (IQR: 1–3) were performed • 76% (62/82) treated successfully without recurrence at median of 33 mo follow-up • Stainless steel hardware (OR: 6.4, 95% CI: 1.70–32.1) and each additional year of age (OR: 1.26, 95% CI: 1.02–1.59) were associated with treatment failure in multivariate analysis
Dubee[b] et al,[54] 2012	50	Median: 11	DAIR	12 wk (2 wk IV + 10 wk PO)	• 96% (48) received oral antibiotics after initial 2-wk IV period • 94% (47) had 1 debridement only • 6% (3) patients experienced treatment failure by median follow-up of 43 mo
Late Infections (>90 d from index surgery to onset infectious symptoms)[d]					
Hedequist[b] et al,[4] 2008	26	Mean (mo): 14 (R: 4–62)	DAIR or removal	Antibiotic detail not provided	• All required hardware removal for successful infection eradication • Mean of 1.7 (R: 0–14) debridements before hardware removal • 6 required revision for curve progression without recurrent infection

(continued on next page)

Table 2
(continued)

Author (Year)	N	Time-To-Onset, Days	Primary Surgical Intervention	Antibiotic Duration	Notes
Ho[c] et al,[99] 2007	22	Mean: 663 (R: 814–1723)	DAIR or removal	Antibiotic detail not provided	• 41% (9) had implant removal at first debridement • Mean of 1.4 debridements (R: 1–2) before implant removal • Of 10 patients who had implant removal at first debridement (including one with onset ≤6 mo after index procedure), 20% (2) required a second debridement
Richards[a] and Emara,[12] 2001	23	Mean (mo): 27	Debridement and removal	IV: 2–14 d PO for 21/23: 1–9 wk	• All had implant removal • 61% (14) had primary closure, 9 (39%) had ≥2 stages before closure • All patients treated with IV antibiotics, 91% (21) with IV and PO antibiotics
Clark[a] and Shufflebarger,[95] 1999	22	Mean (y): 3.1	Debridement and removal	IV: 2 d PO: 7 d	• All had implant removal (inclusion criteria) with primary closure • 82% (18) had solid fusion without curve progression after implant removal; 18% (4) had pseudarthrosis, 2 of whom had revision with titanium implants

Early and Late Infections

Study	N	Time-to-onset	Treatment	Treatment Detail	Outcomes
Messina[a] et al,[92] 2014	23	Median: 16 (R: 8–1052)	DAIR or removal	Median total: 131 d (R: 42–597) Median IV: 45 d Median PO: 165 d	• 83% (19) with onset ≤58 d, 17% (4) with onset ≥168 d • 1 with implant removal at initial surgery • 82% (18 of 22) who underwent DAIR successfully treated without implant removal • Of patients who underwent DAIR, 18% (4) required implant removal for infection: 2 persistent, 2 with recurrence ≥2 y after initial treatment

Abbreviations: 95% CI, 95% confidence interval; DAIR, debridement and instrumentation retention; HR, hazard ratio; IQR, interquartile range; MSSA, methicillin-susceptible *Staphylococcus aureus*; MRSA, methicillin-resistant *Staphylococcus aureus*; NR, not reported; OR, odds ratio; R, range; SAT, suppressive antimicrobial therapy; SD, standard deviation.

Included studies defined early infection as ≤90 days from index surgery and late infection as more than 90 days and had sufficient data on treatment detail, with some exceptions as noted below.

[a] Pediatric only (one study[92] included patients up to 20 years of age).

[b] Fernandez-Gerlinger et al and Dubée et al were prospective studies. All remaining studies were retrospective.

[c] 53 patients included in the study with infections ≤6 months (n = 31) and more than 6 months (n = 22) defined as early and late, respectively. Of the late infections, all 22 occurred more than 90 days from index surgery. Time-to-onset was not reported so time-to-debridement was used.

[d] Time-to-onset in months or years as indicated in parenthesis.

with some preferring to treat for a typical osteomyelitis course of 4 to 6 weeks total duration (ie, IV and oral).

Debridement and Implant Retention Versus Removal

Generally, implant removal is recommended to treat implant-associated or device-associated infections when feasible.[67,96] For early IASI, when bony fusion is unlikely, hardware removal can lead to loss of correction, pseudarthrosis, and instability, requiring reoperation.[97,98] The advent of titanium prostheses, which are less susceptible to biofilm formation than steel and reduces the risk for treatment failure,[41] has likely contributed to the possibility of successful debridement and implant retention (DAIR).[98] For early infections with DAIR, treatment success rates are similar to hardware removal, 76% to 100%, even when ≤12 weeks of antibiotics are provided without suppressive antibiotic therapy (see **Table 2**).[1,40,41,54,72,98] DAIR combined with antibiotics has proven an effective strategy for early IASI.

DAIR has been less successful in late infections with most patients requiring hardware removal.[4] This may be due to the inability to adequately debride bacteria and biofilm from hardware and underlying tissues without hardware removal.[4,43,95] Delayed removal for late infections has been associated with need for multiple irrigation and debridement procedures and increased hospital days and health care costs when compared with removal at first surgery.[4,99] However, removal may not be possible for all patients with late IASI so attempted DAIR may be necessary. Moreover, progressive deformity may still occur in late infections with presumed solid fusion and may not be detected without long-term follow-up after hardware removal.[100,101] DAIR in late infection combined with biofilm-active antibiotics has demonstrated some success in small studies.[49,102]

Deformity Progression After Implant Removal

Implant removal has high morbidity and can lead to loss of correction (deformity progression),[103,104] and must be weighed against other clinical considerations. It is more common in pseudarthrosis but can occur with solid fusion mass (ie, development of a stable structure). Pseudarthrosis is more common with late infections.[104] In addition, pseudarthrosis is associated with infection, though it is unclear if pseudarthrosis increases infection risk or if infection results in pseudarthrosis due to impaired wound healing.[6,104] Deformity progression occurs with IASI with hardware *in situ* but worsens after implant removal.[5] Significant progression (≥10° in ≥1 plane) can occur after implant removal and faster rates of progression have been reported when removed in the first year.[5,99] In a study of 26 patients who underwent implant removal for late infection, 6 (23%) required revision surgery because of curve progression and 4 (15%) developed chronic pain.[4] Need for reoperation may take several years to become apparent.[4]

Intraoperative Pathogen-specific Imaging

Pathogen-specific imaging is being developed for future clinical use and may improve surgical management and treatment outcomes. Many pathogens express highly-specific antigens to which monoclonal (eg, immunodominant staphylococcal antigen A for S aureus)[105] or polyclonal (eg, outer membrane adhesin A for *Yersinia enterocolitica*)[106] pathogen-specific antibodies can be produced and conjugated with a fluorescent or radionuclide label.[106–109] Targeted fluorescent imaging or PET (for radionuclide labels) can then identify sites of infection noninvasively,[107,109] differentiate sterile inflammation from infection,[108] and guide surgical intervention, the latter of which has been demonstrated *in vivo* in staphylococcal implant infections.[107] These technologies may reduce reliance on gross intraoperative appearance, optimize irrigation and debridement, and potentially limit the number of procedures patients are subjected to.[107]

SUMMARY

IASIs are devastating surgical complications with significant impact on particular pediatric patient populations. Although 90 days is used to delineate early from late infections, most early infections occur in the first weeks after index surgery with late infections developing months to years later, likely reflecting unique aspects of their pathophysiology. Further refinement in our understanding of these infections would lead to improved prevention measures and treatment strategies. Implant removal may be necessary in many late infections but thorough debridement combined with biofilm-active antibiotics may increase the likelihood of treatment success when hardware is retained. Further prospective trials are needed to identify the best candidates for hardware preservation. Prolonged antibiotic therapy ($\geq$8 weeks) is usually necessary, but emerging data suggest that oral antibiotics can be the mainstay of therapy and the potential benefits of prolonged antibiotics should be balanced against the risk of adverse events. Emerging technologies, such as pathogen-specific imaging, may advance the field to provide rapid diagnosis, improved surgical outcomes, and valuable monitoring.

CLINICS CARE POINTS

- The mainstays of managemnt for early pediatric implant-associated spinal infection (IASI) are debridement and implant retention with prolonged antibiotic therapy.
- Late IASI typically requires hardware removal but shorter courses of antibiotics may be possible if hardware is removed.
- When a suitable agent is available, the majority of treatment can be completing using oral antibiotics.
- Novel diagnostic and therapeutic options are in development.

DISCLOSURE

The authors have nothing to disclose.

REFERENCES

1. Lamberet A, Violas P, Buffet-Bataillon S, et al. Postoperative spinal implant infections in children: risk factors, characteristics and outcome. Pediatr Infect Dis J 2018;37(6):511–3. https://doi.org/10.1097/INF.0000000000001812.
2. Maesani M, Doit C, Lorrot M, et al. Surgical site infections in pediatric spine surgery: comparative microbiology of patients with idiopathic and nonidiopathic etiologies of spine deformity. Pediatr Infect Dis J 2016;35(1):66–70. https://doi.org/10.1097/INF.0000000000000925.
3. Sponseller PD, Shah SA, Abel MF, et al. Infection rate after spine surgery in cerebral palsy is high and impairs results: multicenter analysis of risk factors and treatment. Clin Orthop Relat Res 2010;468(3):711–6. https://doi.org/10.1007/s11999-009-0933-4.

4. Hedequist D, Haugen A, Hresko T, et al. Failure of attempted implant retention in spinal deformity delayed surgical site infections. Spine 2009;34(1):60–4.

5. Cahill PJ, Warnick DE, Lee MJ, et al. Infection after spinal fusion for pediatric spinal deformity: thirty years of experience at a single institution. Spine 2010; 35(12):1211–7.

6. Master DL, Poe-Kochert C, Son-Hing J, et al. Wound infections after surgery for neuromuscular scoliosis: risk factors and treatment outcomes. Spine (Phila Pa 1976) 2011;36(3):E179–85. https://doi.org/10.1097/BRS.0b013e3181db7afe.

7. Kasliwal MK, Tan LA, Traynelis VC. Infection with spinal instrumentation: review of pathogenesis, diagnosis, prevention, and management. Surg Neurol Int 2013;4(Suppl 5):S392–403. https://doi.org/10.4103/2152-7806.120783.

8. Glotzbecker MP, Riedel MD, Vitale MG, et al. What's the evidence? Systematic literature review of risk factors and preventive strategies for surgical site infection following pediatric spine surgery. J Pediatr Orthop 2013;33(5):479–87.

9. Berrios-Torres SI, Umscheid CA, Bratzler DW, et al. Centers for disease control and prevention guideline for the prevention of surgical site infection, 2017. JAMA Surg 2017;152(8):784–91. https://doi.org/10.1001/jamasurg.2017.0904.

10. Tan T, Lee H, Huang MS, et al. Prophylactic postoperative measures to minimize surgical site infections in spine surgery: systematic review and evidence summary. Spine J 2020;20(3):435–47. https://doi.org/10.1016/j.spinee.2019.09.013.

11. Li Y, Glotzbecker M, Hedequist D. Surgical site infection after pediatric spinal deformity surgery. Curr Rev Musculoskelet Med 2012. https://doi.org/10.1007/s12178-012-9111-5.

12. Richards BS, Emara KM. Delayed infections after posterior TSRH spinal instrumentation for idiopathic scoliosis: revisited. Spine 2001;26(18):1990–5.

13. Di Silvestre M, Bakaloudis G, Lolli F, et al. Late-developing infection following posterior fusion for adolescent idiopathic scoliosis. Eur Spine J 2011;20(1):121–7.

14. Anderson PA, Savage JW, Vaccaro AR, et al. Prevention of surgical site infection in spine surgery. Neurosurgery 2017;80(3S):S114–23. https://doi.org/10.1093/neuros/nyw066.

15. Aleissa S, Parsons D, Grant J, et al. Deep wound infection following pediatric scoliosis surgery: incidence and analysis of risk factors. Can J Surg 2011; 54(4):263–9. https://doi.org/10.1503/cjs.008210.

16. Brook I, Frazier EH. Aerobic and anaerobic microbiology of wound infection following spinal fusion in children. Pediatr Neurosurg 2000;32(1):20–3.

17. Kim JI, Suh KT, Kim SJ, et al. Implant removal for the management of infection after instrumented spinal fusion. J Spinal Disord Tech 2010;23(4):258–65. https://doi.org/10.1097/BSD.0b013e3181a9452c.

18. Weinstein MA, McCabe JP, Cammisa FP Jr. Postoperative spinal wound infection: a review of 2,391 consecutive index procedures. J Spinal Disord 2000; 13(5):422–6. https://doi.org/10.1097/00002517-200010000-00009.

19. Ho C, Sucato DJ, Richards BS. Risk factors for the development of delayed infections following posterior spinal fusion and instrumentation in adolescent idiopathic scoliosis patients. Spine (Phila Pa 1976) 2007;32(20):2272–7. https://doi.org/10.1097/BRS.0b013e31814b1c0b.

20. Garg S, LaGreca J, Hotchkiss M, et al. Management of late (> 1 y) deep infection after spinal fusion: a retrospective cohort study. J Pediatr Orthop 2015; 35(3):266–70.

21. Bhattacharya M, Wozniak DJ, Stoodley P, et al. Prevention and treatment of Staphylococcus aureus biofilms. Expert Rev Anti Infect Ther 2015;13(12): 1499–516. https://doi.org/10.1586/14787210.2015.1100533.

22. Archer NK, Mazaitis MJ, Costerton JW, et al. Staphylococcus aureus biofilms: properties, regulation, and roles in human disease. Virulence 2011;2(5): 445–59. https://doi.org/10.4161/viru.2.5.17724.

23. Hall CW, Mah TF. Molecular mechanisms of biofilm-based antibiotic resistance and tolerance in pathogenic bacteria. FEMS Microbiol Rev 2017;41(3): 276–301. https://doi.org/10.1093/femsre/fux010.

24. Donlan RM. Biofilm formation: a clinically relevant microbiological process. Clin Infect Dis 2001;33(8):1387–92. https://doi.org/10.1086/322972.

25. Mandell JB, Orr S, Koch J, et al. Large variations in clinical antibiotic activity against Staphylococcus aureus biofilms of periprosthetic joint infection isolates. J Orthop Res 2019;37(7):1604–9. https://doi.org/10.1002/jor.24291.

26. Stavrakis AI, Loftin AH, Lord EL, et al. Current animal models of postoperative spine infection and potential future advances. Front Med (Lausanne) 2015;2: 34. https://doi.org/10.3389/fmed.2015.00034.

27. Gordon O, Miller RJ, Thompson JM, et al. Rabbit model of Staphylococcus aureus implant-associated spinal infection. Dis Model Mech 2020;13(7): dmm045385. https://doi.org/10.1242/dmm.045385.

28. Park HY, Zoller SD, Hegde V, et al. Comparison of two fluorescent probes in pre-clinical non-invasive imaging and image-guided debridement surgery of Staphylococcal biofilm implant infections. Sci Rep 2021;11(1):1622. https://doi.org/10.1038/s41598-020-78362-7.

29. Zoller SD, Park HY, Olafsen T, et al. Multimodal imaging guides surgical management in a preclinical spinal implant infection model. JCI Insight 2019;4(3): e124813. https://doi.org/10.1172/jci.insight.124813.

30. Galetta MS, Kepler CK, Divi SN, et al. Consensus on Risk Factors and Prevention in SSI in Spine Surgery. Clin Spine Surg 2020;33(5):E213–25. https://doi.org/10.1097/BSD.0000000000000867.

31. Olsen MA, Nepple JJ, Riew KD, et al. Risk factors for surgical site infection following orthopaedic spinal operations. J Bone Joint Surg Am 2008;90(1): 62–9. https://doi.org/10.2106/JBJS.F.01515.

32. Ballard MR, Miller NH, Nyquist A-C, et al. A multidisciplinary approach improves infection rates in pediatric spine surgery. J Pediatr Orthop 2012;32(3):266–70.

33. Mackenzie WG, Matsumoto H, Williams BA, et al. Surgical site infection following spinal instrumentation for scoliosis: a multicenter analysis of rates, risk factors, and pathogens. J Bone Joint Surg Am 2013;95(9):800–6. https://doi.org/10.2106/JBJS.L.00010. S1–S806.

34. Coe JD, Arlet V, Donaldson W, et al. Complications in spinal fusion for adolescent idiopathic scoliosis in the new millennium. A report of the Scoliosis Research Society Morbidity and Mortality Committee. Spine (Phila Pa 1976) 2006;31(3):345–9. https://doi.org/10.1097/01.brs.0000197188.76369.13.

35. Labbe A-C, Demers A-M, Rodrigues R, et al. Surgical-site infection following spinal fusion: a case-control study in a children's hospital. Infect Control Hosp Epidemiol 2003;24(8):591–5.

36. Linam WM, Margolis PA, Staat MA, et al. Risk factors associated with surgical site infection after pediatric posterior spinal fusion procedure. Infect Control Hosp Epidemiol 2009;30(2):109–16. https://doi.org/10.1086/593952.

37. Mackenzie WGS, McLeod L, Wang K, et al. Team approach: preventing surgical site infections in pediatric scoliosis surgery. JBJS Rev 2018;6(2):e2. https://doi.org/10.2106/JBJS.RVW.16.00121.

38. Ryan SL, Sen A, Staggers K, et al, Texas Children's Hospital Spine Study G. A standardized protocol to reduce pediatric spine surgery infection: a quality improvement initiative. J Neurosurg Pediatr 2014;14(3):259–65. https://doi.org/10.3171/2014.5.PEDS1448.

39. Bratzler DW, Dellinger EP, Olsen KM, et al. Clinical practice guidelines for antimicrobial prophylaxis in surgery. Surg Infect (Larchmt) 2013;14(1):73–156. https://doi.org/10.1089/sur.2013.9999.

40. Bosch-Nicolau P, Rodriguez-Pardo D, Pigrau C, et al. Acute spinal implant infection treated with debridement: does extended antibiotic treatment improve the prognosis? Eur J Clin Microbiol Infect Dis 2019;38(5):951–8. https://doi.org/10.1007/s10096-019-03537-8.

41. Glotzbecker MP, Gomez JA, Miller PE, et al. Management of spinal implants in acute pediatric surgical site infections: a multicenter study. Spine Deform 2016; 4(4):277–82. https://doi.org/10.1016/j.jspd.2016.02.001.

42. Kowalski TJ, Berbari EF, Huddleston PM, et al. The management and outcome of spinal implant infections: contemporary retrospective cohort study. Clin Infect Dis 2007;44(7):913–20.

43. Bose B. Delayed infection after instrumented spine surgery: case reports and review of the literature. Spine J 2003;3(5):394–9.

44. Hu X, Lieberman IH. Revision spine surgery in patients without clinical signs of infection: how often are there occult infections in removed hardware? Eur Spine J 2018;27(10):2491–5.

45. Callanan TC, Abjornson C, DiCarlo E, et al. Prevalence of occult infections in posterior instrumented spinal fusion. Clin Spine Surg 2020;34(1):25–31.

46. Pumberger M, Bürger J, Strube P, et al. Unexpected positive cultures in presumed aseptic revision spine surgery using sonication. Bone Joint J 2019; 101(5):621–4.

47. Burkhard MD, Loretz R, Uçkay I, et al. Occult infection in pseudarthrosis revision after spinal fusion. Spine J 2021;21(3):370–6.

48. Hollern DA, Woods BI, Shah NV, et al. Risk factors for pseudarthrosis after surgical site infection of the spine. Int J Spine Surg 2019;13(6):507–14.

49. Koder K, Hardt S, Gellert MS, et al. Outcome of spinal implant-associated infections treated with or without biofilm-active antibiotics: results from a 10-year cohort study. Infection 2020;48(4):559–68. https://doi.org/10.1007/s15010-020-01435-2.

50. Mok JM, Pekmezci M, Piper SL, et al. Use of C-reactive protein after spinal surgery: comparison with erythrocyte sedimentation rate as predictor of early postoperative infectious complications. Spine 2008;33(4):415–21. https://doi.org/10.1097/BRS.0b013e318163f9ee.

51. Divi SN, Kepler CK, Segar AH, et al. Role of imaging, tissue sampling, and biomarkers for diagnosis of SSI in spine surgery. Clin Spine Surg 2020;33(5): E199–205.

52. Kang B-U, Lee S-H, Ahn Y, et al. Surgical site infection in spinal surgery: detection and management based on serial C-reactive protein measurements. J Neurosurg Spine 2010;13(2):158–64.

53. Pepys MB, Hirschfield GM. C-reactive protein: a critical update. J Clin Invest 2003;111(12):1805–12. https://doi.org/10.1172/JCI18921.

54. Dubee V, Lenoir T, Leflon-Guibout V, et al. Three-month antibiotic therapy for early-onset postoperative spinal implant infections. Clin Infect Dis 2012; 55(11):1481–7. https://doi.org/10.1093/cid/cis769.

55. Beiner JM, Grauer J, Kwon BK, et al. Postoperative wound infections of the spine. Neurosurg Focus 2003;15(3):1–5.

56. Korge A, Fischer R, Kluger P, et al. The importance of sonography in the diagnosis of septic complications following spinal surgery. Eur Spine J 1994;3(6): 303–7.

57. Mazzie JP, Brooks MK, Gnerre J. Imaging and management of postoperative spine infection. Neuroimaging Clin 2014;24(2):365–74.

58. Stradiotti P, Curti A, Castellazzi G, et al. Metal-related artifacts in instrumented spine. Techniques for reducing artifacts in CT and MRI: state of the art. Eur Spine J 2009;18(1):102–8. https://doi.org/10.1007/s00586-009-0998-5.

59. Palestro CJ. Radionuclide imaging of musculoskeletal infection: a review. J Nucl Med 2016;57(9):1406–12.

60. Gemmel F, Dumarey N, Palestro CJ. Radionuclide imaging of spinal infections. Eur J Nucl Med Mol Imaging 2006;33(10):1226–37.

61. Palestro, C.J., Radionuclide imaging of osteomyelitis. Semin Nucl Med, 45 (1), 2015, 32-46.

62. Ngcelwane, M., Kruger, T. and Bomela, L., Positron emission tomography in the diagnosis of spine infection and infected implants, Orthop Proc, 95 (Supp 14), 2013, 76.

63. Nakahara M, Ito M, Hattori N, et al. 18F-FDG-PET/CT better localizes active spinal infection than MRI for successful minimally invasive surgery. Acta Radiol 2015;56(7):829–36.

64. Gordon O, Ruiz-Bedoya CA, Ordonez AA, et al. Molecular imaging: a novel tool to visualize pathogenesis of infections In Situ</em> mBio 2019;10(5): e00317–9. https://doi.org/10.1128/mBio.00317-19.

65. Ordonez AA, Wang H, Magombedze G, et al. Dynamic imaging in patients with tuberculosis reveals heterogeneous drug exposures in pulmonary lesions. Nat Med 2020;26(4):529–34. https://doi.org/10.1038/s41591-020-0770-2.

66. Atkins BL, Athanasou N, Deeks JJ, et al. Prospective evaluation of criteria for microbiological diagnosis of prosthetic-joint infection at revision arthroplasty. J Clin Microbiol 1998;36(10):2932–9.

67. Osmon DR, Berbari EF, Berendt AR, et al. Diagnosis and management of prosthetic joint infection: clinical practice guidelines by the Infectious Diseases Society of America. Clin Infect Dis 2013;56(1):e1–25.

68. Miller JM, Binnicker MJ, Campbell S, et al. A guide to utilization of the microbiology laboratory for diagnosis of infectious diseases: 2018 update by the Infectious Diseases Society of America and the American Society for Microbiology. Clin Infect Dis 2018;67(6):e1–94.

69. Sampedro MF, Huddleston PM, Piper KE, et al. A biofilm approach to detect bacteria on removed spinal implants. Spine (Phila Pa 1976) 2010;35(12): 1218–24. https://doi.org/10.1097/BRS.0b013e3181c3b2f3.

70. McNamara AL, Dickerson EC, Gomez-Hassan DM, et al. Yield of image-guided needle biopsy for infectious discitis: a systematic review and meta-analysis. Am J Neuroradiol 2017;38(10):2021–7. https://doi.org/10.3174/ajnr.A5337.

71. Ordonez AA, Wintaco LM, Mota F, et al. Imaging Enterobacterales infections in patients using pathogen-specific positron emission tomography. Sci Transl Med 2021;13(589):eabe9805. https://doi.org/10.1126/scitranslmed.abe9805.

72. Fernandez-Gerlinger MP, Arvieu R, Lebeaux D, et al. Successful 6-week anti-biotic treatment for early surgical-site infections in spinal surgery. Clin Infect Dis 2019;68(11):1856–61. https://doi.org/10.1093/cid/ciy805.

73. Li H-K, Rombach I, Zambellas R, et al. Oral versus intravenous antibiotics for bone and joint infection. N Engl J Med 2019;380(5):425–36.

74. Spellberg B, Lipsky BA. Systemic antibiotic therapy for chronic osteomyelitis in adults. Clin Infect Dis 2012;54(3):393–407.

75. Zaoutis T, Localio AR, Leckerman K, et al. Prolonged intravenous therapy versus early transition to oral antimicrobial therapy for acute osteomyelitis in children. Pediatrics 2009;123(2):636–42. https://doi.org/10.1542/peds.2008-0596.

76. Keren R, Shah SS, Srivastava R, et al. Comparative effectiveness of intravenous vs oral antibiotics for postdischarge treatment of acute osteomyelitis in children. JAMA Pediatr 2015;169(2):120–8. https://doi.org/10.1001/jamapediatrics.2014.2822.

77. Li HK, Agweyu A, English M, et al. An unsupported preference for intravenous antibiotics. PLoS Med 2015;12(5):e1001825.

78. Perlroth J, Kuo M, Tan J, et al. Adjunctive use of rifampin for the treatment of Staphylococcus aureus infections: a systematic review of the literature. Arch Intern Med 2008;168(8):805–19. https://doi.org/10.1001/archinte.168.8.805.

79. Norden CW, Shaffer M. Treatment of experimental chronic osteomyelitis due to staphylococcus aureus with vancomycin and rifampin. J Infect Dis 1983;147(2):352–7. https://doi.org/10.1093/infdis/147.2.352.

80. Mandell GL. The antimicrobial activity of rifampin: emphasis on the relation to phagocytes. Rev Infect Dis 1983;5(Suppl 3):S463–7. https://doi.org/10.1093/clinids/5.supplement_3.s463.

81. Valour F, Trouillet-Assant S, Riffard N, et al. Antimicrobial activity against intraos-teoblastic Staphylococcus aureus. Antimicrob Agents Chemother 2015;59(4):2029–36. https://doi.org/10.1128/AAC.04359-14.

82. Van der Auwera P, Meunier-Carpentier F, Klastersky J. Clinical study of combi-nation therapy with oxacillin and rifampin for staphylococcal infections. Rev Infect Dis 1983;5(Suppl 3):S515–22. https://doi.org/10.1093/clinids/5.supplement_3.s515.

83. Van der Auwera P, Klastersky J, Thys JP, et al. Double-blind, placebo-controlled study of oxacillin combined with rifampin in the treatment of staphylococcal in-fections. Antimicrob Agents Chemother 1985;28(4):467–72. https://doi.org/10.1128/aac.28.4.467.

84. Euba G, Murillo O, Fernandez-Sabe N, et al. Long-term follow-up trial of oral rifampin-cotrimoxazole combination versus intravenous cloxacillin in treatment of chronic staphylococcal osteomyelitis. Antimicrob Agents Chemother 2009;53(6):2672–6. https://doi.org/10.1128/AAC.01504-08.

85. Karlsen OE, Borgen P, Bragnes B, et al. Rifampin combination therapy in staph-ylococcal prosthetic joint infections: a randomized controlled trial. J Orthop Surg Res 2020;15(1):365. https://doi.org/10.1186/s13018-020-01877-2.

86. Zimmerli W, Widmer AF, Blatter M, et al. Role of rifampin for treatment of ortho-pedic implant-related staphylococcal infections: a randomized controlled trial. Foreign-Body Infection (FBI) Study Group. JAMA 1998;279(19):1537–41. https://doi.org/10.1001/jama.279.19.1537.

87. Liu C, Bayer A, Cosgrove SE, et al. Clinical practice guidelines by the infectious diseases society of america for the treatment of methicillin-resistant Staphylo-coccus aureus infections in adults and children: executive summary. Clin Infect Dis 2011;52(3):285–92. https://doi.org/10.1093/cid/cir034.

88. Diacon AH, Patientia RF, Venter A, et al. Early bactericidal activity of high-dose rifampin in patients with pulmonary tuberculosis evidenced by positive sputum smears. Antimicrob Agents Chemother 2007;51(8):2994–6. https://doi.org/10.1128/AAC.01474-06.

89. Donald PR, Maritz JS, Diacon AH. The pharmacokinetics and pharmacodynamics of rifampicin in adults and children in relation to the dosage recommended for children. Tuberculosis (Edinb) 2011;91(3):196–207. https://doi.org/10.1016/j.tube.2011.02.004.

90. Schaaf HS, Willemse M, Cilliers K, et al. Rifampin pharmacokinetics in children, with and without human immunodeficiency virus infection, hospitalized for the management of severe forms of tuberculosis. BMC Med 2009;7:19. https://doi.org/10.1186/1741-7015-7-19.

91. Billieres J, Uckay I, Faundez A, et al. Variables associated with remission in spinal surgical site infections. J Spine Surg 2016;2(2):128–34. https://doi.org/10.21037/jss.2016.06.06.

92. Messina AF, Berman DM, Ghazarian SR, et al. The management and outcome of spinal implant-related infections in pediatric patients: a retrospective review. Pediatr Infect Dis J 2014;33(7):720–3. https://doi.org/10.1097/INF.0000000000000264.

93. Yen HT, Hsieh RW, Huang CY, et al. Short-course versus long-course antibiotics in prosthetic joint infections: a systematic review and meta-analysis of one randomized controlled trial plus nine observational studies. J Antimicrob Chemother 2019;74(9):2507–16. https://doi.org/10.1093/jac/dkz166.

94. Bernard L, Arvieux C, Brunschweiler B, et al. Antibiotic therapy for 6 or 12 weeks for prosthetic joint infection. N Engl J Med 2021;384(21):1991–2001. https://doi.org/10.1056/NEJMoa2020198.

95. Clark CE, Shufflebarger HL. Late-developing infection in instrumented idiopathic scoliosis. Spine 1999;24(18):1909.

96. Tunkel AR, Hasbun R, Bhimraj A, et al. 2017 Infectious diseases society of america's clinical practice guidelines for healthcare-associated ventriculitis and meningitis. Clin Infect Dis 2017;64(6):e34–65. https://doi.org/10.1093/cid/ciw861.

97. Tominaga H, Setoguchi T, Kawamura H, et al. Risk factors for unavoidable removal of instrumentation after surgical site infection of spine surgery: A retrospective case-control study. Medicine (Baltimore) 2016;95(43):e5118. https://doi.org/10.1097/MD.0000000000005118.

98. Ahmed R, Greenlee JD, Traynelis VC. Preservation of spinal instrumentation after development of postoperative bacterial infections in patients undergoing spinal arthrodesis. Clin Spine Surg 2012;25(6):299–302.

99. Ho C, Skaggs DL, Weiss JM, et al. Management of infection after instrumented posterior spine fusion in pediatric scoliosis. Spine 2007;32(24):2739–44.

100. Farshad M, Sdzuy C, Min K. Late implant removal after posterior correction of AIS with pedicle screw instrumentation—a matched case control study with 10-year follow-up. Spine Deform 2013;1(1):68–71.

101. Potter BK, Kirk KL, Shah SA, et al. Loss of coronal correction following instrumentation removal in adolescent idiopathic scoliosis. Spine 2006;31(1):67–72.

102. Kuehl R, Tschudin-Sutter S, Morgenstern M, et al. Time-dependent differences in management and microbiology of orthopaedic internal fixation-associated infections: an observational prospective study with 229 patients. Clin Microbiol Infect 2019;25(1):76–81. https://doi.org/10.1016/j.cmi.2018.03.040.

103. Muschik M, Luck W, Schlenzka D. Implant removal for late-developing infection after instrumented posterior spinal fusion for scoliosis: reinstrumentation

reduces loss of correction. A retrospective analysis of 45 cases. Eur Spine J 2004;13(7):645–51. https://doi.org/10.1007/s00586-004-0694-4.

104. Khoshbin A, Lysenko M, Law P, et al. Outcomes of infection following pediatric spinal fusion. Can J Surg 2015;58(2):107–13. https://doi.org/10.1503/cjs. 006014.

105. van den Berg S, Bonarius HP, van Kessel KP, et al. A human monoclonal antibody targeting the conserved staphylococcal antigen IsaA protects mice against Staphylococcus aureus bacteremia. Int J Med Microbiol 2015;305(1): 55–64.

106. Wiehr S, Warnke P, Rolle A-M, et al. New pathogen-specific immunoPET/MR tracer for molecular imaging of a systemic bacterial infection. Oncotarget 2016;7(10):10990.

107. Park HY, Zoller SD, Hegde V, et al. Comparison of two fluorescent probes in pre-clinical non-invasive imaging and image-guided debridement surgery of Staphylococcal biofilm implant infections. Sci Rep 2021;11(1):1–13.

108. Pickett JE, Thompson JM, Sadowska A, et al. Molecularly specific detection of bacterial lipoteichoic acid for diagnosis of prosthetic joint infection of the bone. Bone Res 2018;6(1):1–8.

109. Romero Pastrana F, Thompson JM, Heuker M, et al. Noninvasive optical and nuclear imaging of Staphylococcus-specific infection with a human monoclonal antibody-based probe. Virulence 2018;9(1):262–72.

110. Levi AD, Dickman CA, Sonntag VK. Management of postoperative infections after spinal instrumentation. J Neurosurg 1997;86(6):975–80. https://doi.org/10. 3171/jns.1997.86.6.0975.

111. Richards BR, Emara KM. Delayed infections after posterior TSRH spinal instrumentation for idiopathic scoliosis: revisited. Spine (Phila Pa 1976) 2001;26(18): 1990–6. https://doi.org/10.1097/00007632-200109150-00009.

112. Fang A, Hu SS, Endres N, et al. Risk factors for infection after spinal surgery. Spine (Phila Pa 1976) 2005;30(12):1460–5. https://doi.org/10.1097/01.brs. 0000166532.58227.4f.

113. Farley FA, Li Y, Gilsdorf JR, et al. Postoperative spine and VEPTR infections in children: a case-control study. J Pediatr Orthop 2014;34(1):14–21.

114. Bode LG, Kluytmans JA, Wertheim HF, et al. Preventing surgical-site infections in nasal carriers of Staphylococcus aureus. N Engl J Med 2010;362(1):9–17.

115. Kalmeijer M, Coertjens H, van Nieuwland-Bollen P, et al. Surgical site infections in orthopedic surgery: the effect of mupirocin nasal ointment in a double-blind, randomized, placebo-controlled study. Clin Infect Dis 2002;35(4):353–8.

116. Ning J, Wang J, Zhang S, et al. Nasal colonization of Staphylococcus aureus and the risk of surgical site infection after spine surgery: a meta-analysis. Spine J 2020;20(3):448–56. https://doi.org/10.1016/j.spinee.2019.10.009.

117. Vitale MG, Riedel MD, Glotzbecker MP, et al. Building consensus: development of a Best Practice Guideline (BPG) for surgical site infection (SSI) prevention in high-risk pediatric spine surgery. J Pediatr Orthop 2013;33(5):471–8.

118. Webster J, Osborne S. Preoperative bathing or showering with skin antiseptics to prevent surgical site infection. Cochrane Database Syst Rev 2015;(2):CD004985.

119. Hatlen T, Song K, Shurtleff D, et al. Contributory factors to postoperative spinal fusion complications for children with myelomeningocele. Spine (Phila Pa 1976) 2010;35(13):1294–9. https://doi.org/10.1097/BRS.0b013e3181bf8efe.

120. Barker FG. Efficacy of prophylactic antibiotic therapy in spinal surgery: a meta-analysis. Neurosurgery 2002;51(2):391–401.

121. Milstone AM, Maragakis LL, Townsend T, et al. Timing of preoperative antibiotic prophylaxis: a modifiable risk factor for deep surgical site infections after pediatric spinal fusion. Pediatr Infect Dis J 2008;27(8):704–8. https://doi.org/10.1097/INF.0b013e31816fca72.

122. Urquhart JC, Collings D, Nutt L, et al. The effect of prolonged postoperative antibiotic administration on the rate of infection in patients undergoing posterior spinal surgery requiring a closed-suction drain: a randomized controlled trial. J Bone Joint Surg Am 2019;101(19):1732–40. https://doi.org/10.2106/JBJS.19.00009.

123. Takemoto RC, Lonner B, Andres T, et al. Appropriateness of twenty-four-hour antibiotic prophylaxis after spinal surgery in which a drain is utilized: a prospective randomized study. J Bone Joint Surg Am 2015;97(12):979–86.

124. Savage JW, Weatherford BM, Sugrue PA, et al. Efficacy of surgical preparation solutions in lumbar spine surgery. J Bone Joint Surg Am 2012;94(6):490–4.

125. Darouiche RO, Wall MJ Jr, Itani KM, et al. Chlorhexidine–alcohol versus povidone–iodine for surgical-site antisepsis. N Engl J Med 2010;362(1):18–26.

126. Sidhwa F, Itani KM. Skin preparation before surgery: options and evidence. Surg Infect 2015;16(1):14–23.

127. Swenson BR, Hedrick TL, Metzger R, et al. Effects of preoperative skin preparation on postoperative wound infection rates: a prospective study of 3 skin preparation protocols. Infect Control Hosp Epidemiol 2009;30(10):964.

128. Armaghani SJ, Menge TJ, Lovejoy SA, et al. Safety of topical vancomycin for pediatric spinal deformity: nontoxic serum levels with supratherapeutic drain levels. Spine (Phila Pa 1976) 2014;39(20):1683–7. https://doi.org/10.1097/BRS.0000000000000465.

129. Evaniew N, Khan M, Drew B, et al. Intrawound vancomycin to prevent infections after spine surgery: a systematic review and meta-analysis. Eur Spine J 2015;24(3):533–42.

130. Nascimento TLd, Finger G, Sfreddo E, et al. Double-blind randomized clinical trial of vancomycin in spinal arthrodesis: no effects on surgical site infection. J Neurosurg Spine 2020;32(3):473. https://doi.org/10.3171/2019.6.Spine19120.

131. Xie L, Zhu J, Luo S, et al. Do dose-dependent microbial changes occur during spine surgery as a result of applying intrawound vancomycin powder?: a systematic literature review. Asian Spine J 2018;12(1):162.

132. Ghobrial GM, Cadotte DW, Williams K, et al. Complications from the use of intrawound vancomycin in lumbar spinal surgery: a systematic review. Neurosurg Focus 2015;39(4):E11.

133. Cheng M-T, Chang M-C, Wang S-T, et al. Efficacy of dilute betadine solution irrigation in the prevention of postoperative infection of spinal surgery. Spine 2005;30(15):1689–93.

134. Chang F-Y, Chang M-C, Wang S-T, et al. Can povidone-iodine solution be used safely in a spinal surgery? Eur Spine J 2006;15(6):1005–14.

135. Norman G, Atkinson RA, Smith TA, et al. Intracavity lavage and wound irrigation for prevention of surgical site infection. Cochrane Database Syst Rev 2017;10(10):CD012234.

136. Hyldig N, Birke-Sorensen H, Kruse M, et al. Meta-analysis of negative-pressure wound therapy for closed surgical incisions. Br J Surg 2016;103(5):477.

137. Nordmeyer M, Pauser J, Biber R, et al. Negative pressure wound therapy for seroma prevention and surgical incision treatment in spinal fracture care. Int Wound J 2016;13(6):1176–9.

Antiviral Therapeutics in Pediatric Transplant Recipients

William R. Otto, MD[a], Abby Green, MD[b],*

KEYWORDS

- Immunocompromised host • Viral infection • Antiviral • Solid organ transplant
- Hematopoietic stem cell transplant • Herpesvirus • Pediatrics

KEY POINTS

- Viral infections occur frequently in immunocompromised pediatric transplant recipients and can cause substantial morbidity and mortality.
- Cytomegalovirus and other herpesviruses may cause primary infection, donor-derived infection, or reactivation of prior infection in transplant recipients; strategies for prevention of end-organ disease are essential to mitigate morbidity.
- Few antiviral agents exist for the prophylaxis and treatment of viral infections.
- Prophylactic, surveillance, and treatment strategies used for pediatric transplant recipients are frequently extrapolated from studies done primarily in adult patients.
- Novel antiviral strategies, including drugs with unique mechanisms of action and adoptive T-cell therapy, are being investigated for use in transplant recipients.

INTRODUCTION

Viral infections are among the most common complications in children who have undergone hematopoietic cell transplantation (HCT) or solid organ transplantation (SOT), and are a significant source of morbidity and mortality. These infections include primary viral infections, most commonly caused by respiratory viruses, but also reactivation of prior infection, as is seen with herpesviruses.

Pediatric and adult recipients of HCT and SOT encounter similar viral infections and are treated with common antiviral agents. Paradigms for the prevention and treatment of viral infections differ between HCT and SOT recipients based on timing and depth of immune suppression around transplantation. Patients with lymphocyte dysfunction

[a] Division of Infectious Diseases, Department of Pediatrics, The Children's Hospital of Philadelphia, 3401 Civic Center Boulevard, Philadelphia, PA 19104-4399, USA; [b] Division of Infectious Diseases, Department of Pediatrics, Washington University, 425 S. Euclid Avenue, McDonnell Pediatric Research Building, #5105, St Louis, MO 63106, USA
* Corresponding author.
E-mail address: abby.green@wustl.edu

Infect Dis Clin N Am 36 (2022) 125–146
https://doi.org/10.1016/j.idc.2021.11.004
0891-5520/22/© 2021 Elsevier Inc. All rights reserved.

are at the highest risk for viral infection.[1,2] In HCT recipients, lymphocyte depletion occurs in the pre-engraftment phase after chemotherapy conditioning and continues through ~100 days or more after transplant.[2] After lymphocyte engraftment, patients who develop graft-versus-host disease (GVHD) require additional T-cell immunosuppression to minimize symptoms, placing them at continued risk for viral infection. Recipients of SOT are at the highest risk for viral infection or reactivation in the early and intermediate post-transplant period (up to 6 months) when immunosuppression is maximized.[1] Subsequently, episodes of graft rejection are managed with additional lymphocyte suppressive medications, increasing the risk of viral infection.

During these periods of increased risk in both HCT and SOT recipients, antiviral agents are used for prophylaxis and treatment of infection (**Table 1**). However, few antiviral drugs with high-efficacy, low-toxicity profiles exist for use in immunocompromised children (**Table 2**). Published pediatric data are limited and many practice recommendations are extrapolated from studies in adult patients. Thus, the use of antiviral agents in children is often off-label. Here we review antiviral drugs used to prevent and treat common viral infections in immunocompromised children, including herpesviruses, human adenoviruses , and respiratory viruses (**Fig. 1**). We also discuss common practices with both approved and off-label indications for antiviral therapeutics in pediatric transplant recipients.

HERPESVIRUS INFECTIONS

Herpesviruses are major pathogens in immunocompromised children and are particularly noteworthy because of their ability to establish latent infections. In transplant recipients, immunosuppressive agents can suppress cell-mediated immunity, enabling reactivation of latent herpesviruses. Herpesvirus reactivation may manifest as asymptomatic viremia or may present as symptomatic disease. The most clinically problematic herpesvirus in immunocompromised hosts is cytomegalovirus (CMV), though

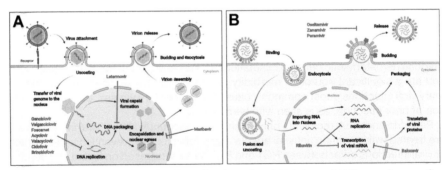

Fig. 1. *Viral life cycles and mechanism of action of antiviral drugs.* (*A*) Herpesviruses: after initial infection, viral DNA enters the nucleus for replication and transcription. The nucleoside/nucleotide analogs block viral DNA replication by inhibiting the viral DNA polymerase. Letermovir acts to block the CMV terminase, preventing DNA packaging, whereas maribavir inhibits the viral UL97 kinase, preventing encapsidation of viral proteins. Letermovir and maribavir are only active against CMV. (*B*) Influenza viruses: after initial binding and endocytosis, the viral particles undergo fusion and uncoating, followed by importation of viral RNA into the nucleus. Viral RNA then undergoes replication and transcription into mRNA. Ribavirin may act to inhibit the viral RNA polymerase to prevent these processes. Baloxavir is a cap-endonuclease inhibitor that blocks mRNA transcription. After viral RNA and mRNA exit the nucleus, progeny virions are then formed and released. The neuraminidase inhibitors block the release of progeny virions. (*Figures created with Biorender.com.*)

herpes simplex virus (HSV), varicella-zoster virus (VZV), or Epstein-Barr virus (EBV) also can cause significant disease.

CMV Infection

CMV is one of the most common opportunistic infections that affect HCT and SOT recipients. Approximately 60% to 80% of the population is infected with CMV by adulthood.[3] Horizontal transmission through person-to-person contact is the most common route of acquisition for primary infection, though CMV can also be transmitted through blood products or organs from infected donors. Subsequent CMV reactivation after organ transplantation can then lead to asymptomatic viremia or tissue-invasive CMV disease. CMV has also been linked to graft rejection, GVHD, and increased risk of other opportunistic infections, making prevention of CMV a priority for improving transplant outcomes.[4]

Epidemiology and risk factors

The incidence of CMV infection and disease among transplant recipients has steadily declined as preventative strategies have evolved, with an associated improvement in mortality.[5,6] HCT recipients at the highest risk for CMV infection are those with T-cell dysfunction, which is affected by conditioning regimen, transplant method, and immunosuppressive therapies used for GVHD. Conditioning regimens with strong lymphodepleting effects, such as those containing fludarabine or alemtuzumab, are associated with high rates of CMV infection.[7] Cord blood and haploidentical transplant recipients, which are associated with delayed T-cell engraftment, are also at high risk for CMV reactivation.[8]

CMV infection after SOT can occur in both the early (<30 days) and the late (>6 months) post-transplant phases.[7] In recipients of SOT, the type of transplanted organ impacts the risk of CMV reactivation and disease due to variation in immunosuppressive regimens used for different organs. Liver, heart, and kidney transplant recipients have a lower risk of CMV infection, whereas risk is higher in lung or small bowel transplant recipients.[9]

In the transplant setting, both donor and recipient serostatus strongly influence the risk of CMV infection or reactivation (**Table 1**). For that reason, universal screening of donor and recipient is recommended during the pretransplant evaluation for both SOT and HCT.[4,10] Notably, children are less likely to have had prior CMV infection than adults, and thus are at higher risk for acquiring CMV from their donor.

Among adult HCT recipients, seropositivity is associated with increased mortality, and upward of 30% to 80% of seropositive recipients will have CMV reactivation post-transplant.[7] The rate of CMV infection in seronegative patients is significantly lower, ranging from 0% to 12%. The high rates of CMV infection reflect the severe and prolonged immunosuppression associated with allogeneic HCT, as rates of CMV infection in seropositive recipients of autologous HCT are 0% to 33%.[7]

Seronegative SOT recipients (R−) who receive an organ from a seropositive donor (D+) comprise the highest risk donor-recipient combination for the development of primary infection and, ultimately, CMV disease.[9] Seropositive recipients (R+) are at risk of CMV reactivation after initiation of immunosuppression. However, the risk is not limited solely to seropositive donors and recipients, and in one multicenter cohort of pediatric lung transplant recipients approximately 7% of D-/R-recipients developed primary CMV infection in the first 12 months after transplant.[11]

Clinical manifestations and diagnosis of CMV infection

Broadly speaking, CMV manifests in one of two forms: CMV infection or CMV disease. CMV infection is defined as the detection of viral antigens or nucleic acid in a body fluid

Table 1
Antiviral drug indications and dosing

Drug	Indication	Route	Age	Dose
Ganciclovir	Induction therapy for CMV syndrome or CMV disease	IV	All ages	5 mg/kg every 12 h
	Maintenance therapy for CMV syndrome or CMV disease	IV	All ages	5 mg/kg every 24 h
	Prophylaxis against CMV infection	IV	All ages	Induction dosing for 7 d, followed by maintenance dosing
Valganciclovir	CMV disease (mild to moderate)	Oral	All ages	7 x BSA x CrCl (maximum dose 900 mg)
	Prophylaxis against CMV infection	Oral	≥4 mo to 16 y	7 x BSA x CrCl (maximum dose 900 mg)
Foscarnet	Induction therapy for CMV syndrome or CMV disease	IV	All ages	60 mg/kg every 12 h
	Maintenance therapy for CMV syndrome or CMV disease	IV	All ages	90 mg/kg once daily
	Prophylaxis against CMV infection	IV	All ages	Induction dosing for 7 d, followed by maintenance dosing
	HSV infection, acyclovir-resistant	IV	All ages	120 mg/kg/d divided every 8 or 12 h
	VZV infection, acyclovir-resistant	IV	All ages	80–120 mg/kg/d divided every 8 or 12 h
Cidofovir	Induction therapy for CMV syndrome or CMV disease	IV	All ages	5 mg/kg every week for 2 consecutive weeks, with hyperhydration ± probenecid
	Maintenance therapy for CMV syndrome or CMV disease	IV	All ages	5 mg/kg every 2 wk, with hyperhydration ± probenecid
	Adenovirus infection	IV	All ages	5 mg/kg every week, with hyperhydration ± probenecid
	HSV infection, acyclovir-resistant and foscarnet-resistant	IV	All ages	5 mg/kg every week for 2 wk, then every 2 wk, with hyperhydration ± probenecid
	VZV infection, acyclovir-resistant	IV	All ages	5 mg/kg every week, with hyperhydration ± probenecid
Letermovir	Prophylaxis against CMV infection	IV, Oral	≥18 y	480 mg every 24 h
Acyclovir	HSV infection (severe or disseminated disease)	IV	All ages	10 mg/kg every 8 h
	HSV infection (mild disease)	Oral	All ages	1000 mg/d, in 3–5 divided doses
	HSV encephalitis	IV	≥4 mo	500 mg/m2 every 8 h, or 10–15 mg/kg every 8 h
	Prophylaxis against HSV infection	IV	All ages	5 mg/kg every 8 h
		Oral	≥2 y	600–1000 mg/d, in 3–5 divided doses
	Varicella or varicella-zoster	IV	<2 y	10 mg/kg every 8 h
		IV	≥2 y	500 mg/m² every 8 h, or 10 mg/kg every 8 h

Drug	Indication	Route	Age	Dose
Valacyclovir	HSV infection (mild localized infection disease)	Oral	≥2 y	20 mg/kg every 12 h (maximum dose 1000 mg)
	Prophylaxis against HSV infection	Oral	≥2 y	<40 kg: 250 mg every 12 h ≥40 kg: 500 mg every 12–24 h
	Varicella or varicella-zoster	Oral	≥2 y	20 mg/kg every 8 h (maximum dose 1000 mg)
	Prophylaxis against VZV infection	Oral	≥2 y	<40 kg: 250 mg every 12 h ≥40 kg: 500 mg every 12–24 h
	VZV postexposure prophylaxis	Oral	≥2 y	<40 kg: 500 mg every 8 h ≥40 kg: 1000 mg every 8 h
Oseltamivir	Treatment of influenza A and B infection	Oral	0–8 mo	3 mg/kg every 12 h
		Oral	9–11 mo	3.5 mg/kg every 12 h
		Oral	1–12 y	≤15 kg: 30 mg every 12 h 15–≤23 kg: 45 mg every 12 h 23–≤40 kg: 60 mg every 12 h >40 kg: 75 mg every 12 h
		Oral	≥13 y	75 mg every 12 h
	Prophylaxis against influenza A and B infection	Oral Oral	≥3 mo	Same as treatment dose, except given once daily
Baloxavir	Treatment of influenza A and B infection Prophylaxis against influenza A and B infection	Oral	≥12 y	40–80 kg: 40 mg >80 kg: 80 mg
Peramivir	Treatment of influenza A and B infection	IV	≥2 y	12 mg/kg (maximum dose 600 mg)
Zanamivir	Treatment of influenza A and B infection	Inhaled	≥7 y	10 mg every 12 h
	Prophylaxis against influenza A and B infection	Inhaled	≥5 y	10 mg every 24 h
Ribavirin	Treatment of RSV infection	Inhaled	All ages	2000 mg every 8 h
		Oral	All ages	20 mg/kg/d divided 3 times per day (maximum dose 600 mg)

Data from the American Academy of Pediatrics. Non-HIV Antiviral Drugs. In: DW K, ed. Red Book: 2021–2024 Report of the Committee on Infectious Diseases; American Academy of Pediatrics; 2021:930–48; and Lexicomp Online. Pediatric and Neonatal Lexi-Drugs Online. July 30, 2021 ed. Waltham, MA: UpToDate, Inc; 2021 or tissue specimen.[12] Detection of CMV may represent primary infection, reactivation of prior infection, or reinfection. Detection of CMV in blood is also specifically defined as viremia (if detected by viral culture), antigenemia (if detected using a pp65 antigen assay), or DNAemia (if detected using nucleic acid amplification techniques).[12] The latter is the most common contemporary method of CMV detection.

CMV disease is defined as the presence of clinical symptoms and is subdivided into 2 specific forms, CMV syndrome and end-organ disease. CMV syndrome involves the detection of CMV in the blood as well as 2 of the following symptoms[12]:

- Fever for at least 2 days
- New or increased malaise or fatigue
- Leukopenia or neutropenia
- Thrombocytopenia
- Presence of $\geq$5% atypical lymphocytes
- Elevation of alanine aminotransferase or aspartate aminotransferase

CMV syndrome can be difficult to distinguish from other transplant-related causes of fever, malaise, transaminitis, or cytopenias.

Tissue-invasive CMV disease can take many forms, depending on the affected organ system. The end-organ disease is diagnosed by the presence of CMV on histopathology, culture, virus isolation, immunohistochemistry, or DNA hybridization of biopsy tissue.[12] Importantly, the presence of clinical symptoms and detectable CMV in blood or serum is not sufficient to definitively diagnose CMV disease—a tissue diagnosis is needed to prove the diagnosis. Definitive tissue diagnosis may not be able to be obtained in critically ill patients, in which case empirical treatment should not be delayed.

Prevention of CMV infection and disease

Prevention of CMV in the post-transplant period has generally taken one of two forms: prophylaxis with antiviral drugs or pre-emptive strategies (Table 1). In the former, antiviral drugs are given to at-risk patients after transplantation, usually for a prespecified period. With pre-emptive therapy, patients undergo serial screening for CMV infection, usually with quantitative polymerase chain reaction (PCR) assays. If there is evidence of CMV replication, identified by an increase in CMV copy number, treatment with antiviral therapy is then initiated.

Each strategy has positive and negative features.[4,13] Universal prophylaxis decreases CMV infection and disease but is costly due to increased antiviral medication use and number of drug-related adverse events even in patients who may not have developed CMV infection or disease.[14] Pre-emptive therapy enables stimulation of natural CMV immunity post-transplant and may allow for quicker immune reconstitution in HCT.[13] However, logistical difficulties related to serial screening and the unknown indirect effects of early CMV DNAemia on the transplanted graft pose a challenge. In addition, the optimal threshold to trigger initiation of pre-emptive therapy has not been defined.[4] It is not uncommon for a hybrid approach to be taken, wherein patients receive antiviral prophylaxis for a set period, followed by surveillance for the development of CMV DNAemia after discontinuation of prophylaxis.[13] No clinical trials have yet evaluated the comparative efficacy of prophylaxis, pre-emptive therapy, or surveillance after prophylaxis strategies in children. Importantly, effective prevention of CMV infection has altered the epidemiology of CMV infection, to the point where many episodes of CMV infection and disease occur later after transplant, commonly after completion of CMV prophylaxis.[15]

Antiviral prophylaxis in HCT. Historically, universal prophylaxis was used less frequently in HCT because of risks of myelosuppression with ganciclovir and valganciclovir, though it is used more frequently with the approval of new antiviral agents.[13] Three recent systematic reviews and a corresponding meta-analysis have shown that antiviral prophylaxis is effective in reducing both CMV infection and CMV disease but not all-cause mortality.[16–18]

Ganciclovir and its oral prodrug, valganciclovir, provide strong anti-CMV activity, and have been shown to prevent CMV infection and disease in early trials in adult HCT.[17] Pharmacokinetic studies have demonstrated that equal or higher drug concentrations can be achieved with valganciclovir compared with intravenous ganciclovir.[19,20] However, the use of these agents is limited by adverse events such as neutropenia, which is reported in 25% to 62% of patients in clinical trials.[16]

Letermovir shows great promise as a drug for CMV prophylaxis, both in its ability to prevent CMV infection and its favorable side-effect profile. Placebo-controlled trials in adult HCT recipients showed that letermovir was effective at preventing CMV infection, and was associated with a decrease in all-cause mortality.[21,22] Although this finding was not confirmed in a subsequent meta-analysis, studies are ongoing.[17] The primary side effects of letermovir are gastrointestinal, with minimal hematologic or renal toxicity reported. Letermovir does not have antiviral activity against other herpesviruses, so patients receiving letermovir should also receive prophylaxis against HSV or VZV if indicated. A phase 2 trial evaluating the safety and tolerability of letermovir prophylaxis for CMV in pediatric HCT recipients is currently ongoing (NCT03940586).

Other drugs have been studied as potential prophylactic agents for CMV in HCT. Neither acyclovir nor valacyclovir significantly reduced CMV infection or disease compared with placebo,[16,17] consistent with their lower level of activity against CMV *in vitro*.[13] Maribavir, an oral benzimidazole riboside with potent anti-CMV activity *in vitro*, did not prevent CMV disease compared with placebo in phase 3 studies in both adult liver transplant and HCT recipients.[23,24] Another oral agent, brincidofovir, did not improve rates of CMV infection at 24 weeks in adult HCT recipients compared with placebo and resulted in more significant adverse events.[25,26] Foscarnet has not been studied as a prophylactic agent in controlled trials in HCT and its use is limited by renal toxicity.[10]

Antiviral prophylaxis in SOT. Universal prophylaxis is frequently used in SOT, and prophylaxis after SOT has been shown to reduce CMV infection and disease, with positive outcomes regarding graft survival, incidence of opportunistic infections, and mortality.[13,27] The prophylaxis regimen and duration of prophylaxis are determined by the transplanted organ and the serostatus of the donor and recipient (see **Table 1**).

Valganciclovir is the most frequently used prophylactic agent, though acyclovir, valacyclovir, and ganciclovir have also been studied for universal prophylaxis. Oral ganciclovir was more effective than acyclovir in preventing CMV infection and disease.[28] Valganciclovir has been shown to be equivalent to ganciclovir in multiple studies.[28,29] However, subgroup analyses in one study revealed that liver transplant recipients given valganciclovir prophylaxis had increased incidence of tissue invasive CMV,[29] and valganciclovir has not been approved for prophylaxis in that population.

Pre-emptive therapy in HCT and SOT. The basic principles of pre-emptive therapy are similar in HCT and SOT, though much of the data are derived from studies in HCT patients. Patients are monitored with serial (weekly) blood PCR testing. When a test is positive at a defined viral threshold (eg, 1000 copies per mL), antiviral therapy is initiated. Threshold levels are determined by each treatment team, given variability across PCR assays. Treatment is generally continued for a minimum of 2 weeks, with at least one negative CMV test required before discontinuation of therapy. If CMV is still detected after 2 weeks of therapy, then a transition to maintenance therapy can be executed. A prolonged duration of therapy may be required in patients with prolonged positivity or slow clearance of CMV.[10] After discontinuation of therapy, patients resume surveillance testing. A second episode of CMV infection can be treated with the same drug initially, though alternative agents should be used if resistance is identified or suspected (see the following section "Management of resistant CMV infection and disease").

Ganciclovir is the most commonly used initial treatment in pre-emptive therapy.[10] Valganciclovir has also been used as pre-emptive therapy, though there have been few controlled trials in HCT or SOT.[30] Foscarnet has also been shown to be effective as pre-emptive therapy in multiple small, randomized trials in adult HCT recipients.[31,32] Maribavir is also under investigation as pre-emptive therapy in both HCT and SOT recipients.

Treatment of CMV Infection and Disease

Ganciclovir and valganciclovir are the first-line therapeutic agents for the treatment of CMV infection and disease (Table 1).[4,10] For treatment of CMV disease, either ganciclovir or valganciclovir can be used as initial therapy, as valganciclovir was shown to be noninferior to ganciclovir in a randomized, controlled trial in adult SOT recipients.[33] However, ganciclovir is preferred in cases of severe, life-threatening CMV disease, or when absorption of valganciclovir may be diminished (as in gastrointestinal CMV disease). After clinical improvement, patients can be transitioned to oral valganciclovir. Foscarnet can be used as an alternative first-line agent if ganciclovir cannot be given because of adverse effects.[10,27]

Antiviral therapy should be continued until resolution of clinical disease and clearance of CMV DNAemia. However, the absence of CMV DNA in the blood may not reflect clinical response in tissue-invasive disease. Longer courses of treatment may be needed in cases of gastrointestinal disease, pneumonitis, or CNS disease, based on clinical response.[4]

Management of resistant CMV infection and disease

Concern for antiviral resistance arises when a patient develops refractory CMV infection, which is defined as increasing or persistent CMV DNAemia after ≥ 2 weeks of antiviral therapy.[34] Worsening symptoms or progression of organ-specific disease despite adequate therapy might also indicate the presence of resistant CMV.[4,10,34] Resistant/refractory CMV infection can occur after prolonged exposure to antiviral agents.[4,10] Subtherapeutic drug levels may also contribute to the development of resistance. In single-center studies in pediatric HCT, antiviral resistance was present in less than 10% of cases.[35,36] Similarly, low levels of resistance have been reported in case series of CMV infection in SOT recipients.[36]

Molecular assays are used to identify specific mutations that confer resistance to each antiviral drug (Table 2). There are no clinical trial data to guide the management of resistant CMV infections, and the treatment principles for resistant infections are based on expert opinion.[4,37] For alterations in UL97 that confer low-level ganciclovir resistance, such as the C592 G mutation, high-dose ganciclovir (10 mg/kg twice daily) may be effective.[37] If high-level ganciclovir resistance is present, treatment-dose foscarnet can be used.[38] If a mutation confers resistance to both ganciclovir and foscarnet, then cidofovir may be used, though efficacy is uncertain.[37]

Maribavir has shown promise in the treatment of resistant infections. In a phase 3 trial, adults treated with maribavir were more likely to have clearance of CMV DNAemia

Table 2
Key antiviral drugs, their mechanisms of action, and toxicities

Drug	Mechanism of Action	Key Toxicities
Ganciclovir[94]	Acyclic nucleoside analog of guanosine, undergoes triphosphorylation and then targets the viral DNA polymerase to inhibit viral DNA synthesis by competitively inhibiting incorporation of dGTP into DNA	Cytopenias Renal dysfunction
Valganciclovir[95]	Prodrug of ganciclovir, rapidly converted to ganciclovir by intestinal and hepatic enzymes after oral administration	Cytopenias Renal dysfunction
Foscarnet	Pyrophosphate analog, directly inhibits CMV DNA replication by binding to the DNA polymerase	Renal dysfunction Electrolyte wasting
Cidofovir	Monophosphate nucleotide analog, phosphorylated to its diphosphate form and then inhibits the viral DNA polymerase by competitively inhibiting incorporation of dCTP into DNA	Renal dysfunction
Letermovir	Inhibits CMV viral terminase complex, preventing packaging of DNA before encapsidation of viral genome	Gastrointestinal symptoms
Maribavir	Inhibits phosphorylation of nuclear lamins by UL97 kinase, preventing formation of viral capsid and nuclear egress of viral particles; also impacts viral gene expression and DNA synthesis	Dysgeusia Nausea and vomiting
Acyclovir[96]	Acyclic guanosine analog, undergoes triphosphorylation and then targets the viral DNA polymerase to inhibit viral DNA synthesis by competitively inhibiting incorporation of dGTP into DNA	Renal dysfunction Anemia Neutropenia Nausea and vomiting Rare neurologic toxicity
Valacyclovir[97]	Prodrug of acyclovir; after oral administration, rapidly converted to acyclovir via first-pass intestinal and hepatic metabolism	Headache Nausea and vomiting Acute renal failure Thrombotic thrombocytopenic purpura/Hemolytic uremic syndrome
Oseltamivir	Competitive inhibitor of influenza neuraminidase, preventing release of new virions	Nausea and vomiting

(continued on next page)

Table 2
(continued)

Drug	Mechanism of Action	Key Toxicities
Baloxavir	Cap-endonuclease inhibitor, inhibits endonuclease subdomain of the viral RNA polymerase, preventing transcription of viral mRNA	Diarrhea
Peramivir	Competitive inhibitor of influenza neuraminidase, preventing release of new virions	
Zanamivir	Competitive inhibitor of influenza neuraminidase, preventing release of new virions	Cough Sore throat
Ribavirin	Guanosine analog, multiple mechanisms of action have been proposed, including inhibition of the viral polymerase of RNA viruses	Hemolytic anemia

after 8 weeks compared to those treated with alternative therapies, including ganciclovir, valganciclovir, foscarnet, and cidofovir.[39] There are limited data regarding the use of maribavir in children. There are no comparative data supporting the use of letermovir for the treatment of CMV infection.

Virus-specific T-lymphocytes (VSTs) have also been used to provide targeted therapy for refractory CMV infection.[40] CMV-specific T-cells are selected from donors and then undergo *ex vivo* expansion before infusion into the infected patients. VSTs can be harvested from the patient's HCT donor, or patients may be given "off-the-shelf" HLA-matched products from third-party VST banks. Several small-scale studies have reported that both donor VSTs and off-the-shelf products can effectively treat refractory CMV disease.[41,42] However, data are limited and VSTs are not frequently used.

HSV Infection

HSV1 and HSV2 infections in transplant recipients are frequently caused by reactivation of prior infection, though primary infection is possible and typically more severe. HSV establishes latency in the dorsal root ganglia and can reactivate in states of physiologic stress or immune suppression. Donor-derived infections are rare because the virus is generally not present in the transplanted organ.[43]

Epidemiology and Risk Factors

The risk of HSV reactivation is related to a patient's degree of immunosuppression.[43] Infection frequently occurs in the first 4 weeks after HCT. HSV reactivation occurs less frequently in adult SOT, and in one large cohort of adult SOT recipients, 6.7% developed HSV infection within 1-year post-transplant, with a median onset of 66 days after SOT.[44]

Clinical Manifestations of HSV Infection

HSV infections in immunocompromised patients can present similarly to infection in immunocompetent hosts. Severe local infections, such as gingivostomatitis, esophagitis, or cutaneous disease, can occur.[45] Highly immunocompromised patients such as HCT recipients are at risk for the development of disseminated disease with end-organ involvement and may be at risk for prolonged symptoms or a more severe disease course.[43,46] Immunocompromised patients are also at risk for frequent HSV reactivations, and reactivation flares may be prolonged.[45]

Prevention of HSV Infection

HSV prophylaxis with acyclovir or valacyclovir was shown to be effective in reducing HSV reactivation and disease in one meta-analysis that included 22 randomized controlled trials of antiviral prophylaxis in adult HCT recipients.[18] Antiviral prophylaxis against HSV is now the standard of care in seropositive HCT recipients.[46] A meta-analysis of 12 randomized trials examining HSV reactivation following SOT in adults found that the use of acyclovir prophylaxis significantly reduced HSV disease.[47] Owing to the relative protection against HSV conferred by anti-CMV agents, HSV prophylaxis is given to seropositive patients who are not receiving prophylaxis against CMV.

Treatment of HSV Infection

Intravenous acyclovir is the primary drug to treat HSV infection (**Table 3**). For more severe infections such as gingivostomatitis, meningoencephalitis, hepatitis, or pneumonitis, intravenous acyclovir is the preferred treatment. For mild disease or localized infections, oral valacyclovir is adequate.[48] The duration of treatment is dependent on the severity of infection; for mild infections treatment of 7 to 10 days is likely sufficient, whereas severe infections are usually treated for 14 to 21 days. In immunocompromised patients, treatment is generally continued until immunosuppression resolves, though patients may be transitioned to a prophylactic regimen after the treatment course is completed.

HSV that is resistant to acyclovir is rare; in one large study of adult HCT recipients, acyclovir-resistant HSV occurred in 0.4% of patients.[49] Resistance testing is onerous and requires viral culture and phenotypic evaluation. However, isolates should be susceptible to foscarnet and cidofovir, both of which do not require the viral thymidine kinase for prodrug metabolism, thus are the preferred agents for acyclovir-resistant HSV.[43,46]

		Risk of CMV	
Serostatus	**Organ**	**Reactivation**	**Recommendation**
D−/R−	All Organs	Low	Prophylaxis not recommended
D+/R−	HCT	Intermediate	100 d
	Kidney, liver, or heart	High	3–6 mo[a]
	Lung	High	6–12 mo
D−/R+	HCT	High	100 d
	Kidney, liver, or heart	Intermediate	3–6 mo
	Lung	High	6–12 mo[b]
D+/R+	HCT	High	100 d
	Kidney, liver, or heart	Intermediate	3–6 mo
	Lung	High	6–12 mo[b]

Table 3
CMV reactivation risk and prophylaxis regimens in transplant

Abbreviations: D+, donor seropositive; D−, donor seronegative; HCT, hematopoietic stem cell transplantation; R+, recipient seropositive; R−, recipient seronegative
[a] Valganciclovir is not approved for use as prophylaxis in liver transplantation[29]
[b] CMV immune globulin is sometimes given to high-risk lung transplant recipients, in addition to antiviral prophylaxis[4]

VZV Infection

Children who have not completed vaccination before transplant are at risk for developing primary infection. As with HSV, VZV develops latency in nerve ganglia and can reactivate with stress or immunosuppression. VZV reactivation is commonly symptomatic and can be severe and/or disseminated in immunocompromised hosts. Donor-derived infections are rare, but have been reported.[50]

Epidemiology and Risk Factors

The development of VZV infection post-transplant is associated with serostatus pretransplant and the patient's overall level of immunosuppression. VZV infection has been reported to occur in 10% to 68% of pediatric and adult patients following HCT, particularly before T-cell engraftment and in patients who develop GVHD.[46,51] In adult SOT, VZV is uncommon; 2.1% developing infection at 1 year after transplant and 4.0% overall in one cohort.[44] Heart and lung transplant recipients have higher rates of VZV compared with other organ transplants. In children, the incidence is thought to be similar to that in adults.[50]

Clinical Manifestations

The clinical presentation of primary varicella and zoster in SOT and HCT recipients is similar to that of the general pediatric population, though immunocompromised children are at increased risk of severe disease.[46,50] Primary VZV infection can present as a pruritic vesicular rash that evolves into crusted scabs or, less commonly, as hemorrhagic lesions.[52] However, atypical infection without a notable rash can occur in immunocompromised children.[46] Severe disease with dissemination to the liver, lungs, or other organs can occur in immunocompromised children. VZV reactivation, or zoster, manifests as itchy or painful groups of skin lesions that are conventionally localized to specific sensory dermatomes, though may present atypically in immunocompromised hosts including in a disseminated fashion similar to primary varicella.

Prevention and Treatment of VZV Infection

Antiviral prophylaxis with acyclovir or valacyclovir is effective in reducing the incidence of VZV disease in adult HCT and SOT recipients.[46,47,50] Prophylaxis is generally given to seropositive HCT recipients for at least 1 year after transplant,[46] though long-term use in SOT is uncommon.[50] Antiviral prophylaxis against CMV also offers protection against VZV, and patients who receive CMV prophylaxis do not require additional VZV prophylaxis.[18,46,47,50]

When VZV infection occurs in immunocompromised children, early treatment is prudent to prevent dissemination and end-organ involvement. Intravenous acyclovir therapy is recommended for use in immunocompromised patients because of the risk of disseminated disease (Table 1).[52] Oral acyclovir should not be used because of poor bioavailability, though some experts advocate for use of oral valacyclovir in patients deemed to be at low risk for dissemination.[52] The duration of antiviral treatment is similar to that of HSV infection. Following the primary treatment course, patients generally receive antiviral prophylaxis until their immunocompromised state has resolved.

ADENOVIRUS INFECTIONS

Human adenoviruses (HAdVs) cause infections of the respiratory and gastrointestinal tracts, and conjunctivitis in healthy children. Infection in immunocompromised children is predominantly *de novo* infection, though HAdV infection from donor tissues has also been described in SOT.[53]

Epidemiology and Risk Factors

In pediatric HCT recipients, HAdVs range from 12% to 42%.[53,54] Risk factors that have been identified in HCT include a T-cell–depleted graft, an unrelated donor, severe GVHD, or severe lymphopenia.[54,55] The correlation between more profound immunosuppression and risk of infection is reflected in the variability of HAdV incidence in pediatric SOT, which ranges from 4% to 38% in liver transplant to greater than 50% in intestinal or heart, lung, or heart-lung transplant.[56]

Clinical Manifestations

In immunocompromised patients, HAdV infection can present with severe localized infection, including gastroenteritis/colitis, pneumonia, hepatitis, nephritis, or cystitis.[53] HAdV can also cause disseminated disease characterized by severe sepsis and multi-organ-system involvement.[57] Mortality can exceed 50% in disseminated disease.[53,57]

Prevention and Treatment of Adenovirus Infection

No evidence exists to support the use of antiviral drugs for prophylaxis of HAdV infection, and prophylaxis is not currently recommended for patients undergoing HCT or SOT.[55,56]

In HCT, pre-emptive treatment is recommended for patients at risk for HAdV infection and disease, and antiviral treatment may be initiated if HAdV is detected in the blood.[55] For SOT recipients, asymptomatic infections are generally not treated.[53,56] If symptomatic disease is present, antiviral therapy and reduction of immunosuppression are the first steps in management.[56]

Clinical trials or comparative effectiveness studies have not been conducted to evaluate antiviral treatment for HAdV infections resulting in no approved agents for the treatment of HAdV infections. Cidofovir, a nucleoside analog of cytosine, is the most frequently used antiviral drug to treat HAdV infection (Table 1).[55,56] The optimal dose of cidofovir is unknown, although the most frequently used dosing is 5 mg/kg weekly. An alternative lower dose of 1 mg/kg 3 times per week has been used to mitigate toxicity.[58] Owing to significant nephrotoxicity, hyperhydration is necessary and probenecid is given to decrease kidney tissue drug levels by competitively inhibiting cidofovir reuptake in the kidney. Toxicity and poor *in vivo* efficacy are major limiting factors for the use of cidofovir. Other drugs have been evaluated, including brincidofovir, ganciclovir, and ribavirin, but none are routinely used.

RESPIRATORY VIRUSES

Antiviral therapies are not available for the vast majority of respiratory viral infections that occur in pediatric transplant patients. Influenza virus and respiratory syncytial virus (RSV) are two exceptions. In this section, we discuss the presentation of influenza and RSV in pediatric transplant recipients as well as antiviral agents available to treat them.

Influenza

Influenza infection results in a spectrum of symptoms in pediatric transplant recipients from mild congestion to respiratory failure. Influenza has also been associated with graft rejection, particularly in lung transplant recipients, though current reports are conflicting and the pathophysiology behind this association is unclear.[59,60]

Epidemiology and Risk Factors

In transplant recipients, influenza virus infection mirrors the seasonality observed in immune-competent hosts with increased incidence in colder months. Symptomatic infection is more common in recipients of lung or heart transplants compared with liver and kidney recipients. Infection occurs more frequently in younger patients and during the first year after SOT, reflecting increased risks of infection during periods of substantial immunosuppression.[61,62] Influenza infection is associated with increased hospitalization, need for mechanical ventilation, and death among adult SOT recipients,[63] but does not appear to substantially impact mortality in pediatric SOT recipients.[61,62]

Clinical Manifestations

Influenza infection causes a similar clinical syndrome in transplant recipients compared with healthy children. Most patients present with fever and cough. Additional symptoms include rhinorrhea, headache, pharyngitis, myalgias, and gastrointestinal distress.[63] In both SOT and HCT recipients, severe complications of influenza infection are more common than in the general population.[64,65] Substantial complications observed in a recent large multicenter cohort of transplant recipients included lower respiratory tract infection (LRTI), hospitalization, and ICU admission,[63] though lower rates of severe disease were observed in the small group of pediatric patients evaluated.

Prevention and Treatment of Influenza Infection

In contrast to herpesviruses, antiviral agents are not routinely used to prevent acquisition of influenza, rather rigorous infection prevention measures such as handwashing, masking, and avoidance of sick contacts are used. Inpatient infection prevention measures are particularly important given the risk of nosocomial infection in this population.

Pre-exposure prophylaxis. Vaccination is an important preventative measure even among immunocompromised patients. Although serologic response to vaccination is variable among transplant recipients and lower than that in healthy controls, immunized transplant recipients have fewer complications of influenza infection than those who are unimmunized.[66,67] Among adult and pediatric transplant recipients, those who received an annual influenza vaccine were less likely to present with a LRTI and less likely to require ICU admission.[63]

Antiviral agents. Neuraminidase (NA) inhibitors are effective against influenza A and B and are approved for the treatment of influenza infection (Table 1). Oseltamivir is an oral agent with pharmacokinetic data available for all pediatric age groups. Zanamivir (inhaled) and peramivir (intravenous) are effective NA inhibitors that are less well studied in transplant recipients and children. Baloxavir is orally available and recently was approved for the treatment of uncomplicated influenza in patients older than 12 years.[68] An international clinical trial investigating the utility of baloxavir to treat high-risk adolescent and adult outpatients (eg, with comorbid asthma or diabetes mellitus) with influenza infection showed similar efficacy of single-dose baloxavir to treatment courses of oseltamivir, though transplant recipients were excluded from this trial.[69]

Postexposure prophylaxis. Although immunization is the most well-studied and effective form of preventing illness related to influenza infection, prophylaxis may be effective in select transplant recipients.[70,71] A more well-defined preventative paradigm is that of postexposure prophylaxis in patients at high risk for complications of influenza infection. In numerous randomized, placebo-controlled trials, NA inhibitors were effective in preventing influenza illness in patients who had close contact (household or nosocomial) with an infected individual.[72,73] Recommendations for SOT and HCT recipients include prophylaxis with oseltamivir or zanamivir within 48 hours of exposure.[74,75]

Treatment of influenza. Treatment with oseltamivir or zanamivir is recommended for all pediatric transplant recipients with symptoms compatible with influenza infection, concurrent with diagnostic evaluation.[74] Initiation of treatment within 48 hours of symptom onset is associated with decreased mortality and ICU admission.[63,64] More data are available regarding the efficacy of oseltamivir in pediatric transplant recipients, although IV formulations (zanamivir or peramivir) may be considered in critically ill patients or those unable to tolerate oral medications. Although early treatment is associated with improved outcomes, symptomatic transplant recipients should receive antiviral therapy even if they present for care beyond the first 48 hours of illness.[74] Treatment with antivirals should be at least 5 days and longer durations may be used in cases of prolonged viral shedding, which is more common in transplant recipients.[76]

Respiratory syncytial virus. In transplant recipients, RSV can cause highly morbid lower respiratory tract disease. Substantial efforts have been made toward preventing the progression of RSV disease to LRTI in transplant recipients in order to mitigate morbidity and mortality.

Epidemiology and Risk Factors

Most children have been infected with RSV by age 2 years, though reinfection can occur at any point. The case fatality rate of immune-competent children with RSV is less than 0.5%, but has been reported to be up to 50% in pediatric HCT recipients.[77,78] Risk factors for the development of LRTI or severe RSV disease among pediatric transplant recipients include age less than 2 years, daycare attendance, lung or heart/lung transplantation, underlying lung disease, and HCT.[79]

Clinical Manifestations and Diagnosis of RSV Infection

RSV may present as a nonspecific URI with rhinorrhea, cough, fever, and wheeze, and in healthy children is self-resolving within 1 to 2 weeks. Progression to LRTI manifests as bronchiolitis or pneumonia, which can progress to respiratory failure. In adult HCT recipients, up to 74% with RSV infection progress to LRTI though contemporary reports of pediatric HCT recipients suggest only ~20% progression to LRTI.[80,81] Risk factors for progression to LRTI in HCT recipients are not well defined in pediatrics, but coinfections and pulmonary comorbidities are associated with progression to LRTI.[80,82] Among SOT recipients, lung transplantation and lung disease are associated with increased severity of disease, although not consistently across all studies.[74,83]

PREVENTION AND TREATMENT OF RSV INFECTION

Prophylaxis. RSV is transmitted through contact with secretions of an infected individual including through droplets and contaminated fomites. Contact precautions and isolation procedures should be used to prevent transmission of infection to transplant recipients. Palivizumab is an RSV-specific humanized monoclonal antibody, which targets the F glycoprotein of RSV, thereby inhibiting viral replication. Palivizumab is effective in preventing hospitalization for RSV infection and progression to LRTI in high-risk children less than 2 years of age, particularly those with lung disease of prematurity and congenital heart disease.[84,85] Owing to substantial cost, the American

Association of Pediatrics has generated guidelines for the use of RSV prophylaxis that suggest the use of palivizumab in immunosuppressed children under 2 years of age. Single-center studies have shown minimal benefit in reducing RSV infection in pediatric HCT recipients through the use of palivizumab.[86] Very little data exist on the efficacy of palivizumab as prophylaxis in the pediatric SOT population. Current guidelines from AST suggest the use of palivizumab only in the youngest and most high-risk SOT recipients.[74]

Prevention and treatment of LRTI. Few options are available for the treatment of RSV infection, but prevention of RSV progression to LRTI can mitigate severe disease and complications of RSV infection in pediatric transplant patients. Inhaled ribavirin has been studied both as a pre-emptive treatment in patients with URI and definitive treatment of established LRTI (Table 1). Early studies of inhaled ribavirin for the prevention of progression to LRTI in pediatric HCT recipients were promising: no treated patients in several single-center studies developed LRTI.[87,88] More recent evaluations have shown a benefit in the prevention of LRTI progression as well as in mortality among those who received ribavirin.[89] A large meta-analysis of HCT recipients treated with ribavirin suggested a trend toward decreased LRTI and decreased RSV-related mortality among patients treated with inhaled ribavirin.[90] Ribavirin also is available as an oral formulation, and studies are mixed regarding a benefit of pre-emptive therapy in small studies of HCT and SOT recipients with RSV URI.[91,92]

Although institutional practice varies, treatment of HCT patients with ribavirin as a pre-emptive or treatment strategy is commonly used. The cost of inhaled ribavirin is significant and, given the modest benefit of pre-emptive treatment, contemporary practices vary in SOT recipients infected with RSV.[93] The AST recommends preemptive treatment with inhaled ribavirin for RSV-infected pediatric lung transplant recipients, and treatment of other SOT recipients with LRTI should be considered depending on additional risk factors.[74]

SUMMARY

Viral infections are a major cause of morbidity and mortality in pediatric transplant patients. Antiviral drugs are used to prevent and treat these infections, but therapeutic options are limited. Future research is needed to further development of antiviral drugs and their use in children.

CLINICS CARE POINTS

- Viral infections are common causes of morbidity and mortality in pediatric transplant patients.
- Antiviral treatment options are limited, and preventative measures are essential.
- Much of the antiviral treatment guidelines used in pediatric patients are extrapolated from data gathered in adult patients.

DISCLOSURE

This work was supported by funding from the National Institutes of Health (K08 CA212299), the Children's Discovery Institute and the Washington University School of Medicine.

REFERENCES

1. Fishman JA. Infection in solid-organ transplant recipients. New Engl J Med 2007; 357:2601–14.
2. Srinivasan A, Wang C, Srivastava DK, et al. Timeline, epidemiology, and risk factors for bacterial, fungal, and viral infections in children and adolescents after allogeneic hematopoietic stem cell transplantation. Biol Blood Marrow Transplant 2013;19:94–101.
3. American Academy of Pediatrics. Cytomegalovirus infection. In: Kimberlin DW, Brady MT, Jackson MA, et al, editors. Red book: 2021 report of the committee on infectious diseases. American Academy of Pediatrics; 2021. p. 310–7.
4. Kotton CN, Kumar D, Caliendo AM, et al. The Third International Consensus Guidelines on the management of cytomegalovirus in solid-organ transplantation. Transplantation 2018;102:900–31.
5. Gooley TA, Chien JW, Pergam SA, et al. Reduced mortality after allogeneic hematopoietic-cell transplantation. N Engl J Med 2010;363:2091–101.
6. Nicastro E, Giovannozzi S, Stroppa P, et al. Effectiveness of preemptive therapy for cytomegalovirus disease in pediatric liver transplantation. Transplantation 2017;101:804–10.
7. Styczynski J. Who Is the patient at risk of CMV recurrence: a review of the current scientific evidence with a focus on hematopoietic cell transplantation. Infect Dis Ther 2018;7:1–16.
8. Sauter C, Abboud M, Jia X, et al. Serious infection risk and immune recovery after double-unit cord blood transplantation without antithymocyte globulin. Biol Blood Marrow Transplant 2011;17:1460–71.
9. Martin JM, Danziger-Isakov LA. Cytomegalovirus risk, prevention, and management in pediatric solid organ transplantation. Pediatr Transplant 2011;15:229–36.
10. Ljungman P, de la Camara R, Robin C, et al. Guidelines for the management of cytomegalovirus infection in patients with haematological malignancies and after stem cell transplantation from the 2017 European Conference on Infections in Leukaemia (ECIL 7). Lancet Infect Dis 2019;19:e260–72.
11. Danziger-Isakov LA, Worley S, Michaels MG, et al. The risk, prevention, and outcome of cytomegalovirus after pediatric lung transplantation. Transplantation 2009;87:1541–8.
12. Ljungman P, Boeckh M, Hirsch HH, et al. Definitions of cytomegalovirus infection and disease in transplant patients for use in clinical trials. Clin Infect Dis 2017;64: 87–91.
13. Haidar G, Boeckh M, Singh N. Cytomegalovirus infection in solid organ and hematopoietic cell transplantation: state of the evidence. J Infect Dis 2020;221: S23–31.
14. Florescu DF, Qiu F, Schmidt CM, et al. A direct and indirect comparison meta-analysis on the efficacy of cytomegalovirus preventive strategies in solid organ transplant. Clin Infect Dis 2014;58:785–803.
15. Limaye AP, Bakthavatsalam R, Kim HW, et al. Impact of cytomegalovirus in organ transplant recipients in the era of antiviral prophylaxis. Transplantation 2006;81: 1645–52.
16. Chen K, Cheng MP, Hammond SP, et al. Antiviral prophylaxis for cytomegalovirus infection in allogeneic hematopoietic cell transplantation. Blood Adv 2018;2: 2159–75.
17. Gagelmann N, Ljungman P, Styczynski J, et al. Comparative efficacy and safety of different antiviral agents for cytomegalovirus prophylaxis in allogeneic

hematopoietic cell transplantation: a systematic review and meta-analysis. Biol Blood Marrow Transplant 2018;24:2101–9.

18. Beyar-Katz O, Bitterman R, Zuckerman T, et al. Anti-herpesvirus prophylaxis, pre-emptive treatment or no treatment in adults undergoing allogeneic transplant for haematological disease: systematic review and meta-analysis. Clin Microbiol Infect 2020;26:189–98.

19. Winston DJ, Baden LR, Gabriel DA, et al. Pharmacokinetics of ganciclovir after oral valganciclovir versus intravenous ganciclovir in allogeneic stem cell transplant patients with graft-versus-host disease of the gastrointestinal tract. Biol Blood Marrow Transplant 2006;12:635–40.

20. Einsele H, Reusser P, Bornhauser M, et al. Oral valganciclovir leads to higher exposure to ganciclovir than intravenous ganciclovir in patients following allogeneic stem cell transplantation. Blood 2006;107:3002–8.

21. Chemaly RF, Ullmann AJ, Ehninger G. CMV prophylaxis in hematopoietic-cell transplantation. New Engl J Med 2014;371:576–7.

22. Marty FM, Ljungman P, Chemaly RF, et al. Letermovir prophylaxis for cytomegalovirus in hematopoietic-cell transplantation. N Engl J Med 2017;377:2433–44.

23. Winston DJ, Saliba F, Blumberg E, et al. Efficacy and safety of maribavir dosed at 100 mg orally twice daily for the prevention of cytomegalovirus disease in liver transplant recipients: a randomized, double-blind, multicenter controlled trial. Am J Transplant 2012;12:3021–30.

24. Marty FM, Ljungman P, Papanicolaou GA, et al. Maribavir prophylaxis for prevention of cytomegalovirus disease in recipients of allogeneic stem-cell transplants: a phase 3, double-blind, placebo-controlled, randomised trial. Lancet Infect Dis 2011;11:284–92.

25. Marty FM, Winston DJ, Rowley SD, et al. CMX001 to prevent cytomegalovirus disease in hematopoietic-cell transplantation. N Engl J Med 2013;369:1227–36.

26. Marty FM, Winston DJ, Chemaly RF, et al. A randomized, double-blind, placebo-controlled phase 3 trial of oral brincidofovir for cytomegalovirus prophylaxis in allogeneic hematopoietic cell transplantation. Biol Blood Marrow Transplant 2019;25:369–81.

27. Razonable RR, Humar A. Cytomegalovirus in solid organ transplant recipients-Guidelines of the American Society of Transplantation Infectious Diseases Community of Practice. Clin Transplant 2019;33:e13512.

28. Hodson EM, Ladhani M, Webster AC, et al. Antiviral medications for preventing cytomegalovirus disease in solid organ transplant recipients. Cochrane Database Syst Rev 2013;(2):CD003774.

29. Paya C, Humar A, Dominguez E, et al. Efficacy and safety of valganciclovir vs. oral ganciclovir for prevention of cytomegalovirus disease in solid organ transplant recipients. Am J Transplant 2004;4:611–20.

30. Chawla JS, Ghobadi A, Mosley J 3rd, et al. Oral valganciclovir versus ganciclovir as delayed pre-emptive therapy for patients after allogeneic hematopoietic stem cell transplant: a pilot trial (04-0274) and review of the literature. Transpl Infect Dis 2012;14:259–67.

31. Reusser P, Einsele H, Lee J, et al. Randomized multicenter trial of foscarnet versus ganciclovir for preemptive therapy of cytomegalovirus infection after allogeneic stem cell transplantation. Blood 2002;99:1159–64.

32. Moretti S, Zikos P, Van Lint MT, et al. Forscarnet vs ganciclovir for cytomegalovirus (CMV) antigenemia after allogeneic hemopoietic stem cell transplantation (HSCT): a randomised study. Bone Marrow Transplant 1998;22:175–80.

33. Asberg A, Humar A, Rollag H, et al. Oral valganciclovir is noninferior to intravenous ganciclovir for the treatment of cytomegalovirus disease in solid organ transplant recipients. Am J Transplant 2007;7:2106–13.

34. Chemaly RF, Chou S, Einsele H, et al. Definitions of resistant and refractory cytomegalovirus infection and disease in transplant recipients for use in clinical trials. Clin Infect Dis 2019;68:1420–6.

35. Choi SH, Hwang JY, Park KS, et al. The impact of drug-resistant cytomegalovirus in pediatric allogeneic hematopoietic cell transplant recipients: a prospective monitoring of UL97 and UL54 gene mutations. Transpl Infect Dis 2014;16:919–29.

36. Kim YJ, Boeckh M, Cook L, et al. Cytomegalovirus infection and ganciclovir resistance caused by UL97 mutations in pediatric transplant recipients. Transpl Infect Dis 2012;14:611–7.

37. El Chaer F, Shah DP, Chemaly RF. How I treat resistant cytomegalovirus infection in hematopoietic cell transplantation recipients. Blood 2016;128:2624–36.

38. Avery RK, Arav-Boger R, Marr KA, et al. Outcomes in transplant recipients treated with foscarnet for ganciclovir-resistant or refractory cytomegalovirus infection. Transplantation 2016;100:e74–80.

39. Avery RK, Alain S, Alexander BD, Blumberg EA, Chemaly RF, Cordonnier C, Duarte RF, Florescu DF, Kamar N, Kumar D, Maertens J, Marty FM, Papanicolaou GA, Silveira FP, Witzke O, Wu J, Sundberg AK, Fournier M; SOLSTICE Trial Investigators. Maribavir for Refractory Cytomegalovirus Infections With or Without Resistance Post-Transplant: Results from a Phase 3 Randomized Clinical Trial. Clin Infect Dis. 2021 Dec 2:ciab988. doi:10.1093/cid/ciab988. Epub ahead of print. PMID: 34864943.

40. Houghtelin A, Bollard CM. Virus-specific T cells for the immunocompromised patient. Front Immunol 2017;8:1272.

41. Feuchtinger T, Opherk K, Bethge WA, et al. Adoptive transfer of pp65-specific T cells for the treatment of chemorefractory cytomegalovirus disease or reactivation after haploidentical and matched unrelated stem cell transplantation. Blood 2010;116:4360–7.

42. Prockop S, Doubrovina E, AN H, et al. Third party CMV-specific cytotoxic T cells for treatment of antiviral resistant CMV infection after hematopoietic stem cell transplant [abstract]. Blood 2016;128:61.

43. Lee DH, Zuckerman RA, Practice ASTIDCo. Herpes simplex virus infections in solid organ transplantation: Guidelines from the American Society of Transplantation Infectious Diseases Community of Practice. Clin Tansplant 2019;33:e13526.

44. Martin-Gandul C, Stampf S, Hequet D, et al. Preventive strategies against cytomegalovirus and incidence of alpha-herpesvirus infections in solid organ transplant recipients: A Nationwide Cohort Study. Am J Transplant 2017;17:1813–22.

45. American Academy of Pediatrics. Herpes Simplex. In: Kimberlin DW, Brady MT, Jackson MA, et al, editors. Red book: 2021 report of the committee on infectious diseases. American Academy of Pediatrics; 2021. p. 437–49.

46. Styczynski J, Reusser P, Einsele H, et al. Management of HSV, VZV and EBV infections in patients with hematological malignancies and after SCT: guidelines from the Second European Conference on Infections in Leukemia. Bone Marrow Transplant 2009;43:757–70.

47. Fiddian P, Sabin CA, Griffiths PD. Valacyclovir provides optimum acyclovir exposure for prevention of cytomegalovirus and related outcomes after organ transplantation. J Infect Dis 2002;186(Suppl 1):S110–5.

48. Bomgaars L, Thompson P, Berg S, et al. Valacyclovir and acyclovir pharmacokinetics in immunocompromised children. Pediatr Blood Cancer 2008;51:504–8.

49. Ariza-Heredia EJ, Chemaly RF, Shahani LR, et al. Delay of alternative antiviral therapy and poor outcomes of acyclovir-resistant herpes simplex virus infections in recipients of allogeneic stem cell transplant - a retrospective study. Transpl Int 2018;31:639–48.

50. Pergam SA, Limaye AP, Practice ASTIDCo. Varicella zoster virus in solid organ transplantation: guidelines from the American Society of Transplantation Infectious Diseases Community of Practice. Clin Transplant 2019;33:e13622.

51. Vermont CL, Jol-van der Zijde EC, Hissink Muller P, et al. Varicella zoster reactivation after hematopoietic stem cell transplant in children is strongly correlated with leukemia treatment and suppression of host T-lymphocyte immunity. Transpl Infect Dis 2014;16:188–94.

52. American Academy of Pediatrics. Varicella-Zoster Virus Infections. In: Kimberlin DW, Brady MT, Jackson MA, et al, editors. Red book: 2021 report of the committee on infectious diseases. American Academy of Pediatrics; 2021. p. 869–83.

53. Lion T. Adenovirus infections in immunocompetent and immunocompromised patients. Clin Microbiol Rev 2014;27:441–62.

54. Fisher BT, Boge CLK, Petersen H, et al. Outcomes of human adenovirus infection and disease in a retrospective cohort of pediatric hematopoietic cell transplant recipients. J Pediatr Infect Dis Soc 2019;8:317–24.

55. Matthes-Martin S, Feuchtinger T, Shaw PJ, et al. European guidelines for diagnosis and treatment of adenovirus infection in leukemia and stem cell transplantation: summary of ECIL-4 (2011). Transpl Infect Dis 2012;14:555–63.

56. Florescu DF, Schaenman JM, Practice ASTIDCo. Adenovirus in solid organ transplant recipients: Guidelines from the American Society of Transplantation Infectious Diseases Community of Practice. Clin Transplant 2019;33:e13527.

57. Munoz FM, Piedra PA, Demmler GJ. Disseminated adenovirus disease in immunocompromised and immunocompetent children. Clin Infect Dis 1998;27:1194–200.

58. Ganapathi L, Arnold A, Jones S, et al. Use of cidofovir in pediatric patients with adenovirus infection. F1000Res 2016;5:758.

59. Martin-Gandul C, Mueller NJ, Pascual M, et al. The Impact of infection on chronic allograft dysfunction and allograft survival after solid organ transplantation. Am J Transplant 2015;15:3024–40.

60. Liu M, Mallory GB, Schecter MG, et al. Long-term impact of respiratory viral infection after pediatric lung transplantation. Pediatr Transplant 2010;14:431–6.

61. Danziger-Isakov L, Steinbach WJ, Paulsen G, et al. A multicenter consortium to define the epidemiology and outcomes of pediatric solid organ transplant recipients with inpatient respiratory virus infection. J Pediatr Infect Dis Soc 2019;8:197–204.

62. Liu M, Worley S, Arrigain S, et al. Respiratory viral infections within one year after pediatric lung transplant. Transpl Infect Dis 2009;11:304–12.

63. Kumar D, Ferreira VH, Blumberg E, et al. A 5-Year Prospective Multicenter Evaluation of Influenza Infection in Transplant Recipients. Clin Infect Dis 2018;67:1322–9.

64. Kumar D, Michaels MG, Morris MI, et al. Outcomes from pandemic influenza A H1N1 infection in recipients of solid-organ transplants: a multicentre cohort study. Lancet Infect Dis 2010;10:521–6.

65. Ljungman P, de la Camara R, Perez-Bercoff L, et al. Outcome of pandemic H1N1 infections in hematopoietic stem cell transplant recipients. Haematologica 2011;96:1231–5.

66. Manuel O, Pascual M, Hoschler K, et al. Humoral response to the influenza A H1N1/09 monovalent AS03-adjuvanted vaccine in immunocompromised patients. Clin Infect Dis 2011;52:248–56.
67. Ryan AL, Wadia UD, Jacoby P, et al. Immunogenicity of the inactivated influenza vaccine in children who have undergone allogeneic haematopoietic stem cell transplant. Bone Marrow Transplant 2020;55:773–9.
68. Hayden FG, Sugaya N, Hirotsu N, et al. Baloxavir Marboxil for Uncomplicated Influenza in Adults and Adolescents. N Engl J Med 2018;379:913–23.
69. Ison MG, Portsmouth S, Yoshida Y, et al. Early treatment with baloxavir marboxil in high-risk adolescent and adult outpatients with uncomplicated influenza (CAPSTONE-2): a randomised, placebo-controlled, phase 3 trial. Lancet Infect Dis 2020;20:1204–14.
70. Jaiswal SR, Bhagwati G, Soni M, et al. Prophylactic oseltamivir during major seasonal influenza H1N1 outbreak might reduce both H1N1 and associated pulmonary aspergillosis in children undergoing haploidentical transplantation. Transpl Infect Dis 2020;22:e13309.
71. Ison MG, Szakaly P, Shapira MY, et al. Efficacy and safety of oral oseltamivir for influenza prophylaxis in transplant recipients. Antivir Ther 2012;17:955–64.
72. Hayden FG, Atmar RL, Schilling M, et al. Use of the selective oral neuraminidase inhibitor oseltamivir to prevent influenza. N Engl J Med 1999;341:1336–43.
73. Hayden FG, Gubareva LV, Monto AS, et al. Inhaled zanamivir for the prevention of influenza in families. Zanamivir Family Study Group. N Engl J Med 2000;343:1282–9.
74. Manuel O, Estabrook M, American Society of Transplantation Infectious Diseases Community of P. RNA respiratory viral infections in solid organ transplant recipients: Guidelines from the American Society of Transplantation Infectious Diseases Community of Practice. Clin Transplant 2019;33:e13511.
75. Tomblyn M, Chiller T, Einsele H, et al. Guidelines for preventing infectious complications among hematopoietic cell transplantation recipients: a global perspective. Biol Blood Marrow Transplant 2009;15:1143–238.
76. Khanna N, Steffen I, Studt JD, et al. Outcome of influenza infections in outpatients after allogeneic hematopoietic stem cell transplantation. Transpl Infect Dis 2009;11:100–5.
77. Fisher BT, Alexander S, Dvorak CC, et al. Epidemiology and potential preventative measures for viral infections in children with malignancy and those undergoing hematopoietic cell transplantation. Pediatr Blood Cancer 2012;59:11–5.
78. Tam J, Papenburg J, Fanella S, et al. Pediatric Investigators Collaborative Network on Infections in Canada Study of Respiratory Syncytial Virus-associated Deaths in Pediatric Patients in Canada, 2003-2013. Clin Infect Dis 2019;68:113–9.
79. Science M, Akseer N, Asner S, et al. Risk stratification of immunocompromised children, including pediatric transplant recipients at risk of severe respiratory syncytial virus disease. Pediatr Transplant 2019;23:e13336.
80. El-Bietar J, Nelson A, Wallace G, et al. RSV infection without ribavirin treatment in pediatric hematopoietic stem cell transplantation. Bone Marrow Transplant 2016;51:1382–4.
81. Chemaly RF, Dadwal SS, Bergeron A, et al. A phase 2, randomized, double-blind, placebo-controlled trial of presatovir for the treatment of respiratory syncytial virus upper respiratory tract infection in hematopoietic-cell transplant recipients. Clin Infect Dis 2020;71:2777–86.

82. Chemaly RF, Ghantoji SS, Shah DP, et al. Respiratory syncytial virus infections in children with cancer. J Pediatr Hematol Oncol 2014;36:e376–81.
83. Bridevaux PO, Aubert JD, Soccal PM, et al. Incidence and outcomes of respiratory viral infections in lung transplant recipients: a prospective study. Thorax 2014;69:32–8.
84. Palivizumab, a humanized respiratory syncytial virus monoclonal antibody, reduces hospitalization from respiratory syncytial virus infection in high-risk infants. The IMpact-RSV Study Group. Pediatrics 1998;102:531–7.
85. Pignotti MS, Carmela Leo M, Pugi A, et al. Consensus conference on the appropriateness of palivizumab prophylaxis in respiratory syncytial virus disease. Pediatr Pulmonol 2016;51:1088–96.
86. Teusink-Cross A, Davies SM, Danziger-Isakov L, et al. Restrictive palivizumab use does not lead to increased morbidity and mortality in pediatric hematopoietic stem cell transplantation patients. Biol Blood Marrow Transplant 2016;22:1904–6.
87. Adams R, Christenson J, Petersen F, et al. Pre-emptive use of aerosolized ribavirin in the treatment of asymptomatic pediatric marrow transplant patients testing positive for RSV. Bone Marrow Transplant 1999;24:661–4.
88. Adams RH. Preemptive treatment of pediatric bone marrow transplant patients with asymptomatic respiratory syncytial virus infection with aerosolized ribavirin. Biol Blood Marrow Transplant 2001;7(Suppl):16S–8S.
89. Shah DP, Ghantoji SS, Shah JN, et al. Impact of aerosolized ribavirin on mortality in 280 allogeneic haematopoietic stem cell transplant recipients with respiratory syncytial virus infections. J Antimicrob Chemother 2013;68:1872–80.
90. Shah JN, Chemaly RF. Management of RSV infections in adult recipients of hematopoietic stem cell transplantation. Blood 2011;117:2755–63.
91. Gueller S, Duenzinger U, Wolf T, et al. Successful systemic high-dose ribavirin treatment of respiratory syncytial virus-induced infections occurring pre-engraftment in allogeneic hematopoietic stem cell transplant recipients. Transpl Infect Dis 2013;15:435–40.
92. Trang TP, Whalen M, Hilts-Horeczko A, et al. Comparative effectiveness of aerosolized versus oral ribavirin for the treatment of respiratory syncytial virus infections: A single-center retrospective cohort study and review of the literature. Transpl Infect Dis 2018;20:e12844.
93. Beaird OE, Freifeld A, Ison MG, et al. Current practices for treatment of respiratory syncytial virus and other non-influenza respiratory viruses in high-risk patient populations: a survey of institutions in the Midwestern Respiratory Virus Collaborative. Transpl Infect Dis 2016;18:210–5.
94. Ganciclovir injection. Lenoir (NC): Exela Pharma Sciences; 2017.
95. Valcyte (valganciclovir). San Francisco (CA): Genentech, Inc.; 2020.
96. Zovirax (acyclovir sodium). Brentford (England): GlaxoSmithKline; 2005.
97. Valtrex (valacyclovir hydrochloride) Caplets. (Brentford) England: GlaxoSmithKline; 2008.

Contemporary Treatment of Resistant Gram-Negative Infections in Pediatric Patients

Samantha A. Basco, PharmD, BCPS[a],
Jennifer E. Girotto, PharmD, BCPPS, BCIDP[b],*

KEYWORDS

- Antimicrobial stewardship • Resistance • Pharmacotherapy

KEY POINTS

- Pediatric patients differ from adult patients with regard to pharmacokinetics, although pharmacodynamic goals remain the same. Pediatric patients often require higher or more frequent dosing of antibiotics.
- Beta-lactamases are the most common mechanism of resistance among gram-negative infections.
- AmpC enzymes may be inducible in certain organisms, making repeat susceptibility testing or knowledge of previous antibiotic exposure important.
- Prolonged infusions of several beta-lactam antibiotics are promising methods to overcome some resistance mechanisms owing to beta-lactams time-dependent antimicrobial activity.
- Newer agents including cefiderocol, meropenem–vaborbactam, imipenem–relebactam, and ceftolozane–tazobactam are promising options for resistant gram-negative infections in adults, but more data is needed in pediatric patients to ensure pharmacodynamic goals are reached.

INTRODUCTION

Resistant gram-negative infections have become increasingly problematic, even in children. Resistant gram-negative infections in children are associated with a 68% increase in the overall hospital length of stay and a 138% increase in critical care duration.[1] Rates of Enterobacterales resistance in pediatrics, especially carbapenem resistance, have been increasing since at least 1999.[2] Resistance patterns for gram-negative infections in pediatric patients vary by organism, source of infection, and patient location.[3,4] From 2015 to 2017 as compared with 2011 to 2014, the

[a] University of Connecticut, Storrs CT and Connecticut Children's, Hartford, CT, USA;
[b] University of Connecticut School of Pharmacy, Connecticut Children's, Hartford, CT, USA
* Corresponding author.
E-mail address: Jgirotto@connecticutchildrens.org

Infect Dis Clin N Am 36 (2022) 147–171
https://doi.org/10.1016/j.idc.2021.11.007
0891-5520/22/© 2021 Elsevier Inc. All rights reserved.

id.theclinics.com

National Healthcare Safety Network reported that carbapenem resistance increased in pediatric critical care isolates from 1.1% to 2.4% for *Escherichia coli*, 3.0% to 3.4% for *Enterobacter* spp., and 1.8% to 3.3% for *Klebsiella* spp.[3,4]

As resistance continues to evolve, it is important to understand hospital-specific resistance patterns and ensure that pediatric patients receive prompt and appropriate therapy. The Surviving Sepsis Campaign's pediatric guidelines suggest administration of an active antibiotic within 3 hours for sepsis and 1 hour in cases of septic shock.[5] Although only alluded to in the guidelines, the dosing of these medications is very important for pediatric patients. Clinicians should consider pediatric-specific pharmacokinetics and evaluate whether antibiotic choices will result in goal pharmacodynamic exposures. This article reviews the mechanisms of resistance and potential treatment options for resistant gram-negative infections in pediatric patients.

RESISTANCE MECHANISMS

Gram-negative organisms have developed several mechanisms of resistance to currently available antibiotic classes. Among these are beta-lactamase enzymes and efflux pumps and porins, with beta-lactamases being the most clinically relevant to identify as strategies to overcome these enzymes are well-established.

RESISTANCE TO BETA-LACTAMS

Beta-lactams are one of the most important and commonly used antibiotic classes for systemic gram-negative infections. One of the most common mechanisms of resistance to this class is hydrolysis by beta-lactamases. We highlight the common beta-lactamases that have the greatest impact on pediatric infections.

AmpC-PRODUCING ENTEROBACTERALES

AmpC enzymes are a common cephalosporinase that are most often a clinical issue for some Enterobacterales species. When AmpC is produced, it can result in resistance to most of the beta-lactams except for carbapenems, cefiderocol, ceftazidime–avibactam, and in some situations cefepime and piperacillin–tazobactam.[6] Therefore, it is important to determine if the specific Enterobacterales organism is likely to harbor chromosomal *ampC* or instead if *ampC* is only rarely obtained from a plasmid. *Enterobacter* spp., *Klebsiella aerogenes, Serratia marcescens,* and *Citrobacter freundii* are examples of organisms that have chromosomal *ampC* expression.[6,7] A cohort study including 399 adult patients found that 38% of *Enterobacter* spp., 15% of *S marcescens*, and 1% of *Citrobacter* spp. expressed *ampC*.[8] By contrast, *Klebsiella pneumoniae* and *Proteus mirabilis* need to acquire this resistance mechanism via a plasmid.[7,9] *AmpR*, a transcriptional regulator involved in the expression of *ampC*, may become conformationally changed after exposure to beta-lactam antibiotics. This change results in increased expression of *ampC*. Some gram-negative species, including *E coli* and *Acinetobacter baumanii,* do not harbor the *ampR* gene; thus, even if acquired via plasmid, AmpC production is not inducible in these organisms.[7]

In a 2014 analysis of *Enterobacter* spp. bloodstream infections in pediatric patients, carbapenems, cefepime, and ciprofloxacin were reported as the most likely antibiotics to be active.[10] Additionally, newer agents including ceftazidime-avibactam and cefiderocol have also shown activity against AmpC-producing organisms. Cefiderocol appears to be minimally affected by AmpC enzymes, whereas the addition of avibactam, a newer beta-lactamase inhibitor, is able to prevent degradation of ceftazidime by AmpC and thus restores activity for ceftazidime.[11,12]

In recent years, as an effort to protect the carbapenems, a few case controlled and retrospective studies in adult patients have provided initial evidence that piperacillin–tazobactam may be considered for infections caused by AmpC-producing Enterobacterales.[13,14] This strategy may be successful because piperacillin is a weak inducer of AmpC enzymes, whereas tazobactam may provide some inhibition. The MERINO II trial, a well-designed, prospective adult trial comparing piperacillin–tazobactam (4.5 g given every 6 hours) with meropenem (1 g given every 8 hours) for bloodstream infections caused by likely chromosomal AmpC-producing *Enterobacter* spp., *K aerogenes, S marcescens, Providencia* spp., *Morganella* spp., or *C freundii* was recently completed. A total of 72 patients (38 received piperacillin–tazobactam, 34 received meropenem) were evaluated. Twenty-nine percent of piperacillin–tazobactam patients experienced death, microbiologic or clinical failure, or microbiologic relapse compared with 21% of meropenem patients (95% confidence interval, -12% to 28%). However, this study was unable to recruit as many participants as was planned; therefore, an additional larger study would be beneficial.[15]

Cefepime is another potential carbapenem-sparing option for AmpC-producing Enterobacterales. In 2013, Tamma and colleagues[8] reported no difference in 30-day mortality in adults who received definitive therapy using cefepime versus meropenem for the treatment of AmpC-producing Enterobacterales infections (bacteremia, pneumonia, intra-abdominal infections). The was a propensity score matched cohort study that included 32 matched pairs. Importantly, the majority of cefepime minimum inhibitory concentrations (MICs) were reported as 1 μg/mL or less.[8] Another study in adults published in 2020 provides additional evidence that cefepime may be useful in AmpC-producing Enterobacterales bacteremia. In this propensity score adjusted, multivariate analysis, they reported no difference in 30-day mortality in 189 patients (n = 57 cefepime vs n = 132 carbapenem) who received cefepime or a carbapenem as definitive therapy for Enterobacterales bacteremia with species that commonly produce AmpC (*Enterobacter* spp, *Serratia* spp, *C freundii, Providencia* spp. and *Morganella morganii*).[14] Despite these encouraging results, it is important to note that these data are from small studies in adults and to consider the impact of different MICs— the first study included primarily cefepime MICs of 1 μg/mL or less, whereas the second study did not report MICs. There remains concern that an inoculum effect may result in increasing MICs. Specifically, cefepime MICs have been reported in vitro to greatly increase (eg, from 1 μg/mL to >256 μg/mL) in the setting of high inocula (10^7 cfu/mL) of AmpC-producing *K pneumoniae*.[16]

Although fluoroquinolones are not directly affected by AmpC production, coresistance is possible. When organisms are susceptible to fluoroquinolones, they have been shown to be an effective option for AmpC-producing Enterobacterales infections. The American Academy of Pediatrics also supports their use in the treatment of a multidrug-resistant organism or where they are the only oral option for treatment.[17] One of the first case series to report the use of ciprofloxacin for sepsis in infants was a report of 6 preterm neonates (24–29 weeks gestational age) with *Enterobacter cloacae* sepsis. Bacteremia resolved in all of the infants.[18] There are very limited data comparing fluoroquinolones to beta-lactams for serious AmpC infections. One recent retrospective review comparing fluoroquinolone versus beta-lactam definitive therapy in AmpC-producing Enterobacterales bacteremia in adults did not demonstrate a significant difference in clearance, mortality, or readmission between the 2 groups. The study did, however, report a nonstatistically significant but numerically longer average duration of therapy (12 days vs 8 days) when a fluoroquinolone was used.[19]

In summary, carbapenems remain an option for serious AmpC-producing Entero-bacterales. The newer agents cefiderocol and ceftazidime–avibactam may be effective, but there are limited data for these infections in pediatric patients at this time. Other options that can be considered as carbapenem-sparing agents include fluoroquinolones, cefepime, and possibly piperacillin–tazobactam. Most would reserve them for low inoculum infections with sensitive organisms and low MICs (important dosing considerations discussed elsewhere in this article); cefepime seems to be the most promising option for bacteremia with sensitive organisms. As discussed elsewhere in this article, there are significant pharmacokinetic differences in children, so it is crucial, in pediatric patients especially, to consider if the agent is reaching pharmacodynamic targets.

EXTENDED SPECTRUM BETA-LACTAMASES

Extended spectrum beta-lactamases (ESBLs) include TEM-3, SHV-2, and CTX-M and are most commonly reported in E coli and Klebsiella spp.[6] Data from a meta-analysis of studies published from 1996 through 2013 that included pediatric patients outside of the United States with laboratory-confirmed bloodstream infections reported an overall 9% prevalence of ESBL-producing organisms with a 2.3% annual increase over the study period. Cases were more common in neonatal patients with an ESBL prevalence of 11% compared with 5% in pediatric patients more than 28 days old. There were also significant differences in ESBL prevalence by region: 44% Asia/India, 21% Asia, 17% Africa, 9% Europe, 5% Oceania, and 4% South America (no studies from North America).[20] Data in North America, where the ESBL prevalence is much lower, are limited, but Logan and colleagues[21,22] reported the types of ESBLs identified in resistant Enterobacterales isolates from pediatric patients from 2011 to 2016 at 3 Chicago hospitals. Of 356 suspected or confirmed ESBL-producing isolates, 68% carried a bla_{CTX-M} gene, whereas 10.7% carried only $bla_{TEM-ESBL}$ or $bla_{SHV-ESBL}$ genes. Of 38 isolates with only TEM- or SHV-type ESBL resistance, 34.2% were also resistant to fluoroquinolones, 44.7% were resistant to gentamicin, 52.6% were resistant to tobramycin, and 44.7% were resistant to trimethoprim–sulfamethoxazole. Also concerning was that 58% were resistant to 3 or more classes of antibiotics.[22]

Clinical debate continues regarding the need for ESBL testing as part of clinical management. Neither the Clinical and Laboratory Standards Institute (CLSI) nor the European Committee on Antimicrobial Susceptibility Testing recommend ESBL testing, but instead rely on lowered MIC susceptibility breakpoints, with the assumption that ESBL-producing isolates will be reported as resistant.[23,24] Recently, data from a large clinical trial provides evidence that the recognition of ESBL-producing organisms remains clinically relevant, because noncarbapenem beta-lactam treatment failures have been seen, even when using antibiotics susceptible in vitro for these infections in adults.[25]

Carbapenems are the gold standard for treatment of infections caused by ESBL-producing Enterobacterales (ESBL-E). In recent years, carbapenem-sparing options have been evaluated in adults; however, studies comparing treatment options for ESBL-E infections in pediatrics are scarce. One of the most important adult studies was published in 2018, the MERINO trial, in which Harris and colleagues reported a 30-day mortality rate of 12.3% in 188 patients who received piperacillin–tazobactam (4.5 g every 6 hours) compared with a 3.7% rate in 191 patients treated with meropenem (1 g every 8 hours) for ceftriaxone nonsusceptible E coli and Klebsiella spp. bloodstream infections.[25] It is important to note that the dosing for piperacillin–tazobactam was the adult maximum dose, whereas the dosing of meropenem in the study, 1 g every 8 hours, is below the recommended dosing for systemic ESBL-E infections in adults, which is 2 g every 8 hours.[26] Despite the difference in the dosing, a subanalysis demonstrated a less pronounced difference in mortality in organisms with a lower MIC for piperacillin–tazobactam.[27] Most recently, in a study of nonbacteremic urinary tract infections, including pyelonephritis, caused by ESBL-E there was no significant difference in recurrence, resolution of symptoms at 7 days, or mortality within 30 days between groups treated with a carbapenem or piperacillin–tazobactam.[28] Therefore, piperacillin–tazobactam may be an option for nonbacteremic ESBL-E infections, particularly urinary tract infections, but carbapenems are preferred for ESBL-E bacteremia and other serious infections.

Additional studies evaluating cefepime instead of a carbapenem for ESBL-E bloodstream infections have revealed trends toward worse outcomes in patients treated with cefepime.[29,30] Wang and colleagues[31] evaluated 14-day mortality in patients 12 years of age and older (the number of pediatric patients included was not reported) with ESBL-E bacteremia who received either cefepime (1–2 g every 8 hours) or a carbapenem (ertapenem 1 g every 24 hours, imipenem–cilastatin 0.5 g every 6 hours, and meropenem 1 g every 8 hours) and found a trend toward worse outcomes in the cefepime group (41% vs 20%; hazard ratio, 2.87; 95% confidence interval, 0.88–9.41). Five of the 7 patients treated with cefepime who died had bacteremia with organisms with cefepime MICs of 4 μg/mL, which lies within the CLSI susceptible dose-dependent range for Enterobacterales.[31] Therefore, evidence continues to suggest that cefepime should not be used for infections caused by ESBL-E.

Ceftazidime–avibactam and cefiderocol have reported high activity against ESBL-E.[32–34] Specifically for ceftazidime–avibactam, 1 study reported a greater than 99% susceptibility among 8461 ESBL-producing isolates from pediatric patients and another reported $MIC_{50/90}$ of 0.12 μg/mL and 0.25 μg/mL, respectively.[32,33] Importantly, although ESBL-E are susceptible to ceftazidime–avibactam and cefiderocol, they are last-resort agents that should be reserved for those infections where other agents, including carbapenems, are not options.

CARBAPENEMASES

Carbapenemases are one of the most concerning beta-lactamase resistance types. The most prevalent carbapenemase is the *K pneumoniae* carbapenemase (KPC). Logan and colleagues[35] reported that a history of multidrug-resistant organisms (i.e., resistant to ≥3 antibiotic classes) and recurrent infections were factors associated with pediatric KPC-producing organisms (n = 18) in Chicago between 2008 to 2014.[35]

In recent years, ceftazidime–avibactam, meropenem–vaborbactam, and imipenem–relebactam have taken over as the drugs of choice for systemic infections with KPC-producing organisms.[26] Ceftazidime–avibactam is preferred in pediatric patients because it has the most published data and is approved by the US Food and Drug Administration (FDA) for use in this population. It is important to note that these agents should be considered over traditional therapies (e.g., colistin, high-dose prolonged infusion meropenem), because they have shown mortality benefit in adults.[36,37] Additionally, cefiderocol is also approved for treatment of KPC-producing infections. The pediatric case reports using these newer agents are summarized in **Table 1**.[38–50]

Oxacillinase (OXA) carbapenemases hydrolyze oxacillin and carbapenems and are generally not inhibited by clavulanic acid.[6] The clinically relevant OXA enzymes are most frequently isolated from *Acinetobacter* spp., with the exception of OXA-48, which is most frequently isolated from *K pneumoniae*.[51] Treatment studies of OXA

Table 1
Pediatric case reports and series for multidrug-resistant infections using newer therapies[38-50]

Reference	Resistance	Patients	Infection	Directed Therapies
Iosifidis et al.,[38] 2019	Carbapenem-resistant *Klebsiella* species	8 patients (13 d–4.5 years old)	7/8 possible/proven bloodstream infection	Ceftazidime–avibactam doses of either 25 or 50 mg/kg q8h
Rodriguez et al.,[39] 2018	KPC *Serratia marcescens*	16 years old	Appendicitis and abscess	Ceftazidime–avibactam 2.5 g over 3 h q8h (with metronidazole, gentamicin that was changed to tigecycline)
Vargas et al.,[40] 2019	*Klebsiella pneumoniae* resistant to all antibiotics except colistin and ceftazidime–avibactam	14 years old	Septic shock	Ceftazidime–avibactam 2.5 g q8h (with linezolid and meropenem)
Rup et al.,[41] 2020	*K pneumoniae* resistant to all antibiotics except fosfomycin	3 years old	Sepsis and pneumonia	Ceftazidime–avibactam 62.5 mg/kg q8h, aztreonam, and fosfomycin
Coskun and Atici,[42] 2020	Carbapenem resistant *K pneumoniae* sensitive only to tigecycline	27-wk gestational age 25 days old	Urinary tract infection	Ceftazidime–avibactam 40 mg/kg ceftazidime and 10 mg/kg avibactam q8h
Yasmin et al.,[43] 2020	New Deli Metallo-beta-lactamase and *K pneumoniae* carbapenemase	4 years old	Bloodstream infection	Ceftazidime–avibactam 50 mg/kg 3 h infusion q8h and aztreonam 50 mg/kg q8h[a]

Study	Organism	Age	Condition	Treatment
Cowart and Ferguson,[44] 2021	Stenotrophomonas	11 years old	Cystic fibrosis	Ceftazidime–avibactam 50 mg/kg (ceftazidime component) over 2 h q8h, aztreonam 66 mg/kg over 4 h q8h, and minocycline 2 mg/kg q12h[b] dosing of ceftazidime–avibactam changed to 200 mg/kg/d initially as q8h but once access available as continuous infusion
Alamarat et al,[45] 2020	ESBL-producing K pneumoniae (0.5 μg/mL) and multidrug-resistant Pseudomonas (4 μg/mL)	15 years old	Chronic osteomyelitis	Cefiderocol 2 g over 3 h q8h (initially with aztreonam but stopped owing to liver issues)
Gainey et al.,[46] 2020	Pan-resistant Achromobacter	10 years old	Cystic fibrosis	Cefiderocol 60 mg/kg over 3 h q8h, meropenem/vaborbactam 2 g over 3 h q8h and bacteriophage therapy
Aitken et al.,[47] 2016	Multidrug resistant P aeruginosa (MIC 6 μg/mL; repeat infection 8 μg/mL)	9 years old	Bloodstream infection in neutropenic patient	Ceftolozane/tazobactam 50 mg/kg (1500 mg) over 3 h q8h[c], tobramycin and ciprofloxacin; repeat infection ceftolozane 40 mg/kg over 3 h q6h

(continued on next page)

Table 1
(continued)

Reference	Resistance	Patients	Infection	Directed Therapies
Zikri and El Masri,[48] 2019	Multidrug-resistant *P aeruginosa* (MIC 3 μg/mL); resistant to all beta-lactams and intermediate to ciprofloxacin, amikacin, and gentamicin, sensitive only to colistin	14 years old	Combined immunodeficiency syndrome diagnosed with septic shock and bilateral bronchopneumonia	Ceftolozane/tazobactam 1000/500 mg (44/22 mg/kg) (infusion time not provided) q8h with amikacin and colistin
Martin-Cazana et al.,[49] 2019	Multidrug resistant *P aeruginosa* (MIC 2 μg/mL) (resistant to ceftazidime, cefepime, aztreonam, fluoroquinolones; meropenem)	5 years old	Endocarditis and persistent bacteremia	Ceftolozane/tazobactam 50 mg/kg over 3 h q8h[d] and tobramycin
Hanretty et al.,[50] 2018	*K pneumoniae* carbapenemase (MIC 0.094 μg/mL)	4 years old	Sepsis	Meropenem/vaborbactam 40 mg/kg over 3 h q6h

[a] Therapeutic drug monitoring (TDM) performed to ensure optimal drug concentrations of 100% T > MIC for ceftazidime and aztreonam, while avibactam remained above 2.5 μg/mL for about 50% of the interval.

[b] TDM performed to achieve goal concentrations.

[c] Concentrations at 1.5, 3, and 5 hours after the start of infusion on day 3 resulted in a calculated half-life of 1.3 hours and trough of 5.2 μg/mL; follow-up levels and calculations was half-life of 1.4 hours and trough of 18.1 μg/mL. The authors considered the difference of achieving 2 times the MIC for the entire dosing interval to be associated with the positive clinical outcome.

[d] For steady-state concentrations maximum concentration was 72.9 ng/mL; the minimum concentration was 2.6 ng/mL.

carbapenemase-producing carbapenem-resistant Enterobacterales (CP-CRE) are limited. Data from a murine thigh model suggest that ceftazidime could be an option for OXA-48.[52] Further, avibactam has activity against OXA-48; importantly, vaborbactam does not.[53,54] Ceftolozane–tazobactam has variable activity against OXA-48.[55] Ceftazidime–avibactam should be considered for the rare infections owing to isolated OXA-48 CP-CRE.[26]

Metallo-beta-lactamases (MBLs) are another group of carbapenemases that have a zinc ion at the active site instead of serine.[56] MBLs are clinically different from the other carbapenemases as they spare aztreonam.[6] Although rare in the United States, MBLs are common throughout Asia and in parts of Africa. MBLs include New Delhi MBLs, Verona integron-encoded MBLs, and imipenemase enzymes.[57] Case reports of treatments of these organisms have been published in pediatric patients (see **Table 1**). In adult patients, ceftazidime–avibactam in combination with aztreonam or cefiderocol is recommended, whereas the combination therapy of ceftazidime–avibactam with aztreonam is preferred in pediatric patients owing to the established dosing and safety of each of these medications in this population.[26] The combination of aztreonam with avibactam is not currently commercially available, but would be sufficient and ideal in these infections.

Although specific therapies directed at individual carbapenemases are described elsewhere in this article, multiple carbapenemases can be coexpressed. For example, a patient's carbapenemase may contain both MBLs and OXA-48.[58,59] In this situation, aztreonam would treat the MBL, but be hydrolyzed by the OXA-48, limiting its usefulness as monotherapy. When a CP-CRE coproduces a serine beta-lactamase and an MBL, the culture and susceptibility results are likely to come back as resistant to both agents. In this instance, E-tests can be stacked to determine if a "zone of hope," or a gradient area of bacterial inhibition, exists to help guide therapy.[60–63]

PUMPS AND PORINS

Efflux pumps and porin proteins are also important mechanisms of resistance in gram-negative organisms. The overexpression of efflux pumps across the cell wall of gram-negative bacteria allows for survival of these organisms by transporting antibiotic out of the cell.[61] For many multidrug-resistant *Pseudomonas aeruginosa* strains, it is thought that a combination of pumps, porins, and other resistance mechanisms result in multidrug resistance.[62,63,64,65] It is important to consider local susceptibilities when targeting therapies against *P aeruginosa* infections. When usual first line agents of ceftazidime, cefepime, piperacillin–tazobactam, or meropenem are not feasible, ceftazidime–avibactam and ceftolozane–tazobactam, have the most evidence in pediatric patients (see **Table 1**).

PEDIATRIC PHARMACOKINETICS AND PHARMACODYNAMICS

Pharmacokinetics describe how the body affects drugs (ie, absorption, distribution, metabolism, elimination), and pharmacodynamics describe how the drug affects the body (ie, response, duration). Although pharmacodynamic goals, such as bacteriostatic versus bactericidal exposures, do not differ based on the age of the patient, the pharmacokinetics (eg, volume of distribution and clearance) do vary significantly among various age populations. In healthy patients the estimated glomerular filtration rate varies significantly based on age. For example, healthy adults aged 30 years have a mean baseline estimated glomerular filtration rate of 100 mL/min/1.73 m^2, which is about 20% slower than children, which can be approximately 127 mL/min/1.73 m^2.[66,67] Because of this difference in clearance, suboptimal exposures are

Table 2
Pharmacokinetic and susceptibility data by antibiotic

Antibiotic	Patients	Pharmacokinetics	Susceptibility breakpoints[23]
Cefepime[77]	2.1 mo–16 y (n = 35)	V_d 0.41 ± 0.2 L/kg; $t_{1/2}$ 1.8 ± 0.6 h	Enterobacterales spp. ≤2 μg/mL (S), 4–8 μg/mL (susceptible dose-dependent range), ≥16 μg/mL (R) P aeruginosa and Acinetobacter spp. ≤8 μg/mL (S), 16 μg/mL (I), ≥32 μg/mL (R)
Piperacillin–tazobactam[82]	0.1–18 y, >2.5 kg (n = 50)	Median V_d 0.33 L/kg (0.21–0.86), median $t_{1/2}$ of 0.9 h (0.15–4.2 h)	Enterobacterales, P aeruginosa and Acinetobacter spp. ≤16/4 μg/mL (S), 32/4–64/4 μg/mL (I), ≥128/4 μg/mL (R)
Ertapenem[87]	3 mo–16 y (n = 83)	V_d 0.21 ± 0.05 L/kg in those <2 y, 0.21 ± 0.06 L/kg in those 2–12 y, 0.17 ± 0.02 L/kg patients >12 y; $t_{1/2}$ 2.9 ± 0.7 h <2 y, 3.0 ± 0.9 h in patients 2–12 y, 4.0 ± 0.8 h >12 y	Enterobacterales ≤0.5 μg/mL (S), 1 μg/mL (I), ≥2 μg/mL (R)
Meropenem[88]	2 mo–12 y (n = 63)	V_d 0.5 ± 0.1 L/kg 2–5 mo, 0.6 ± 0.2 L/kg 6–23 mo, 0.5 ± 0.2 L/kg 2–5 y, 0.4 ± 0.1 L/kg 6–12 y; $t_{1/2}$ 1.6 ± 0.6 h in those 2–5 mo, 1.3 ± 0.4 h 6–23 mo, 1.0 ± 0.4 h 2–5 y, 0.8 ± 0.2 h 6–12 y	Enterobacterales ≤1 μg/mL (S), 2 μg/mL intermediate (I), ≥4 μg/mL (R) P aeruginosa and Acinetobacter spp. ≤2 μg/mL (S), 4 μg/mL (I), ≥8 μg/mL (R)
Cefiderocol	No published pediatric data	No data	Enterobacterales, P aeruginosa, and Acinetobacter spp. ≤4 μg/mL (S), 8 μg/mL (I), and ≥16 μg/mL (R)
Ceftazidime–avibactam[94]	6.5–17.3 y (n = 16)	Ceftazidime $t_{1/2}$ 1.6 h (0.9–1.8 h) in those 6–11 y, 1.7 h (0.9–2.8 h) 12–17.3 y Avibactam $t_{1/2}$ 1.7 h (0.9–2.0 h) 6–11 y, 1.6 h (0.9–2.8 h) 12–17.3 y	Enterobacterales and P aeruginosa ≤8/4 (S) and ≥16/4 (R)

Drug	Population	PK data	Breakpoints
Ceftolozane–tazobactam[97]	Enrolled patients 7 d to < 18 y (n=37)	Ceftolozane mean V_d ranges for pediatric ages V_d for pediatric ages 0.27 - 0.33 L/kg for 2y–<18 y; 0.28-0.34 L/kg for 3 mo–<2 y; 0.34-0.39 7 d - < 3mo;mean t 1/2 ranges for pediatric ages 1.3 - 1.5 h 2 y–<18y; 1.3 - 1.6 for 3 mo–<2y; 1.7-3.1 h for 7 d - <3 mo.Tazobactam mean V_d for pediatric ages 0.48 - 0.74 L/kg for 2y–<18 y; 0.42-0.57 L/kg for 3 mo–<2 y; 0.34-0.67 7 d - < 3mo;mean t 1/2 for pediatric ages 0.54 - 0.77 h for 2y–<18 y; 0.54-0.81 h for 3 mo–<2y; 0.88-3.0 h for 7 d - < 3mo;	Enterobacterales ≤2/4 (S), 4/4 (I) and ≥8/4 (R); P aeruginosa ≤4/4 (S), 8/4 (I), ≥16/4 (R)
Meropenem–vaborbactam[50]	4-year-old boy	V_d 0.59 L/kg, $t_{1/2}$ 0.5 h	Enterobacterales ≤4/8 (S), 8/8 (I), ≥16/8 (R)
Imipenem/relebactam	No published pediatric data	no data	Enterobacterales[a] ≤1/4 (S), 2/4 (I), ≥4/4 (R); P aeruginosa ≤2/4 (S), 4/4 (I), ≥8/4 (R)
Ciprofloxacin[111]	1 d–24 y (n = 37)	Mean $t_{1/2}$ 16.6 h (10.5–24.5 h) in patients 0–28 d, 6.16 h (3.24–12.8 h) in patients 28 d–23 mo, 4.16 h (1.82–19.9 h) in those 2–11 y, 3.32 h (2.40–4.89 h) in patients 12–24 y	Enterobacterales ≤0.25 µg/mL (S), 0.5 µg/mL (I), ≥1 µg/mL (R); P aeruginosa ≤0.5 µg/mL (S), 1 µg/mL (I), ≥2 µg/mL (R)
Levofloxacin (IV)[110]	6 mo–16 y (n = 80)	V_d 1.56 ± 0.30 L/kg patients 0.5–2 y, 1.50 ± 0.21 L/kg in patients 2–5 y, 1.57 ± 0.44 L/kg patients 5–10 y, 1.44 ± 0.35 L/kg patients 10–12 y, 1.56 ± 0.53 h patients 12–16 y $t_{1/2}$ 4.1 ± 1.3 h in those 0.5–2 y, 4.0 ± 0.8 h in 2–5 y, 4.8 ± 0.8 h in those 5–10 y, 5.4 ± 0.8 h 10–12 y, 6.0 ± 2.1 h 12–16 y	Enterobacterales ≤0.5 µg/mL (S), 1 µg/mL (I), ≥2 µg/mL (R); P aeruginosa ≤1 µg/mL (S), 2 µg/mL (I), ≥4 µg/mL (R)

(I), intermediate; (R), resistant; (S), susceptible; $t_{1/2}$, half-life; V_d, volume of distribution.

a These breakpoints do not apply to Morganella spp., Proteus spp., and Providencia spp.

possible if pediatric patients with normal renal function are provided the same or proportional doses as adult patients. Therefore, pharmacodynamic dosing for antibiotics need to be considered differently for pediatric patients.

Antibiotic pharmacodynamics are divided into 2 major categories: time dependent or concentration dependent. Time-dependent antibiotics are those for which antimicrobial activity is related to the time the free antibiotic concentration remains above the MIC, usually expressed as %fT>MIC. Traditionally, bactericidal pharmacodynamic goals have been about 40% for carbapenems and 50% to 60% for cephalosporins and penicillins.[68] Some recent studies suggest that up to 100% fT>MIC and potentially 4 to 6 times the MIC at the trough is needed for serious gram-negative infections, including bacteremia.[69–72] Data are scarce for these higher goals, but these targets likely require continuous infusions combined with therapeutic drug monitoring. Importantly, when considering different infusion regimens for acute infections, it is recommended that these continuous or prolonged infusions begin after an initial traditional dose (eg, a loading dose) to ensure there is no initial delay in achieving therapeutic concentrations.

Often, limited attention has been paid to concurrent use of beta-lactamase inhibitors. Initial evaluations suggest that tazobactam requires 80% to 85%.[73] The goal for tazobactam is estimated to be about 44% and 35% f%T>MIC of 0.5 µg/mL and 1 µg/mL, respectively, for bactericidal activity.[74] Avibactam is unique; it is a reversible beta-lactamase inhibitor, allowing it to be reused throughout the dosing interval, but studies suggest that for full efficacy it needs to remain above a threshold concentration 0.25 to 0.50 µg/mL for the entire dosing interval.[75] Therefore, to optimize these agents, one should strongly consider the use of prolonged or continuous infusions.

PROLONGED INFUSIONS

Clinical outcomes in pediatric patients for optimized pharmacodynamic therapy regimens are limited. Recently, a study was conducted comparing the outcomes of standard (n = 293) versus prolonged (n = 258) infusions in pediatric patients who received cefepime (50 mg/kg every 8 hours, max 2000 mg/dose), piperacillin-tazobactam (100 ,g/kg every 8 hours, maximum of 4000 mg/dose of piperacillin component), or meropenem (20–40 mg/kg every 8 hours, maximum 2000 mg/dose).[76] The prolonged infusions were 3 hours for meropenem and 4 hours for cefepime and piperacillin–tazobactam, whereas standard infusions were 0.25 to 0.50 hours. The indication for antibiotics was not assessed for the majority of patients in this study; only 21 patients had gram-negative bacteremia. No differences were reported for duration of treatment or blood culture clearance. All-cause mortality was not significantly different for the whole population (1.2% prolonged vs 3.8% standard; $P = .054$), but did meet statistical significance for those in the critical care unit (2.1% prolonged vs 19.6% standard; $P = .006$).[76] Importantly, this study is the first within the pediatric population to demonstrate clinical improvement in outcomes using pharmacodynamically optimized dosing in children, which mirrors extensive adult data.

Beta-Lactams

Cefepime
Pediatric pharmacokinetics and susceptibility data for cefepime are reported in **Table 2**.[77] Kohlmann and colleagues[78] evaluated the MIC distributions for cefepime for both wild-type Enterobacterales and AmpC derepressed mutants. Specifically, wild-type E cloacae complex had an $MIC_{50/90}$ of 0.064 µg/mL and 2 µg/mL, and the mutants had an $MIC_{50/90}$ of 0.25 µg/mL and 8 µg/mL.[78] In adult patients, dosing

specific for the susceptible dose-dependent category is defined for cefepime. Concerningly, as discussed by Nielsen and colleagues,[79] the CLSI does not provide any guidance for pediatric patients. Therefore, it is imperative to understand the expected pediatric pharmacodynamic exposures.

Monte Carlo simulations suggest that higher doses, more frequent administration, and extended infusions may be necessary to reach pharmacodynamic targets for cefepime, especially when treating infections caused by organisms with higher MICs. A 5000-patient Monte Carlo simulation in a population of 2- and 12-year-old children modeled various doses and infusions of cefepime with a pharmacodynamic target of at least 90% of simulations achieving 50%fT>MIC.[80] For 150 mg/kg/day of cefepime, continuous infusions reached the target for MICs up to 16 μg/mL, every 8-hour dosing met this goal for MICs up to 8 μg/mL as a 3-hour infusion or for MICs up to 4 μg/mL for 0.5-hour infusions. Importantly, when simulating 100 mg/kg/day of cefepime the target attainment was much lower, meeting goals for continuous infusion at MICs of up to 8 μg/mL, 3-hour infusion every 8 hours for MICs up to 2 μg/mL, and a 0.5-hour infusion every 8 hours for MIC of 0.5 μg/mL.[80] Another study evaluated cefepime 30 mg/kg or 50 mg/kg given every 8 hours or every 12 hours as an 0.5-hour infusion or every 8 hours a 3-hour infusion for Enterobacterales with a median age of 1 month (including preterm and term neonates).[81] Assuming a 90% target for their goal of at least 60%fT>MIC, preterm neonates met targets for MICs at 8 μg/mL for both doses every 12 hours as 0.5-hour infusions, whereas in term neonates this goal was met only for the higher dose regimen. For those older than 30 days, exposures dropped significantly and even at a 50 mg/kg/dose prolonged infusion for 3 hours was needed every 8 hours to achieve 90% target attainment. For MICs of 4 μg/mL, at least a 90% chance of target attainment was achieved by 50 mg/kg/dose every 6 hours as a 0.5-hour infusion or every 8 hours administered as a 3-hour infusion.[81]

Based on the data from these models and the clinical outcome data including cefepime, doses of 150 mg/kg/day every 8 hours as 0.5-hour infusions may reach traditional pharmacodynamic targets for MICs of up to approximately 4 μg/mL. In cases of critical illness or when increased MICs are suspected or confirmed, the use of 150 mg/kg/day as a continuous or prolonged 3-hour infusion every 8 hours is preferred.

Piperacillin–tazobactam

The pediatric pharmacokinetics for piperacillin–tazobactam are summarized in **Table 2**.[82] In Denmark, 165 P aeruginosa isolates from pediatric patients with cancer (from 2004 to 2013) had a MIC$_{50/90}$ distribution for piperacillin–tazobactam of 2 μg/mL and 4 μg/mL.[83] There have been multiple pharmacodynamic evaluations for piperacillin–tazobactam. Cies and colleagues[84] performed a 5000-patient Monte Carlo analysis simulating 1- to 6 year-old boys. The study assessed the likelihood of at least 90% of simulations reaching goal 50%fT>MIC for piperacillin.[84] Piperacillin at 50 mg/kg every 4 hours, 80 mg/kg every 8 hours, and 100 mg/kg every 6 hours at various infusion durations were studied. Only the 400 mg/kg/day every 6 hours or as a continuous infusion achieved goal exposures for MICs of 16 μg/mL; no dosing resulted in goal exposures for higher MICs.[84] Another Monte Carlo simulation (n = 12; 9 months and 11 years old) used 5040 simulations with a similar target (50%fT>MIC).[85] They reported 4-hour infusions of 80 mg/kg and 100 mg/kg every 8 hours or 0.5- to 3-hour infusions of the same dose modeled every 6 hours all achieved pharmacodynamic goals at least 90% of simulations.[85] A third Monte Carlo study (6000 patient) also reported a continuous or 3- to 4-hour infusion with dosing regimens of 300 mg/kg/day for patients with normal renal clearances, and 400 mg/kg/day for patients with augmented renal clearance, were needed to achieve traditional pharmacodynamic goals at an MIC of 16 µg/mL.[86] This study suggested that the 4-hour infusions may produce adequate exposures for intermediate MICs of 32 µg/mL in those with normal and augmented renal function.[82] The most recent study (1000 patient simulation) modeled patients 2 months to 6 years of age with 480 mg/kg/d as 3-hour infusions every 6 hours, 4-hour infusions of 390 mg/kg/day every 8 hours, or continuous infusions of 300 or 400 mg/kg/d. All simulated dosing regimens were predicted to achieve at least 90% likelihood of attaining 50%fT>MIC at the susceptibility breakpoint MIC of 16 µg/mL.[86]

The current data suggest that traditional doses of 240 mg/kg/day of piperacillin–tazobactam are not likely to be sufficient for treatment of gram-negative infections in children when these bacteria have MICs that approach the breakpoints and that continuous or extended infusions of at least 3-hours with doses of 300 to 400 mg/kg/day should be considered for serious gram-negative infections, especially in institutions where MICs routinely approach the breakpoint or are unknown.

Carbapenems

There are 3 carbapenems that are considered for use in pediatric patients: ertapenem, meropenem, and imipenem. The pharmacokinetics of these are summarized in **Table 2**.[87,88] Upon review of the literature no pediatric pharmacodynamic evaluations have been found for ertapenem, and dose escalation of imipenem raises concerns for seizures. Therefore, the rest of this section focuses on meropenem. The $MIC_{50/90}$ for ESBL producing Enterobacterales to meropenem was 0.03/0.03 mg/L and the$MIC_{50/90}$ for P aeruginosa are 0.5/8 mg/L in pediatric patients.[33]

There have been multiple Monte Carlo evaluations for meropenem dosing in pediatrics. The first was conducted by Courter and colleagues,[80] where doses were simulated for a 5000-patient population of 2- and 12-year-old children. In this study doses of 20 mg/kg and 40 mg/kg every 8 hours as 0.5-hour infusions would only have 90% likelihood of reaching targets of 40% T>MIC for MICs up to 1 µg/mL and 2 µg/mL, respectively.[80] Three-hour infusions (20 and 40 mg/kg) were needed to meet target goals for higher MICs of 4 µg/mL (20 mg/kg) and 8 µg/mL (40 mg/kg).[80] The next study used meropenem concentrations and associated pharmacokinetics from 14 pediatric patients with a median age of 6 years. The data from these patients were then incorporated into a 10,000-patient Monte Carlo evaluation that targeted MICs of 1 µg/mL and 4 µg/mL as the susceptibility breakpoints for Enterobacterales and P aeruginosa, respectively.[89] In this study, they reported that meropenem doses of 20 mg/kg and 40 mg/kg every 8 hours were not expected to achieve goal pharmacodynamic targets (at either breakpoint) and that 20 mg/kg as a 3-hour infusion would be predicted to achieve a 90% likelihood of bactericidal goal even at the 4 µg/mL target.[89] The final simulation used common organisms in Japanese survey and their MICs (vast majority <1 µg/mL) combined with pharmacokinetic data from 40 pediatric Japanese patients with a mean age 6.6 ± 4.1 years receiving 19.2 ± 8.2 mg/kg over 0.5 or 1 hour.[90] The researchers simulated a 10,000-patient Monte Carlo simulation for weights of 10 kg, 20 kg, and 30 kg. When reviewing the data with goals of 90% target attainment, regimens modeled only achieved greater than 90% target attainment for E coli with an MIC_{90} of 0.03 µg/mL. For all other organisms, they reported a lesser likelihood of target attainment. For example, for P aeruginosa (MIC_{90} 1 µg/mL) the percent target attainment was 76% to 87% for the 10- to 30-kg patients modeled, even when 40 mg/kg every 8 hours was evaluated.[90]

When evaluating the clinical outcome and simulation evidence, traditional meropenem dosing with standard infusion may provide effective exposures. Prolonged infusions, potentially with higher dosing, should be considered if higher MICs are likely, such as those needed for *P aeruginosa* and in cases of critical illness.

Cefiderocol

Cefiderocol acts as a siderophore, which binds ferric (free) iron, allowing passage of the drug across the bacterial cell wall to exhibit bactericidal activity by inhibiting cell wall synthesis via penicillin binding proteins. Cefiderocol is only FDA approved in adults. Data from other beta-lactams were incorporated into a Monte Carlo evaluation to determine initial study doses in pediatric patients. Using targets of 75% $fT>MIC$ for MICs up to 4 µg/mL to ensure at least 90% of patients the following doses were proposed for clinical study: gestational age less than 32 weeks, 30 mg/kg if less than 2 months or 40 mg/kg if 2 to less than 3 months and 32 weeks gestational age or greater, 40 mg/kg if less than 2 months or 60 mg/kg if 2 to less than 3 months. A dose of 60 mg/kg with a max of 2000 mg is being used for patients 3 months to less than 18 years.[91] These doses identified in the model are being evaluated every 8 hours (with infusion rates of 1 hour in those < 3 months old or over 3 hours in older infants, children, and adolescents) in a pharmacokinetic study to confirm the model.[91,92] The MIC_{90} for cefiderocol against Enterobacterales, *Klebsiella* spp., *E coli*, *Serratia* spp., and *P aeruginosa* were 0.5 µg/mL, whereas the MIC_{90} for *Citrobacter* spp. and *A baumanii* were 1 µg/mL and 2 µg/mL, respectively, in a large 2015/2016 surveillance study from laboratories across North America and Europe.[93]

There have only been 2 cases describing the use of cefiderocol in pediatric patients as included in **Table 1**.[45,46] At this point, cefiderocol should only be considered for a pediatric patient when no other therapy is available or as a part of a clinical trial.

New Beta-Lactam and Beta-Lactamase Inhibitors

Ceftazidime–avibactam

Ceftazidime–avibactam, a third-generation cephalosporin combined with a beta-lactamase inhibitor, is FDA approved in pediatric patients 3 months old and greater for complicated intra-abdominal and complicated urinary tract infections.[53] It is effective against KPC and some other CP-CREs. In the ceftazidime–avibactam phase I trial, all doses were administered over 2 hours and goals of 50% $fT>MIC$ for MICs of 8µg/mL and with a threshold concentration of 1 µg/mL were used. The single dose population pharmacokinetic evaluation study reported ceftazidime–avibactam doses of 50 to 12.5 mg/kg up to 2000 to 500 mg were expected to reach pharmacodynamic goals in at least 90% of patients within each cohort.[94] According to a surveillance study from 2016 to 2019, for children less than 18 years old, the ceftazidime–avibactam MIC_{90} and MIC_{50} for Enterobacterales was 0.25 µg/mL and 0.12 µg/mL.[95]

In addition to the clinical trials, ceftazidime–avibactam has the most case reports/series of any of the newer agents in pediatric patients (see **Table 1**). In these reports, it is often unclear if the dose provided is based on the ceftazidime component or the total product. In general, most would use a ceftazidime dose of 50 mg/kg or a total product dose of 62.5 mg/kg as a prolonged infusion and given every 8 hours and it is thought that is what has likely been reported (see **Table 1**).[38–44]

Ceftolozane–tazobactam

Ceftolozane–tazobactam, a fifth-generation cephalosporin/beta-lactamase inhibitor combination, has activity against ESBL producing organisms and, most important, multidrug-resistant *P aeruginosa*. Recent MIC epidemiology data have reported ranges of $MIC_{50/90}$ of 0.25/0.5 µg/mL to 2 µg/mL for Enterobacterales and 0.5/1 µg/mL for *P aeruginosa*.[33,96]

A pediatric phase I study followed by a population pharmacokinetic analysis were performed for ceftolozane–tazobactam.[97,98] In the phase I trial, multiple dosing regimens were included and adapted based on the cohort and initial few patient levels.[97] These data were then incorporated into a population pharmacokinetic analysis to mimic adult exposures as much as possible and to ensure 90% of the simulations attaining $fT>MIC$ of 30% for ceftolozane up to an MIC of 4 μg/mL and tazobactam percent time above the concentration threshold (1 μg/mL) of 20%.[98] Phase II trials for intra-abdominal infections and urinary tract infections use 20 to 10 mg/kg dosing of ceftolozane–tazobactam up to a max of 1000 to 500 mg and administering the maximum dose to all patients 12 years of age and older with all doses administered over 1 hour.[98] It is currently uncertain if this pharmacodynamic parameter of 30% $fT>MIC$ for ceftolozane is sufficient, because at least 1 model suggests that a goal of 40% $fT>MIC$ may be optimal for ceftolozane.[99] Further, similar to adults, double doses (eg, 40–20 mg/kg up to 2000–1000 mg maximum) are likely needed when treating pulmonary infections as only about 50% of ceftolozane reaches epithelial lung fluid.[100]

Several case reports describing the use of ceftolozane–tazobactam in pediatric patients have been published, demonstrating good outcomes with its use (see **Table 1**).[47–49] Dosing and pharmacodynamic goals continue to evolve. At least one patient was suspected of having treatment relapse did improve with a higher daily dose divided every 6 hours.[48] Until more data are available, when the drug is used, beginning dosing at the clinical trial dose of 20 to 10 mg/dose every 8 hours can be considered, but only with therapeutic drug monitoring with doses adjusted as appropriate.

Meropenem–vaborbactam

A phase I study evaluating the pharmacokinetic and safety profile of meropenem–vaborbactam, a carbapenem/beta-lactamase inhibitor, in pediatric patients is underway, which uses a single prolonged infusion (3 h) dose of 40 to 40 mg/kg or for those greater than 33 kg to 60 mg/kg (max of 2000–2000 mg).[101] To date, there has only been 1 published case of a pediatric patient receiving meropenem-vaborbactam (see **Table 1**). That report was for a 4-year-old patient with sepsis owing to KPC-producing K pneumoniae. As stated by the authors of the case, the meropenem half-life and volume of distribution were as expected in a critically ill child. Luckily, the MIC of 0.094 μg/mL made it easy to achieve any pharmacodynamic goals (eg, 40%$fT>MIC$, 100%$fT>MIC$) and the patient improved clinically.[50] Similar to other agents, limited data are available for meropenem–vaborbactam in pediatric patients. In cases where no other options are available, doses similar to meropenem as prolonged infusions (20–40 mg/kg every 8 hours over 3 hours) might be considered, with therapeutic drug monitoring.

Imipenem–relebactam

A global study evaluating pediatric isolates reported 99.7% E coli, 97.7% E cloacae, 95.4% K pneumoniae, and 94.2% P aeruginosa isolates were susceptible to imipenem–relebactam.[102] Phase I and II studies determining the pharmacokinetic and safety profile of imipenem–relebactam in pediatric patients are ongoing.[103,104] The dose being used in these trials is 15 to 7.5 mg/kg imipenem–relebactam, up to a maximum of 500 to 250 mg given every 6 hours.[103] There are currently no pediatric cases reported in the literature using this antibiotic.

Fluoroquinolones

Fluoroquinolones are another useful option in resistant gram negative infections, but in contrast with the aforementioned beta-lactam antibiotics, they have concentration-dependent antibacterial activity, with and area under the curve at 24 hours (AUC_{24})/ MIC$\geq$125 being the minimum bactericidal pharmacodynamic goal for gram-negative organisms.[105] The CLSI susceptibility breakpoints have recently been lowered for both for ciprofloxacin and levofloxacin.[106] The new breakpoints are included in **Table 2**. CLSI data from 2011 to 2013 found for Enterobacterales the MIC_{50} was 0.03 μg/mL or less for ciprofloxacin and 0.12 μg/mL or less for levofloxacin, and for *P aeruginosa* the MIC_{50} was 0.12 μg/mL for ciprofloxacin and 0.5 μg/mL for levoflox-acin.[107] Even with these lower breakpoints, it is very difficult to achieve minimal AUC_{24}/MIC $\geq$125 goal. The minimum AUC_{24} that would be needed even for MICs of 0.25 μg/mL is 32 μg*h/mL, and exposures of 62.5 μg*h/mL and 125 μg*h/mL are needed for higher MICs of 0.5 and 1 μg/mL.

Patients in previous clinical trials (median age, 5.6 years) received a median of cip-rofloxacin 30 mg/kg/day intravenously divided every 8 or 12 hours.[108] The data from these patients were incorporated into a model to determine doses needed to achieve $AUC/_{24}$MIC goal of 125 or greater at least 80% of the time. Dosing was modeled separately for patients with and without sickle cell disease owing to increased clearance and hyperfiltration of renally cleared drugs owing to sickle cell nephropathy.[108] Overall, the authors suggested that doses as low as 10 mg/kg/day would be effective for MICs of 0.06 μg/mL, but that doses used in practice of 30 mg/kg/d would only be sufficient for MICs of 0.25 μg/mL in patients without sickle cell disease who were either less than 6 years old or more than 12 years old. Further, doses higher than have been tested to be safe (37.5 mg/kg/d–90 mg/kg/d) would be needed to achieve pharmaco-dynamic goals for those with sickle cell disease and MICs of 0.25 μg/mL or for any patient with MICs of 0.5 μg/mL or higher.[108] Finally, this study does not mention or clearly account for free drug concentration/protein binding. Therefore, it seems that this study is modeling the AUC_{24}/MIC and not the fAUC. Another study has looked to evaluate the pharmacodynamic exposure of ciprofloxacin in pediatric patients. Specifically, it included 134 pediatric patients (median age, 5.6 years) with acute lymphoblastic leukemia throughout their chemotherapy courses. Overall, 81% of patients achieved goal exposures for MICs of 0.125 μg/mL, although this decrease to 18% and 0% for MICs of 0.25 μg/mL and 0.5 μg/mL, respectively. Interestingly, the ciprofloxacin drug exposures were different in the different phases of cancer therapies (AUC range, 16–29 μg*h/mL).[109]

There are also a few models looking at levofloxacin pharmacodynamic exposures in children. The first included 3 pediatric pharmacokinetic studies for a total of 80 children with concentration data (6 months to 16 years). The goal was to produce similar exposures to those used in adult trials (especially 500 mg/day dosing).[110] The authors predicted exposures similar to those achieved in adult trials (adult AUC with 500 mg/ day 54.6 μg*h/mL) in pediatric patients with doses of 10 mg/kg twice daily in those 6 months to less than 5 years (AUC_{24} of 58.4 μg*h/mL) and 10 mg/kg once daily (max 500 mg; AUC_{24} of 38.4 μg*h/mL) in those 5 to less than 10 years of age and (AUC_{24} of 54.8 μg*h/mL) 10 to 16 years old.[110] Based on these data, this dose would be expected to achieve exposures to reach pharmacodynamic targets for MICs including 0.25 μg/mL. For higher MICs, a higher dose would be needed.

Overall in pediatric patients, even with lower breakpoints, it is important to understand the importance of dosing and local MICs to be able to estimate if patients may be able to achieve adequate exposures with safe dosing. Other considerations relevant to fluoroquinolone use include the reduction in absorption by certain dietary items (dairy, calcium, multivitamins) and administration via tube feedings. These additional factors should be considered when evaluating optimal fluoroquinolone exposure in pediatric patients.

SUMMARY

When treating the increasing number of resistant gram-negative infections in pediatric patients, it is important to understand both the resistance mechanisms of the organism as well as the pharmacodynamic properties of the drug to optimize dosing. Knowing the mechanism of resistance can guide the treating clinician in the best way to overcome the resistance (prolonged infusion, higher or more frequent dosing, agent choice, or multidrug therapy).

DISCLOSURE

Dr J. Girotto is a consultant for Lexi-Comp. Drs J. Girotto and S. Basco have no other potential or actual financial or commercial conflicts of interest.

REFERENCES

1. Haeusler GM, Mechinaud F, Daley AJ, et al. Antibiotic-resistant gram-negative bacteremia in pediatric oncology patients–risk factors and outcomes. Pediatr Infect Dis J 2013;32(7):723–6.
2. Logan LK, Renschler JP, Gandra S, et al. Carbapenem-resistant enterobacteriaceae in children, United States, 1999-2012. Emerg Infect Dis 2015;21(11): 2014–21.
3. Weiner-Lastinger LM, Abner S, Benin AL, et al. Antimicrobial-resistant pathogens associated with pediatric healthcare-associated infections: summary of data reported to the National Healthcare Safety Network, 2015-2017. Infect Control Hosp Epidemiol 2020;41(1):19–30.
4. Lake JG, Weiner LM, Milstone AM, et al. Pathogen distribution and antimicrobial resistance among pediatric healthcare-associated infections reported to the national healthcare safety network, 2011-2014. Infect Control Hosp Epidemiol 2018;39(1):1–11.
5. Weiss SL, Peters MJ, Alhazzani W, et al. Surviving sepsis campaign international guidelines for the management of septic shock and sepsis-associated organ dysfunction in children. Pediatr Crit Care Med 2020;21(2):e52–106.
6. Bush K, Jacoby GA. Updated functional classification of beta-lactamases. Antimicrob Agents Chemother 2010;54(3):969–76.
7. Jacoby GA. AmpC beta-lactamases. Clin Microbiol Rev 2009;22(1):161–82.
8. Tamma PD, Girdwood SC, Gopaul R, et al. The use of cefepime for treating AmpC β-lactamase-producing Enterobacteriaceae. Clin Infect Dis 2013;57(6): 781–8.
9. Pérez-Pérez FJ, Hanson ND. Detection of plasmid-mediated AmpC beta-lactamase genes in clinical isolates by using multiplex PCR. J Clin Microbiol 2002;40(6):2153–62.
10. Chen HL, Lu JH, Wang HH, et al. Clinical analysis of Enterobacter bacteremia in pediatric patients: a 10-year study. J Microbiol Immunol Infect 2014;47(5): 381–6.
11. Ito A, Nishikawa T, Ota M, et al. Stability and low induction propensity of cefiderocol against chromosomal AmpC β-lactamases of Pseudomonas aeruginosa

and Enterobacter cloacae [published correction appears in J Antimicrob Chemother. 2019 Feb 1;74(2):539]. J Antimicrob Chemother 2018;73(11):3049–52.

12. Bonnefoy A, Dupuis-Hamelin C, Steier V, et al. In vitro activity of AVE1330A, an innovative broad-spectrum non-beta-lactam beta-lactamase inhibitor. J Antimicrob Chemother 2004;54(2):410–7.

13. Cheng L, Nelson BC, Mehta M, et al. Piperacillin-Tazobactam versus other antibacterial agents for treatment of bloodstream infections due to AmpC β-lactamase-producing enterobacteriaceae. Antimicrob Agents Chemother 2017; 61(6):e00276.

14. Tan SH, Ng TM, Chew KL, et al. Outcomes of treating AmpC-producing Enterobacterales bacteraemia with carbapenems vs. non-carbapenems. Int J Antimicrob Agents 2020;55(2):105860.

15. Stewart AG, Paterson DL, Young B, et al. Meropenem versus piperacillin-tazobactam for definitive treatment of bloodstream infections caused by AmpC β-lactamase-producing Enterobacter spp, Citrobacter freundii, Morganella morganii, Providencia spp, or Serratia marcescens: a pilot multicenter randomized controlled trial (MERINO-2). Open Forum Infect Dis 2021;8(8):ofab387.

16. Kang CI, Pai H, Kim SH, et al. Cefepime and the inoculum effect in tests with Klebsiella pneumoniae producing plasmid-mediated AmpC-type beta-lactamase. J Antimicrob Chemother 2004;54(6):1130–3.

17. Jackson MA, Schutze GE, Committee on Infectious Diseases. The use of systemic and topical fluoroquinolones. Pediatrics 2016;138(5):e20162706.

18. Bannon MJ, Stutchfield PR, Weindling AM, et al. Ciprofloxacin in neonatal Enterobacter cloacae septicaemia. Arch Dis Child 1989;64(10 Spec No): 1388–91.

19. Gunter SG, Barber KE, Wagner JL, et al. Fluoroquinolone versus nonfluoroquinolone treatment of bloodstream infections caused by chromosomally mediated AmpC-producing enterobacteriaceae. Antibiotics (Basel) 2020;9(6):331.

20. Flokas ME, Karanika S, Alevizakos M, et al. Prevalence of ESBL-producing enterobacteriaceae in pediatric bloodstream infections: a systematic review and meta-analysis. PLoS One 2017;12(1):e0171216.

21. Logan LK, Medernach RL, Domitrovic TN, et al. The clinical and molecular epidemiology of CTX-M-9 group producing enterobacteriaceae infections in children. Infect Dis Ther 2019;8(2):243–54.

22. Logan LK, Rispens JR, Medernach RL, et al. A multicentered study of the clinical and molecular epidemiology of TEM- and SHV-type extended-spectrum beta-lactamase producing enterobacterales infections in children. Pediatr Infect Dis J 2021;40(1):39–43.

23. CLSI. Performance standards for antimicrobial susceptibility testing. 31st edition CLSI supplement M100. Clinical and Laboratory Standards Institute; 2021.

24. The European Committee on Antimicrobial Susceptibility Testing. Breakpoint tables for interpretation of MICs and zone diameters. Version 11.0, 2021. Available at: http://www.eucast.org.

25. Harris PNA, Tambyah PA, Lye DC, et al. Effect of Piperacillin-Tazobactam vs Meropenem on 30-Day Mortality for Patients With E coli or Klebsiella pneumoniae Bloodstream Infection and Ceftriaxone Resistance: A Randomized Clinical Trial. JAMA 2018;320(10):984–94.

26. Tamma PD, Aitken SL, Bonomo RA, et al. Infectious Diseases Society of America guidance on the treatment of extended-spectrum β-lactamase producing enterobacterales (ESBL-E), carbapenem-resistant enterobacterales (CRE), and

Pseudomonas aeruginosa with difficult-to-treat resistance (DTR-P. aeruginosa). Clin Infect Dis 2021;72(7):e169–83.

27. Henderson A, Paterson DL, Chatfield MD, et al. Association between minimum inhibitory concentration, beta-lactamase genes and mortality for patients treated with piperacillin/tazobactam or meropenem from the MERINO study [published online ahead of print, 2020 Oct 27]. Clin Infect Dis 2020;ciaa1479.

28. Sharara SL, Amoah J, Pana ZD, et al. Is piperacillin-tazobactam effective for the treatment of pyelonephritis caused by extended-spectrum β-lactamase-producing organisms? Clin Infect Dis 2020;71(8):e331–7.

29. Lee NY, Lee CC, Huang WH, et al. Cefepime therapy for monomicrobial bacteremia caused by cefepime-susceptible extended-spectrum beta-lactamase-producing Enterobacteriaceae: MIC matters. Clin Infect Dis 2013;56(4):488–95.

30. Chopra T, Marchaim D, Veltman J, et al. Impact of cefepime therapy on mortality among patients with bloodstream infections caused by extended-spectrum-β-lactamase-producing Klebsiella pneumoniae and Escherichia coli. Antimicrob Agents Chemother 2012;56(7):3936–42.

31. Wang R, Cosgrove SE, Tschudin-Sutter S, et al. Cefepime therapy for cefepime-susceptible extended-spectrum β-lactamase-producing enterobacteriaceae bacteremia. Open Forum Infect Dis 2016;3(3):ofw132.

32. Sader HS, Huband MD, Duncan LR, et al. Ceftazidime-avibactam antimicrobial activity and spectrum when tested against gram-negative organisms from pediatric patients: results from the INFORM surveillance program (United States, 2011-2015). Pediatr Infect Dis J 2018;37(6):549–54.

33. Sader HS, Castanheira M, Streit JM, et al. Frequency and antimicrobial susceptibility of bacteria causing bloodstream infections in pediatric patients from United States (US) medical centers (2014-2018): therapeutic options for multidrug-resistant bacteria. Diagn Microbiol Infect Dis 2020;98(2):115108.

34. Golden AR, Adam HJ, Baxter M, et al. In vitro activity of cefiderocol, a novel siderophore cephalosporin, against gram-negative bacilli isolated from patients in Canadian intensive care units. Diagn Microbiol Infect Dis 2020;97(1):115012.

35. Logan LK, Nguyen DC, Scaggs Huang FA, et al. A multi-centered case-case-control study of factors associated with Klebsiella pneumoniae carbapenemase-producing enterobacteriaceae infections in children and young adults. Pediatr Infect Dis J 2019;38(5):490–5.

36. van Duin D, Lok JJ, Earley M, et al. Colistin versus ceftazidime-avibactam in the treatment of infections due to Carbapenem-resistant enterobacteriaceae. Clin Infect Dis 2018;66(2):163–71.

37. Karaiskos I, Daikos GL, Gkoufa A, et al. Ceftazidime/avibactam in the era of carbapenemase-producing Klebsiella pneumoniae: experience from a national registry study. J Antimicrob Chemother 2021;76(3):775–83.

38. Iosifidis E, Chorafa E, Agakidou E, et al. Use of Ceftazidime-avibactam for the treatment of extensively drug-resistant or pan drug-resistant Klebsiella pneumoniae in neonates and children <5 years of age. Pediatr Infect Dis J 2019;38(8):812–5.

39. Rodríguez C, Brengi S, Cáceres MA, et al. Successful management with fosfomycin + ceftazidime of an infection caused by multiple highly-related subtypes of multidrug-resistant and extensively drug-resistant KPC-producing Serratia marcescens. Int J Antimicrob Agents 2018;52(5):737–9.

40. Vargas M, Buonomo AR, Buonanno P, et al. Successful treatment of KPC-MDR septic shock with ceftazidime-avibactam in a pediatric critically ill patient. ID-Cases 2019;18:e00634.

41. Rup AR, Dash AK, Patnaik S. Ceftazidime-avibactam for hospital acquired pneumonia due to extended drug-resistant Klebsiella pneumoniae. Indian J Pediatr 2021;88(3):290–1.

42. Coskun Y, Atici S. Successful treatment of Pandrug-resistant Klebsiella pneumoniae infection with Ceftazidime-avibactam in a preterm infant: a case report. Pediatr Infect Dis J 2020;39(9):854–6.

43. Yasmin M, Fouts DE, Jacobs MR, et al. Monitoring ceftazidime-avibactam and aztreonam concentrations in the treatment of a bloodstream infection caused by a multidrug-resistant Enterobacter sp. carrying both Klebsiella pneumoniae Carbapenemase-4 and New Delhi Metallo-β-Lactamase-1. Clin Infect Dis 2020;71(4):1095–8.

44. Cowart MC, Ferguson CL. Optimization of Aztreonam in combination with ceftazidime/avibactam in a cystic fibrosis patient with chronic Stenotrophomonas maltophilia Pneumonia using therapeutic drug monitoring: a case study. Ther Drug Monit 2021;43(2):146–9.

45. Alamarat ZI, Babic J, Tran TT, et al. Long-term compassionate use of cefiderocol to treat chronic osteomyelitis caused by extensively drug-resistant Pseudomonas aeruginosa and extended-spectrum-β-lactamase-producing Klebsiella pneumoniae in a pediatric patient. Antimicrob Agents Chemother 2020;64(4): e01872.

46. Gainey AB, Burch AK, Brownstein MJ, et al. Combining bacteriophages with cefiderocol and meropenem/vaborbactam to treat a pan-drug resistant Achromobacter species infection in a pediatric cystic fibrosis patient. Pediatr Pulmonol 2020;55(11):2990–4.

47. Aitken SL, Kontoyiannis DP, DePombo AM, et al. Use of Ceftolozane/Tazobactam in the treatment of multidrug-resistant Pseudomonas aeruginosa bloodstream infection in a pediatric leukemia patient. Pediatr Infect Dis J 2016; 35(9):1040–2.

48. Zikri A, El Masri K. Use of Ceftolozane/tazobactam for the treatment of multidrug-resistant *Pseudomonas aeruginosa* pneumonia in a pediatric patient with combined immunodeficiency (CID): a case report from a tertiary hospital in Saudi Arabia. Antibiotics (Basel) 2019;8(2):67.

49. Martín-Cazaña M, Grau S, Epalza C, et al. Successful ceftolozane-tazobactam rescue therapy in a child with endocarditis caused by multidrug-resistant Pseudomonas aeruginosa. J Paediatr Child Health 2019;55(8):985–7.

50. Hanretty AM, Kaur I, Evangelista AT, et al. Pharmacokinetics of the Meropenem component of Meropenem-Vaborbactam in the treatment of KPC-producing Klebsiella pneumoniae bloodstream infection in a pediatric patient. Pharmacotherapy 2018;38(12):e87–91.

51. Evans BA, Amyes SG. OXA β-lactamases. Clin Microbiol Rev 2014;27(2): 241–63.

52. Wiskirchen DE, Nordmann P, Crandon JL, et al. Efficacy of humanized carbapenem and ceftazidime regimens against Enterobacteriaceae producing OXA-48 carbapenemase in a murine infection model. Antimicrob Agents Chemother 2014;58(3):1678–83.

53. Avycaz (ceftazidime/avibactam) [prescribing information]. Madison, NJ: Allergan USA Inc; 2020.

54. Vabomere (meropenem and vaborbactam) [prescribing information]. Lincolnshire, IL: Melinta Therapeutics Inc; 2020.

55. Stewart A, Harris P, Henderson A, et al. Treatment of Infections by OXA-48-Producing Enterobacteriaceae. Antimicrob Agents Chemother 2018;62(11): e01195.

56. Garau G, Di Guilmi AM, Hall BG. Structure-based phylogeny of the metallo-beta-lactamases. Antimicrob Agents Chemother 2005;49(7):2778–84.

57. Tan X, Kim HS, Baugh K, et al. Therapeutic Options for Metallo-β-Lactamase-Producing Enterobacterales. Infect Drug Resist. 2021;14:125–142

58. Hasassri ME, Boyce TG, Norgan AP, et al. An immunocompromised child with bloodstream infection caused by two Escherichia coli Strains, one harboring NDM-5 and the other harboring OXA-48-like Carbapenemase. Antimicrob Agents Chemother 2016;60(6):3270–5.

59. Davido B, Fellous L, Lawrence C, et al. Ceftazidime-Avibactam and Aztreonam, an interesting strategy to overcome β-lactam resistance conferred by Metallo-β-lactamases in Enterobacteriaceae and Pseudomonas aeruginosa. Antimicrob Agents Chemother 2017;61(9):e01008–17.

60. Avery LM, Nicolau DP. Assessing the in vitro activity of ceftazidime/avibactam and aztreonam among carbapenemase-producing Enterobacteriaceae: defining the zone of hope. Int J Antimicrob Agents 2018;52(5):688–91.

61. Du D, Wang-Kan X, Neuberger A, et al. Multidrug efflux pumps: structure, function and regulation [published correction appears in Nat Rev Microbiol. 2018 Jul 18]. Nat Rev Microbiol 2018;16(9):523–39.

62. Hocquet D, Nordmann P, El Garch F, et al. Involvement of the MexXY-OprM efflux system in emergence of cefepime resistance in clinical strains of Pseudomonas aeruginosa. Antimicrob Agents Chemother 2006;50(4):1347–51.

63. Laohavaleeson S, Lolans K, Quinn JP, et al. Expression of the MexXY-OprM efflux system in Pseudomonas aeruginosa with discordant cefepime/ceftazidime susceptibility profiles. Infect Drug Resist 2008;1:51–5.

64. Ochs MM, McCusker MP, Bains M, et al. Negative regulation of the Pseudomonas aeruginosa outer membrane porin OprD selective for imipenem and basic amino acids. Antimicrob Agents Chemother 1999;43(5):1085–90.

65. Hammami S, Ghozzi R, Burghoffer B, et al. Mechanisms of carbapenem resistance in non-metallo-beta-lactamase-producing clinical isolates of Pseudomonas aeruginosa from a Tunisian hospital. Pathol Biol (Paris) 2009;57(7–8): 530–5.

66. Schwartz GJ, Work DF. Measurement and estimation of GFR in children and adolescents. Clin J Am Soc Nephrol 2009;4(11):1832–43.

67. Fenton A, Montgomery E, Nightingale P, et al. Glomerular filtration rate: new age- and gender- specific reference ranges and thresholds for living kidney donation. BMC Nephrol 2018;19(1):336.

68. Craig WA. Pharmacokinetic/pharmacodynamic parameters: rationale for antibacterial dosing of mice and men. Clin Infect Dis 1998;26(1):1–12.

69. Taccone FS, Laterre PF, Dugernier T, et al. Insufficient β-lactam concentrations in the early phase of severe sepsis and septic shock. Crit Care 2010;14(4):R126.

70. Miglis C, Rhodes NJ, Kuti JL, et al. Defining the impact of severity of illness on time above the MIC threshold for cefepime in gram-negative bacteraemia: a 'Goldilocks' window. Int J Antimicrob Agents 2017;50(3):487–90.

71. Scharf C, Liebchen U, Paal M, et al. The higher the better? Defining the optimal beta-lactam target for critically ill patients to reach infection resolution and improve outcome. J Intensive Care 2020;8(1):86.

72. Guilhaumou R, Benaboud S, Bennis Y, et al. Optimization of the treatment with beta-lactam antibiotics in critically ill patients-guidelines from the French Society

of Pharmacology and Therapeutics (Société Française de Pharmacologie et Thérapeutique-SFPT) and the French Society of Anaesthesia and Intensive Care Medicine (Société Française d'Anesthésie et Réanimation-SFAR). Crit Care 2019;23(1):104.

73. Nicasio AM, VanScoy BD, Mendes RE, et al. Pharmacokinetics-Pharmacodynamics of Tazobactam in combination with piperacillin in an in vitro infection model. Antimicrob Agents Chemother 2016;60(4):2075–80.

74. Melchers MJ, Mavridou E, van Mil AC, et al. Pharmacodynamics of Ceftolozane combined with Tazobactam against Enterobacteriaceae in a neutropenic mouse thigh model. Antimicrob Agents Chemother 2016;60(12):7272–9.

75. Coleman K, Levasseur P, Girard AM, et al. Activities of ceftazidime and avibactam against β-lactamase-producing Enterobacteriaceae in a hollow-fiber pharmacodynamic model. Antimicrob Agents Chemother 2014;58(6):3366–72.

76. Zembles TN, Schortemeyer R, Kuhn EM, et al. Extended infusion of beta-lactams is associated with improved outcomes in pediatric patients. J Pediatr Pharmacol Ther 2021;26(2):187–93.

77. Reed MD, Yamashita TS, Knupp CK, et al. Pharmacokinetics of intravenously and intramuscularly administered cefepime in infants and children. Antimicrob Agents Chemother 1997;41(8):1783–7.

78. Kohlmann R, Bähr T, Gatermann SG. Effect of ampC derepression on cefepime MIC in Enterobacterales with chromosomally encoded inducible AmpC β-lactamase. Clin Microbiol Infect 2019;25(9):1158.e1–4.

79. Nielsen LE, Forrester JB, Girotto JE, et al. One size fits all? Application of susceptible-dose-dependent breakpoints to pediatric patients and laboratory reporting. J Clin Microbiol 2019;58(1):e01446.

80. Courter JD, Kuti JL, Girotto JE, et al. Optimizing bactericidal exposure for beta-lactams using prolonged and continuous infusions in the pediatric population. Pediatr Blood Cancer 2009;53(3):379–85.

81. Shoji K, Bradley JS, Reed MD, et al. Population pharmacokinetic assessment and pharmacodynamic implications of pediatric cefepime dosing for susceptible-dose-dependent organisms. Antimicrob Agents Chemother 2016; 60(4):2150–6.

82. Béranger A, Benaboud S, Urien S, et al. Piperacillin population pharmacokinetics and dosing regimen optimization in critically Ill children with normal and augmented renal clearance. Clin Pharmacokinet 2019;58(2):223–33.

83. Maarbjerg SF, Thorsted A, Kristoffersson A, et al. Piperacillin pharmacokinetics and target attainment in children with cancer and fever: can we optimize our dosing strategy? Pediatr Blood Cancer 2019;66(6):e27654.

84. Cies JJ, Shankar V, Schlichting C, et al. Population pharmacokinetics of piperacillin/tazobactam in critically ill young children. Pediatr Infect Dis J 2014;33(2): 168–73.

85. Nichols K, Chung EK, Knoderer CA, et al. Population pharmacokinetics and pharmacodynamics of extended-infusion piperacillin and Tazobactam in critically Ill children. Antimicrob Agents Chemother 2015;60(1):522–31.

86. Thibault C, Lavigne J, Litalien C, et al. Population pharmacokinetics and safety of piperacillin-tazobactam extended infusions in infants and children. Antimicrob Agents Chemother 2019;63(11):e01260.

87. Abdel-Rahman SM, Kearns GL, Topelberg S, et al. Pharmacokinetics and tolerability of single-dose intravenous ertapenem in infants, children, and adolescents. Pediatr Infect Dis J 2010;29(12):1072–6.

88. Blumer JL, Reed MD, Kearns GL, et al. Sequential, single-dose pharmacokinetic evaluation of meropenem in hospitalized infants and children. Antimicrob Agents Chemother 1995;39(8):1721–5.

89. Kongthavonsakul K, Lucksiri A, Eakanunkul S, et al. Pharmacokinetics and pharmacodynamics of meropenem in children with severe infection. Int J Antimicrob Agents 2016;48(2):151–7.

90. Ikawa K, Morikawa N, Ikeda K, et al. Population pharmacokinetics and pharmacodynamics of meropenem in Japanese pediatric patients. J Infect Chemother 2010;16(2):139–43.

91. Katsube T, Echols R, Wajima T. 739. Prediction of Cefiderocol pharmacokinetics and probability of target attainment in pediatric subjects for proposing dose regimens. Open Forum Infect Dis 2019;6(Suppl 2):S330–1.

92. Safety, tolerability, and pharmacokinetics of Cefiderocol in hospitalized pediatric patients. ClinicalTrials.gov identifier: NCT042159916. Available at: https://clinicaltrials.gov/ct2/show/NCT04215991. Accessed May 16, 2021.

93. Karlowsky JA, Hackel MA, Tsuji M, et al. In vitro activity of Cefiderocol, a Siderophore Cephalosporin, against gram-negative bacilli isolated by clinical laboratories in North America and Europe in 2015-2016: SIDERO-WT-2015. Int J Antimicrob Agents 2019;53(4):456–66.

94. Bradley JS, Armstrong J, Arrieta A, et al. Phase I study assessing the pharmacokinetic profile, safety, and tolerability of a single dose of ceftazidime-avibactam in hospitalized pediatric patients. Antimicrob Agents Chemother 2016;60(10):6252–9.

95. Lin LY, Riccobene T, Debabov D. Antimicrobial activity of ceftazidime-avibactam against contemporary pathogens from urinary tract infections and intra-abdominal infections collected from US children During the 2016-2019 INFORM Surveillance Program. Pediatr Infect Dis J 2021;40(4):338–43.

96. Shortridge D, Duncan LR, Pfaller MA, et al. Activity of ceftolozane-tazobactam and comparators when tested against gram-negative isolates collected from paediatric patients in the USA and Europe between 2012 and 2016 as part of a global surveillance programme. Int J Antimicrob Agents 2019;53(5):637–43.

97. Bradley JS, Ang JY, Arrieta AC, et al. Pharmacokinetics and safety of single intravenous doses of ceftolozane/tazobactam in children with proven or suspected gram-negative infection. Pediatr Infect Dis J 2018;37(11):1130–6.

98. Larson KB, Patel YT, Willavize S, et al. Ceftolozane-Tazobactam population pharmacokinetics and dose selection for further clinical evaluation in pediatric patients with complicated urinary tract or complicated intra-abdominal infections. Antimicrob Agents Chemother 2019;63(6):e02578.

99. Lepak AJ, Reda A, Marchillo K, et al. Impact of MIC range for Pseudomonas aeruginosa and Streptococcus pneumoniae on the ceftolozane in vivo pharmacokinetic/pharmacodynamic target. Antimicrob Agents Chemother 2014;58(10):6311–4.

100. Xiao AJ, Miller BW, Huntington JA, et al. Ceftolozane/tazobactam pharmacokinetic/pharmacodynamic-derived dose justification for phase 3 studies in patients with nosocomial pneumonia. J Clin Pharmacol 2016;56(1):56–66.

101. Dose-finding, Pharmacokinetics, and Safety of VABOMERE in pediatric subjects with bacterial infections (TANGOKIDS). ClinicalTrials.gov identifier: NCT02687906. Available at: https://clinicaltrials.gov/ct2/show/NCT02687906. Accessed May 16, 2021.

102. Karlowsky JA, Lob SH, Young K, et al. In vitro activity of Imipenem/Relebactam against gram-negative bacilli from pediatric patients-study for monitoring anti-microbial resistance trends (SMART) global surveillance program 2015-2017. J Pediatr Infect Dis Soc 2021;10(3):274–81.

103. Safety, tolerability, efficacy and pharmacokinetics of imipenem/cilastatin/rele-bactam (MK-7655A) in pediatric participants with gram-negative bacterial infec-tion (MK-7655A-021). ClinicalTrials.gov identifier: NCT03969901. Available at: https://clinicaltrials.gov/ct2/show/NCT03969901. Accessed May 16, 2021.

104. A pharmacokinetics study of MK-7655A in pediatric participants with gram-negative infections (MK-7655A-020). ClinicalTrials.gov identifier: NCT03230916. Available at: https://clinicaltrials.gov/ct2/show/NCT03230916. Accessed May 16, 2021.

105. Forrest A, Nix DE, Ballow CH, et al. Pharmacodynamics of intravenous ciproflox-acin in seriously ill patients. Antimicrob Agents Chemother 1993;37(5):1073–81.

106. Van TT, Minejima E, Chiu CA, et al. Don't get wound up: revised fluoroquinolone breakpoints for Enterobacteriaceae and Pseudomonas aeruginosa. J Clin Mi-crobiol 2019;57(7):e02072.

107. CLSI. Fluoroquinolone breakpoints for Enterobacteriaceae and Pseudomonas aeruginosa. In: CLSI rationale document MR02. 1st edition. Wayne, PA: Clinical and Laboratory Standards Institute; 2019.

108. Facchin A, Bui S, Leroux S, et al. Variability of ciprofloxacin pharmacokinetics in children: impact on dose range in sickle cell patients. J Antimicrob Chemother 2018;73(12):3423–9.

109. Sassen SDT, Mathôt RAA, Pieters R, et al. Population Pharmacokinetics and Pharmacodynamics of ciprofloxacin prophylaxis in pediatric acute lympho-blastic leukemia patients. Clin Infect Dis 2020;71(8):e281–8.

110. Chien S, Wells TG, Blumer JL, et al. Levofloxacin pharmacokinetics in children. J Clin Pharmacol 2005;45(2):153–60.

111. Payen S, Serreau R, Munck A, et al. Population pharmacokinetics of ciprofloxa-cin in pediatric and adolescent patients with acute infections. Antimicrob Agents Chemother 2003;47(10):3170–8.

The Current State and Future Directions of Inpatient Pediatric Antimicrobial Stewardship

Rebecca G. Same, MD

KEYWORDS

- Antibiotic stewardship • Pediatrics • Handshake stewardship • Guidelines
- Implementation science

KEY POINTS

- Antimicrobial review is a key component of inpatient antimicrobial stewardship programs (ASPs). Prospective audit and feedback, especially handshake stewardship, may be the most effective method to reduce excess antibiotic use.
- The development of guidelines and decision-support tools can improve appropriate prescribing and foster collaboration with frontline providers.
- Diagnostic stewardship is emerging as an opportunity for ASPs to impact upstream steps that influence antimicrobial prescribing. Newer syndrome-based rapid diagnostic panels require collaboration among ASPs, microbiologists, and frontline prescribers to realize their potential benefits and avoid the overuse of both tests and antimicrobials.
- Implementation science uses behavioral science and additional research frameworks to help close the gap between evidence-based recommendations and practice changes.
- Telehealth may be an important component of initiatives to extend stewardship from large academic centers to smaller hospitals, but further research is needed into how to optimize these relationships to improve antibiotic use at smaller hospitals.

The introduction of antibiotics was one of the most important medical advances of the 20th century. However, as soon as they were introduced, antibiotics were overused. There have been attempts to control and optimize their use ever since, with formalized hospital antimicrobial stewardship programs (ASPs) becoming more common and better codified over the last 30 years. As antibiotic resistance continues to rise, we have gained a better understanding of the need for stewardship and increasingly rigorous research has revealed the benefits of ASPs and identified optimal practices, though gaps in knowledge about how to best implement stewardship interventions

Department of Pediatrics, Division of Pediatric Infectious Diseases, Washington University School of Medicine in St. Louis, MSC 8116-43-10, 660 S. Euclid Avenue, St. Louis, MO 63110, USA
E-mail address: rsame@wustl.edu

Infect Dis Clin N Am 36 (2022) 173–186
https://doi.org/10.1016/j.idc.2021.12.001
0891-5520/22/© 2021 Elsevier Inc. All rights reserved.

remain. The future of stewardship will include increased inclusion of partners who have sometimes been overlooked by ASPs, such as nurses, and emphasis on implementation (and de-implementation) science as well as expansion to smaller hospitals. This article reviews the ongoing need for inpatient antimicrobial stewardship, the essential components of ASPs, and future directions for pediatric inpatient antimicrobial stewardship.

HISTORY OF ANTIMICROBIAL STEWARDSHIP

When antibiotics were first discovered and came into clinical use in the 1940s, they were hailed as miracle drugs and some predicted the end of infectious diseases (ID). However, it was not long before clinicians began to identify some of the problems associated with antimicrobials. Negative side effects were noted early, including rashes, drug fever, and anaphylaxis.[1] At least as troubling, clinicians noticed that rather than eliminating ID, the widespread use of antibiotics led to a shift in the microbiology of the most serious infections. In a 1960 essay, Maxwell Finland described the changing epidemiology of patients with bacteremia after the introduction of sulfonamides and penicillins.[2] He identified that, while the mortality associated with Streptococcal infections had decreased, there was rising penicillin resistance in Staphylococcal infections and increasing incidence of serious infections caused by pathogens that had previously been relatively unheard of, including *Enterococcus*, *Escherichia coli, Proteus, Pseudomonas,* and *Aerobacter (Klebsiella) aerogenes*. He blamed this changing epidemiology on selective pressure for organisms with acquired or inherent resistance to antibiotics caused by their extensive use. Finland went on to identify many of the same challenges that continue to face stewards in the use of antibiotics, including near universal antibiotic use. He was particularly offended by the widespread use of antibiotics for prophylaxis, which he remarked was "generally futile." He also suggested many of our modern stewardship tools, including restricting the use of antibiotics to indications for which they are known to be beneficial and reserving certain antibiotics.

Early efforts to curb the excess use of antibiotics used education and persuasion, but they had little impact. A point prevalence survey in 1970 revealed that 30% of hospitalized patients were receiving antibiotics, 60% of whom had no clear infection.[3] In 1976, the Joint Commission Standards on Infection Control included a requirement that physicians be involved in antimicrobial usage, leading to calls for a multidisciplinary approach to antimicrobial review that many would recognize as a precursor to antimicrobial stewardship.4 However, there was little uptake of these recommendations.

The advent of new antibiotics in the 1980s led to a feeling of invincibility; new antibiotics seemed to be a plentiful and practical solution to rising resistance.[5] When the Infectious Diseases Society of America (IDSA) released "Guidelines for Improving the Use of Antimicrobial Agents in Hospitals" in 1988, which proposed the restriction of select antimicrobials, providers had little motivation to reduce antibiotic use.[6] Nevertheless, that same year, Briceland published the first description of a successful program to "streamline" antibiotics from combination therapy regimens to monotherapy.[7] They used an audit and feedback approach by a combined ID physician and pharmacist team and showed sustained changes in prescribing practices over the course of their intervention. The primary outcome they tracked was cost savings, which they used to justify the program to hospital leadership.

In the 1990s antibiotic resistance continued to increase as the pipeline of new antibiotics slowed, leading to an increased interest in solutions to antibiotic overuse.[5] Ultimately this led to the development of more robust ASPs in the late 1990s and early

2000s. In 2007, the IDSA released the first guidelines for the development and implementation of an ASP, which were supported by the American Academy of Pediatrics (AAP) and the Pediatric Infectious Diseases Society (PIDS).[8] They framed stewardship as an essential component of patient safety and defined the goal of an ASP: "to optimize clinical outcomes while minimizing unintended consequences of antimicrobial use, including toxicity, the selection of pathogenic organisms (such as *Clostridium difficile*), and the emergence of resistance."

ASPs continue to grow. In 2014 the CDC released the Core Elements of Hospital ASPs, which were updated in 2019 (**Table 1**).[9] Also in 2019, the Centers for Medicare and Medicaid Services began requiring US hospitals to implement ASPs as a condition of participation. The increasing regulatory attention to the need for ASPs has led to their rapid expansion. A 2011 survey of 38 free-standing children's hospitals found that 42% had established a formal ASP while a similar survey of 52 hospitals from 2016 to 2017 found that 94% had established ASPs with dedicated financial resources.[10]

RATIONALE FOR ANTIMICROBIAL STEWARDSHIP

More than 60 years after Finland first lamented the near universal use of antibiotics, the problem of excess antimicrobial use persists. Antibiotic use across children's hospitals is highly variable, with 38% to 72% of children receiving antibiotics during their admission.[11] About half of this use is likely unnecessary and 21% is considered to be suboptimal.[12] Prophylactic antibiotic use remains problematic as well, with 33%

Table 1 Centers for Disease Control and Prevention Core Elements of Hospital Antibiotic Stewardship Programs	
Hospital Leadership Commitment	Senior leadership of the hospital supports antibiotic stewardship with necessary resources, including providing time and financial support.
Accountability	One or more leaders, ideally one pharmacist and one physician, are identified to be responsible for the management and outcomes of the antibiotic stewardship program (ASP).
Pharmacy Expertise	A pharmacist is strongly engaged with the ASP, preferably as a coleader, and empowered to lead ASP interventions.
Action	The ASP implements interventions to improve antimicrobial use, including antimicrobial review through either prior authorization or prospective audit and feedback, development of facility-specific guidelines, and other interventions targeted at specific infections or members of the health care team.
Tracking	The ASP tracks outcomes of importance, including overall antibiotic use as well as clinical outcomes such as *Clostridioides difficile* rates, hospital length of stay, readmissions, and mortality.
Reporting	ASP leaders report outcomes to stakeholders, including hospital leadership, frontline providers, pharmacists, and nurses.
Education	The ASP educates prescribers, pharmacists, nurses, and patients about antimicrobial use and stewardship.

Data from CDC. Core Elements of Hospital Antibiotic Stewardship Programs. Atlanta, GA: US Department of Health and Human Services, CDC; 2019.

of surgical prophylaxis considered inappropriate in a recent point-prevalence survey of antibiotic use in children's hospitals.[13]

Excess antibiotic use continues to contribute to the worsening problem of antimicrobial resistance, with antibiotic use consistently identified as a major risk factor for multidrug-resistant infections in children.[14] Additionally, there is growing recognition of the impact of antibiotic-associated adverse drug events in children. Over 20% of antibiotic courses prescribed to children during their hospitalization result in an antibiotic-associated adverse drug event, with problems ranging from rashes to acute kidney injury to *Clostridioides difficile* infections.[15] Antibiotic use in childhood has also been associated with chronic health problems, including obesity, asthma, and juvenile idiopathic arthritis.[16–18]

Inpatient ASPs can reduce the negative impact of antibiotics by ensuring that children only receive antibiotics when necessary and that the drugs with the narrowest spectrum and lowest likelihood of adverse effects are selected. Pediatric inpatient ASPs have been shown to reduce overall antibiotic use and prescribing errors.[19] Some studies have shown a decrease in antibiotic resistance associated with the implementation of ASPs, but this has been a less consistent finding, likely because the development of resistance is a multifactorial process that may reflect broader epidemiologic trends that can be very difficult to reverse.[20] The primary purpose of antimicrobial stewardship is to ensure optimal prescribing to improve patient outcomes. Additionally, by decreasing both antibiotic expenditures and indirect expenses related to unnecessary antibiotic use, ASPs also reduce health care costs.[21]

ANTIBIOTIC STEWARDSHIP PROGRAM TEAM COMPOSITION

The 2019 update to the CDC Core Elements of Hospital Antimicrobial Stewardship Programs highlights the importance of joint physician/pharmacist leadership of ASPs, which is in line with recommendations from IDSA.[8,9] This reflects recent trends in pediatric ASPs: in 2017 88% of surveyed hospital ASPs reported having a pharmacist devoted to their program compared with only 34% in 2011.[10] Pharmacists offer a unique perspective and skillset that is critical to the success of an ASP. Their comprehensive understanding of antimicrobials, including detailed knowledge of dosing and administration, is critical to improve antimicrobial use within hospitals.[22] In fact, while a joint physician/pharmacist model is preferred, at least one study has shown that ASP programs led by pharmacists without physician support can successfully reduce antimicrobial use.[23]

The IDSA recommends that both the physician and pharmacist leaders of the ASP should have ID specialty training.[8] While ID training is certainly beneficial and is common at larger academic medical centers, the dearth of both ID pharmacists and physicians makes this impractical at many smaller institutions, which nevertheless face a regulatory requirement to have an ASP. Expanding access to ASPs will require creativity in selecting leaders, including the consideration of both pharmacists and physicians without formal ID training.[24] Hospitalists are well situated to act as antimicrobial stewards; there are increasing numbers of hospitalists at many institutions that lack ID physicians and they care for a significant proportion of patients receiving antibiotics.[25] They also often have training in quality improvement (QI) and guideline development that can be applied to stewardship. Many resources are available for ASP leaders without formal ID training to gain the knowledge and skills required to build a successful and impactful ASP, including a toolkit from the AAP and PIDS and collaborative guidance from the Society for Hospital Epidemiology of America, PIDS, and others.[26,27]

In addition to pharmacist and/or physician leaders, core members of an inpatient antimicrobial stewardship team generally include a medical microbiologist and information system or data specialist.[8] Collaboration with the medical microbiology laboratory is crucial to develop local antibiograms to understand local patterns of resistance and inform treatment recommendations, to stay abreast of changes in antimicrobial susceptibility testing and discuss testing for new antimicrobials the ASP may want to add to formulary, and to evaluate and consider new diagnostics. ASPs also work closely with both microbiology and infection prevention teams to identify trends in diagnoses (e.g., surgical site infections) and prescribing (e.g., perioperative prophylaxis) that may be amenable to ASP intervention. Information system specialists can help with the development of clinical decision support tools and order sets embedded in the electronic health record to guide appropriate antibiotic use. Data analysts are essential to tracking the impact of stewardship interventions.

The incorporation of nurses is a much needed addition to many ASP teams.[28] By virtue of their close relationship with patients and position at the bedside, nurses are uniquely situated to contribute to and lead a number of ASP initiatives. A recent series of focus groups and interviews with 61 nurses, 39% of whom worked in a pediatric setting, found that nurses saw participation in antimicrobial stewardship activities as an important extension of their role as patient advocates.[29] They identified gaps in knowledge around antimicrobial use as the primary barrier to their involvement in ASPs. The authors recognized 3 types of nurse-driven ASP interventions that were viewed most favorably: questioning the necessity of urinary cultures, ensuring proper culturing techniques, and encouraging the transition from intravenous (IV) to oral antibiotics. A pilot study of a nurse-driven protocol on a general medicine ward to evaluate the necessity of urine cultures led to a significant decrease in overall urine cultures and a numeric decrease in inappropriate urine cultures, though this did not reach statistical significance.[30] Nursing partnership likely represents a significant untapped resource for ASPs, but it is important to carefully frame the partnership in order for it to succeed. Poor communication and lack of inclusion or education of nursing may lead to a sense of increased work rather than partnership.[31] Nurse-driven initiatives should be truly collaborative and should focus on nurses' expertise in patient safety and role as patient advocates. It may also be helpful to highlight how stewardship can actually improve nursing workload, for instance, that transitioning to oral antibiotics can eliminate the need to administer IV antibiotics.[32]

ANTIMICROBIAL STEWARDSHIP ACTIONS

The CDC Core Elements of Antimicrobial Stewardship identify a number of different actions that stewardship programs should pursue.[9] These include different methods to oversee antibiotic use, facility-specific guidelines, and targeted interventions for common infections (such as community-acquired pneumonia (CAP) and urinary tract infections) or high-risk prescribing (such as outpatient parenteral antibiotic therapy). They also identify the importance of interventions that are directed at different professionals, including provider-based interventions such as "timeouts" to reassess the need for antibiotics, pharmacy-based interventions like requiring the documentation of the indication for antibiotics, microbiology-based interventions as in the selective reporting of antimicrobial susceptibility results, or nursing-based interventions to optimize the collection of cultures. This article will highlight 2 central components of ASPs (the choice between preauthorization and prospective audit and feedback and guideline development) and areas of emerging research (diagnostic stewardship and new evidence to guide the implementation of stewardship interventions).

Preauthorization Versus Prospective Audit and Feedback

There are 2 primary approaches to the management and oversight of antibiotic use in the hospital: prior authorization and prospective audit and feedback, also known as postprescription review.

Prior authorization requires prescribers to obtain approval from a representative of the ASP before using certain antibiotics. This strategy allows people with expertise in antibiotic use to provide early guidance, which may improve empiric therapy for serious conditions, such as sepsis, and reduce unnecessary antibiotic use before it is initiated. This requires timely availability of experts to approve and release restricted antibiotics rapidly to avoid delays in the initiation of therapy, particularly for conditions such as sepsis, whereby timely administration of antibiotics is critically important.[9] Some ASPs that use prior authorization allow for the exemption of a single dose of antibiotics for critically ill patients.

In prospective audit and feedback, antibiotic therapy is reviewed by experts after it is prescribed and recommendations are made to optimize use. Many different versions of prospective audit and feedback can be implemented to meet the needs and capacity of an individual program. ASPs may choose to focus on specific antibiotics, conditions, or to broadly review all prescribed antibiotics. Prospective audit and feedback can be conducted over the phone or through the electronic medical record, but the most effective approach occurs with face-to-face meetings, which is commonly called "handshake stewardship."[33] This strategy can be very resource-intensive, but research shows that ultimately the approach saves money.[21] This interactive model facilitates the education of frontline providers, which may result in better prescribing in the future, lessening the need for ongoing intervention. It also can lead to the development of relationships and collaboration that likely improve the acceptability of recommendations when compared with prior authorization, which does not foster the same collaborative environment.

Prior authorization and prospective audit and feedback are both well-established methods to improve antibiotic prescribing, but prospective audit and feedback may be the more effective of the 2. A quasi-experimental crossover study assigned medical teams to either preprescription authorization (PPA) or postprescription review with feedback (PPRF), which included in-person visits from the ASP team, for the first 4 months and then switched to the other approach for the second 4 months.[34] Antibiotic therapy was more likely to be appropriate on day 1 under the PPA model, but day 3 appropriateness was higher with PPRF. In the group assigned initially to PPRF, antibiotic use declined and then remained steady after switching to PPA, possibly reflecting the ongoing impact of education the group had initially received through PPRF. Median days of antibiotic therapy were lower with PPRF. Prior authorization and prospective audit and feedback can also be combined, with a limited set of antibiotics requiring prior approval to target empiric therapy and broader application of postprescription review.

Clinical Practice Guidelines

One of the cornerstones of stewardship is the development of institutional clinical practice guidelines. Facility-specific guidelines tailor national guidelines to reflect local susceptibilities, formulary, and patient characteristics. They are an important mechanism to convey national guidelines to frontline clinicians, especially because national guidelines can be long, too extensive, and often lag behind the most up-to-date research, making them difficult to apply at the point of care. Local guidelines can also facilitate the communication of new research findings, which may be published in ID journals that may not otherwise be widely distributed.[35] The most straightforward benefit of an institutional guideline is to optimize the management of common infections. Additionally, ASPs can use guideline development to engage provider stakeholders and build consensus. Frontline providers should be involved in identifying which guidelines to prioritize for development and should be included in committees or working groups that help to adapt national recommendations to the individual institution. The inclusion of providers who will use the guidelines is paramount to their success, both because they can provide input on current practices and feasibility of changes and because they can serve as ambassadors to their colleagues, who may more readily accept recommendations from their peers than from a stewardship team.

Multiple studies have demonstrated that the development and implementation of institutional guidelines can improve prescribing.[19] In one study, the implementation of a CAP guideline without a formal ASP but in association with didactic lectures and guideline dissemination resulted in an improvement in ampicillin prescribing from 8% to 44%.[36] In another study, the implementation of a guideline for the management of CAP in conjunction with an ASP resulted in an increase in ampicillin use from 13% to 63%.[37] Addition of QI strategies can further improve guideline adherence, with a third study demonstrating 100% adherence to a CAP guideline with the use of an existing QI framework.[38] There is growing recognition that the development of the guideline alone is inadequate and that the incorporation of EHR clinical decision support tools and monitoring of adherence to guidelines and performance feedback are also important to a guideline's success.[39]

Diagnostic Stewardship: Syndrome-Based Rapid Diagnostic Tests

While antimicrobial stewardship has traditionally focused on the prescribing of antibiotics, upstream steps, such as the appropriate use of diagnostics, are critically important to determining antimicrobial use. Diagnostic stewardship in the ICU is addressed in detail in another article, with emphasis on how improving the use of blood, urine, and tracheal aspirate cultures can improve appropriate antibiotic prescribing. Another important opportunity for diagnostic stewardship is the optimization of the use of rapid syndromic panels, which have expanded significantly. The increasing availability of highly sensitive rapid PCR-based panels presents both challenges and opportunities: identifying a causative organism early presents an opportunity to tailor therapy, but the identification of organisms of unclear significance that may have gone undetected by conventional diagnostics could lead to increased antibiotic prescribing.

Several studies have demonstrated the value of antimicrobial stewardship in the interpretation and implementation of rapid diagnostics, in particular in rapid blood culture identification (BCID) systems. Gram-positive panels that identify the presence or absence of mecA should allow for earlier discontinuation of vancomycin, but in a retrospective study at a large tertiary care children's hospital in which a Gram-positive rapid BCID system was implemented without direct clinical feedback, there was no change in vancomycin use.[40] However, in another study in which the BCID panel was combined with prospective audit and clinical feedback from ASP, unnecessary antibiotic use decreased, including the use of vancomycin, antibiotic therapy for probable contaminants, and nonpenicillin use for Enterococcus, group A Streptococcus, or group B Streptococcus infections.[41] Importantly, the application of results from Gram-negative BCID systems is less straightforward due to the more complicated mechanisms of resistance in Gram-negative organisms. In the same study in which the identification of a Gram-positive organism facilitated antibiotic de-escalation, identification of Gram-negative organisms often resulted in antibiotic escalation, despite low institutional rates of Gram-negative antibiotic resistance.[41]

Respiratory pathogen panels (RPPs) are also commonly used in pediatrics and can have a positive impact on antimicrobial use. Identification of a viral pathogen from an RPP can facilitate early discontinuation of antibiotics in patients with lower respiratory tract infections who would otherwise have been treated with antibiotics for presumed bacterial pneumonia. The implementation of RPPs in pediatric settings has been associated with reductions in the median duration of antibiotic use and chest X-rays, shortened duration of empiric antibiotics, and decreased hospital length of stay.[42–44] The newer BioFire Pneumonia Panel, which is the first multiplexed PCR panel from lower respiratory specimens to identify bacterial causes of pneumonia other than the atypical bacteria included on prior RPPs, presents new opportunities and challenges that ASPs can help navigate. The rapid turnaround time and high negative predictive value for on-panel targets may allow earlier narrowing of broad empiric therapy, much as BCID systems allow for earlier discontinuation of vancomycin.[45] However, to date real-world experience with this test has not been published, and the increased sensitivity relative to culture could also lead to overtreatment. It will be crucial for ASPs to work closely with microbiology laboratories in determining how and when to introduce this test and with frontline providers to optimize the interpretation of the results.[46] Collaboration with microbiologists, frontline providers, and other partners across the health care system is critical to optimize reporting and interpretation of rapid diagnostic tests to ensure that their potential benefits are realized while avoiding overuse of both the tests and antimicrobials.

Implementation Science

The success of stewardship interventions depends on behavior change, which has long been recognized as central to the uptake of any ASP intervention.[47] Nevertheless, gaps remain between the development of guidelines and their successful application to drive and maintain changes in practice. There is growing interest in research to better understand how to close this gap, leading to increased collaboration between stewardship and other disciplines, including both behavioral science and implementation science.[48]

Behavioral science helps elucidate the knowledge, skills, and attitudes that underly current behaviors, which can inform the best way to approach changing current practice. For instance, traditional arguments for reducing unnecessary antibiotic exposure often focus on the risk of antibiotic resistance, but research shows that clinicians tend to perceive antibiotic resistance as a public health problem but do not believe it is relevant to their patients and therefore to their personal practice.[49] Framing the need to reduce antibiotic use around concerns that are perceived to more directly impact their patients, such as the risk of antibiotic-associated adverse events, may have more of an impact for some prescribers.[15] Implementation science incorporates behavioral science along with other research frameworks to understand how to translate evidence-based recommendations into practice. ASP interventions often focus on the de-implementation of established practices, such as recommending shorter durations of therapy for common infections based on newer data that contradicts historical practice. It can be particularly challenging to gain traction for de-implementation.[50] Incorporation of implementation science into stewardship research and practice allows ASPs to tailor their approach to their audience with evidence-based methods informing programs to instigate change, which will ideally increase the likelihood of success and sustainability of ASPs.

REPORTING AND OUTCOMES OF INTEREST

Regardless of the methods used, all ASPs should regularly track and report the outcomes of their interventions to stakeholders, including prescribers, pharmacists, nurses, and hospital leadership. ASPs commonly track process measures, including types of recommendations made by the ASP and their acceptance by frontline providers. They should also assess and report adherence to local guidelines and overall antibiotic use (generally reported as days of therapy per thousand patient days) and the financial impact of the program.[39] While these metrics are important, the ultimate goal of stewardship is to improve patient care, which can be much harder to demonstrate. *C. difficile* rates have often been followed as a clinically relevant metric tied to improved antimicrobial use, but ASPs should also evaluate their impact on other metrics such as the length of hospital stay, readmissions, and mortality.[51]

EDUCATION

At its core, antimicrobial stewardship has always focused on the education of frontline providers with the goal of empowering them to make optimal antibiotic choices for their patients. This education can take many forms, including didactics, dedicated rotations for trainees, or case-based teaching focused on specific prescribing choices during interactions around prior authorization or prospective audit and feedback of antimicrobials. All interactions can benefit from using a consistent framework to help understand antimicrobial prescribing, such as the 4 moments of antibiotic decision-making, which identifies 4 key points in the treatment of infection when providers should pause and reconsider their antibiotic plan: diagnosis; obtaining cultures and choosing empiric therapy; stopping, narrowing, or transitioning to oral antibiotics; and determining treatment duration.[52] Many studies have shown that education geared toward prescribers can have a positive impact on antimicrobial use, especially when combined with the measurement of outcomes and feedback.[53] Newer studies have also evaluated novel vehicles for education, including the use of social media or videogames.[53]

While ASPs have traditionally focused on educating prescribers, there is increasing attention on the need for the education of ASP team members. A 2016 survey of adult ID fellowship directors found that half had a formal stewardship curriculum and that, while 60% reported that their fellows had oversight of antimicrobial approvals, only 13% formally assessed their fellows' competency in antimicrobial stewardship.[54] In response to this gap, the IDSA developed a Core Antimicrobial Stewardship Curriculum for fellows that has grown and expanded since. PIDS also has recommendations for the training and experience that pediatric ID fellows should obtain to become effective antimicrobial stewardship practitioners.[55] Further research is needed into the optimal methods to educate ASP team members and how to assess competency to optimize ASP effectiveness.

ASP education of nonprescribers is also important. As noted previously, nurses cite knowledge gaps about antibiotics and stewardship concepts as a primary barrier to their participation in the stewardship process.[29] Targeted education for nurses and other members of the health care team, including respiratory therapists, should be a priority for ASPs in the future. Team members who do not prescribe antibiotics still have a significant impact on antibiotic use through their influence on decisions about whether and how to obtain diagnostics as well as their relationships with patients, which may be closer than that of prescribers due to their more frequent presence at the bedside. Education and collaboration with nurses and other bedside members of the health care team are crucial to optimize diagnostics and subsequent antimicrobial use and because they are important allies in patient education, which has been a focus of outpatient stewardship but has been largely overlooked in inpatient stewardship programs.

Antimicrobial stewardship has traditionally been centered in major academic centers, but 73% of hospitals in the US have fewer than 200 beds, and most pediatric hospitalizations are in nonchildren's hospitals.[24,56] All hospitals are required by regulatory agencies to have a stewardship program that focuses on all patient populations, including pediatrics, and has implemented the CDC Core Elements, but there are significant challenges in community hospitals that may not have providers and pharmacists with ID or stewardship training. In 2015 only 49% of small hospitals had ASPs that met the CDC Core Elements.[24] Expanding ASP access to smaller community hospitals is critically important, but data on the best ways to do so are limited.

Telehealth is often proposed as a solution, but the specific components that are necessary and beneficial need to be defined, as well as which elements can be performed remotely and which require local partners. A cluster-randomized study in 15 small children's hospitals in the same system evaluated the impact of 3 different levels of stewardship intervention.[57] All hospitals received basic stewardship education and tools directed at local pharmacists, provider access to an ID hotline 24 hours a day and 7 days a week, and an antibiotic utilization report. The next most intensive group also received advanced education for pharmacists, limited prospective audit and feedback, and local restriction of antimicrobials that was overseen by local pharmacists. The most intensive intervention group also received more expanded audit and feedback, ID-controlled antibiotic restriction, and ID review of designated culture results. Only the most intensive intervention group resulted in improvement in antibiotic use (and even in this group the finding did not achieve statistical significance).

These results highlight some of the opportunities and challenges in supporting ASPs at smaller hospitals. In this study identifying local ASP members and access to an ID hotline alone were not adequate to move the needle on antibiotic use or downstream patient outcomes. More frequent and intensive involvement of ID providers may be an important component of ASP outreach to smaller hospitals. This also highlights the importance of tracking metrics of interest to verify that interventions are actually achieving their intended outcomes. Likely, approaches will have to be tailored to local environments and may benefit from the use of QI methods, such as plan/do/study/act cycles, to allow for rapid adaptation based on results and feedback at the local hospital.

SUMMARY

Antibiotic use in hospitalized children is highly variable and often unnecessary, which puts children at risk of antibiotic-associated harms, including adverse drug events, the development of antibiotic resistance, and long-term chronic health problems. Antimicrobial stewardship programs are effective in reducing unnecessary antibiotic use and related costs. Antimicrobial review, pre or postprescription, is central to inpatient ASPs and prospective audit and feedback, especially handshake stewardship, may be the most effective method. The development of guidelines and decision-support tools can also improve appropriate prescribing and foster collaboration with frontline providers. Diagnostic stewardship is emerging as a crucial role for ASPs, in particular of newer rapid diagnostic panels. New research into the optimal ways to implement stewardship interventions has the potential to close the gap between evidence-based recommendations and practice changes. Further research is also needed into how to extend stewardship from large academic centers to smaller hospitals.

CLINICS CARE POINTS

- Inpatient pediatric antimicrobial stewardship programs (ASPs) should be co-led by a physician and pharmacist. Ideally leaders should have infectious diseases (ID) training; in settings where this is not possible, there are many resources for non-ID-trained leaders to gain the knowledge and skills required to build a successful ASP.

- ASPs should conduct antimicrobial review by either prospective audit and feedback, prior authorization, or a combination of the two. Handshake stewardship is an effective way to combine antimicrobial review and education to decrease unnecessary antibiotic use.

- Education is the cornerstone of a successful ASP. Targets for ASP education include frontline providers, infectious diseases fellows and future stewards, and non-prescriber healthcare professionals including nurses.

- ASPs can leverage behavioral science and implementation science to help translate evidence-based recommendations into practice changes.

DISCLOSURE

The author has nothing to disclose.

REFERENCES

1. Finland M, Weinstein L. Complications induced by antimicrobial agents. N Engl J Med 1953;248(6):220–6.
2. Finland M. Treatment of pneumonia and other serious infections. N Engl J Med 1960;263(5):207–21.
3. Scheckler WE, Bennett JV. Antibiotic usage in seven community hospitals. JAMA 1970;213(2):264–7.
4. Counts GW. Review and control of antimicrobial usage in hospitalized patients: a recommended collaborative approach. JAMA 1977;238(20):2170–2.
5. Kazanjian PH. Efforts to regulate antibiotic misuse in hospitals: A history. Infect Control Hosp Epidemiol 2021;1–4. https://doi.org/10.1017/ice.2021.330.
6. Marr JJ, Moffet HL, Kunin CM. Guidelines for improving the use of antimicrobial agents in hospitals: a statement by the Infectious Diseases Society of America. J Infect Dis 1988;157(5):869–76.
7. Briceland LL, Nightingale CH, Quintiliani R, et al. Antibiotic streamlining from combination therapy to monotherapy utilizing an interdisciplinary approach. Arch Intern Med 1988;148(9):2019–22.
8. Dellit TH, Owens RC, McGowan JE Jr, et al. Infectious Diseases Society of America and the Society for Healthcare Epidemiology of America guidelines for developing an institutional program to enhance antimicrobial stewardship. Clin Infect Dis 2007;44(2):159–77.
9. CDC. Core. Elements of hospital antibiotic stewardship programs. Atlanta (GA): US Department of Health and Human Services, CDC; 2019.
10. McPherson C, Lee BR, Terrill C, et al. Characteristics of pediatric antimicrobial stewardship programs: current status of the sharing antimicrobial reports for pediatric stewardship (SHARPS) Collaborative. Antibiotics (Basel) 2018;7(1). https://doi.org/10.3390/antibiotics7010004.
11. Gerber JS, Newland JG, Coffin SE, et al. Variability in antibiotic use at children's hospitals. Pediatrics 2010;126(6):1067–73.

12. Tribble AC, Lee BR, Flett KB, et al. Appropriateness of antibiotic prescribing in U.S. Children's Hospitals: a national point prevalence survey. Clin Infect Dis 2020. https://doi.org/10.1093/cid/ciaa036.

13. Lee BR, Tribble AC, Gerber JS, et al. Inappropriate antibiotic surgical prophylaxis in pediatric patients: a national point-prevalence study. Infect Control Hosp Epidemiol 2020;41(4):477–9.

14. Chiotos K, Tamma PD, Flett KB, et al. Multicenter Study of the risk factors for colonization or infection with carbapenem-resistant enterobacteriaceae in children. Antimicrob Agents Chemother 2017;61(12):e01440-17.

15. Same RG, Hsu AJ, Cosgrove SE, et al. Antibiotic-associated adverse events in hospitalized children. J Pediatr Infect Dis Soc 2021;10(5):622–8.

16. Bailey LC, Forrest CB, Zhang P, et al. Association of antibiotics in infancy with early childhood obesity. JAMA Pediatr 2014;168(11):1063–9.

17. Patrick DM, Sbihi H, Dai DLY, et al. Decreasing antibiotic use, the gut microbiota, and asthma incidence in children: evidence from population-based and prospective cohort studies. Lancet Respir Med 2020;8(11):1094–105.

18. Horton DB, Scott FI, Haynes K, et al. Antibiotic exposure and juvenile idiopathic arthritis: a Case-Control Study. Pediatr 2015;136(2):e333–43.

19. Smith MJ, Gerber JS, Hersh AL. Inpatient antimicrobial stewardship in pediatrics: a systematic review. J Pediatr Infect Dis Soc 2015;4(4):e127–35.

20. Wagner B, Filice GA, Drekonja D, et al. Antimicrobial stewardship programs in inpatient hospital settings: a systematic review. Infect Control Hosp Epidemiol 2014;35(10):1209–28.

21. Parker SK, Hurst AL, Thurm C, et al. Anti-infective acquisition costs for a stewardship program: getting to the bottom line. Clin Infect Dis 2017;65(10):1632–7.

22. Heil EL, Kuti JL, Bearden DT, et al. The essential role of pharmacists in antimicrobial stewardship. Infect Control Hosp Epidemiol 2016;37(7):753–4.

23. Waters CD. Pharmacist-driven antimicrobial stewardship program in an institution without infectious diseases physician support. Am J Health Syst Pharm 2015;72(6):466–8.

24. Stenehjem E, Hyun DY, Septimus E, et al. Antibiotic stewardship in small hospitals: barriers and potential solutions. Clin Infect Dis 2017;65(4):691–6.

25. Mack M, Brancaccio A, Popova K, et al. Stewardship-Hospitalist Collaboration. Infect Dis Clin North Am 2020;34(1):83–96.

26. Cosgrove SE, Hermsen ED, Rybak MJ, et al. Guidance for the knowledge and skills required for antimicrobial stewardship leaders. Infect Control Hosp Epidemiol 2014;35(12):1444–51.

27. Pediatric Infectious Diseases Society. Pediatric ASP Toolkit. Available at: https://pids.org/pediatric-asp-toolkit/. November 23, 2021.

28. Monsees EA, Tamma PD, Cosgrove SE, et al. Integrating bedside nurses into antibiotic stewardship: a practical approach. Infect Control Hosp Epidemiol 2019;40(5):579–84.

29. Carter EJ, Greendyke WG, Furuya EY, et al. Exploring the nurses' role in antibiotic stewardship: A multisite qualitative study of nurses and infection preventionists. Am J Infect Control 2018;46(5):492–7.

30. Fabre V, Pleiss A, Klein E, et al. A Pilot Study to Evaluate the impact of a nurse-driven urine culture diagnostic stewardship intervention on urine cultures in the acute care setting. Jt Comm J Qual Patient Saf 2020;46(11):650–5.

31. Kirby E, Broom A, Overton K, et al. Reconsidering the nursing role in antimicrobial stewardship: a multisite qualitative interview study. BMJ Open 2020;10(10):e042321.

32. Redefining the antibiotic stewardship team: recommendations from the American Nurses Association/Centers for Disease Control and Prevention Workgroup on the role of registered nurses in hospital antibiotic stewardship practices. JAC Antimicrobial Resist 2019;1(2). https://doi.org/10.1093/jacamr/dlz037.

33. Hurst AL, Child J, Pearce K, et al. Handshake stewardship: a highly effective rounding-based antimicrobial optimization service. Pediatr Infect Dis J 2016; 35(10):1104–10.

34. Tamma PD, Avdic E, Keenan JF, et al. What is the more effective antibiotic stewardship intervention: preprescription authorization or postprescription review with feedback? Clin Infect Dis 2017;64(5):537–43.

35. Jenkins TC, Tamma PD. Thinking beyond the "core" antibiotic stewardship interventions: shifting the onus for appropriate antibiotic use from stewardship teams to prescribing clinicians. Clin Infect Dis 2021;72(8):1457–62.

36. Smith MJ, Kong M, Cambon A, et al. Effectiveness of antimicrobial guidelines for community-acquired pneumonia in children. Pediatrics 2012;129(5):e1326–33.

37. Newman RE, Hedican EB, Herigon JC, et al. Impact of a guideline on management of children hospitalized with community-acquired pneumonia. Pediatrics 2012;129(3):e597–604.

38. Ambroggio L, Thomson J, Murtagh Kurowski E, et al. Quality improvement methods increase appropriate antibiotic prescribing for childhood pneumonia. Pediatrics 2013;131(5):e1623–31.

39. Gerber JS, Jackson MA, Tamma PD, et al. Antibiotic Stewardship in Pediatrics. Pediatrics 2021;147(1). https://doi.org/10.1542/peds.2020-040295.

40. Pak D, Kronman M, Brothers A, et al. Rapid diagnostic testing alone does not alter antimicrobial prescribing in children with staphylococcus aureus bloodstream infection. Pediatr Infect Dis J 2020;39(8):E217–8.

41. Juttukonda LJ, Katz S, Gillon J, et al. Impact of a rapid blood culture diagnostic test in a children's hospital depends on gram-positive versus gram-negative organism and day versus night shift. J Clin Microbiol 2020;58(4):1–10.

42. Subramony A, Zachariah P, Krones A, et al. Impact of multiplex polymerase chain reaction testing for respiratory pathogens on healthcare resource utilization for pediatric inpatients. J Pediatr 2016;173:196–201.e2.

43. Lee BR, Hassan F, Jackson MA, et al. Impact of multiplex molecular assay turn-around-time on antibiotic utilization and clinical management of hospitalized children with acute respiratory tract infections. J Clin Virol 2019;110:11–6.

44. Rogers BB, Shankar P, Jerris RC, et al. Impact of a rapid respiratory panel test on patient outcomes. Arch Pathol Lab Med 2015;139(5):636–41.

45. Buchan BW, Windham S, Balada-Llasat JM, et al. Practical Comparison of the BioFire FilmArray Pneumonia panel to routine diagnostic methods and potential impact on antimicrobial stewardship in adult hospitalized patients with lower respiratory tract infections. J Clin Microbiol 2020;58(7). https://doi.org/10.1128/JCM. 00135-20.

46. Nguyen S, Same R. No small thing: clinical implications of rapid syndromic panel-based diagnostic testing in children. Clin Microbiol Newsl 2021;43(17):143–54.

47. Livorsi D, Comer A, Matthias MS, et al. Factors influencing antibiotic-prescribing decisions among inpatient physicians: a qualitative investigation. Infect Control Hosp Epidemiol 2015;36(9):1065–72.

48. Morris AM, Calderwood MS, Fridkin SK, et al. Research needs in antibiotic stewardship. Infect Control Hosp Epidemiol 2019;40(12):1334–43.

49. Stach LM, Hedican EB, Herigon JC, et al. Clinicians' Attitudes Towards an Antimicrobial Stewardship Program at a Children's Hospital. J Pediatr Infect Dis Soc 2012;1(3):190–7.

50. Niven DJ, Mrklas KJ, Holodinsky JK, et al. Towards understanding the de-adoption of low-value clinical practices: a scoping review. BMC Med 2015; 13:255.

51. Lee BR, Goldman JL, Yu D, et al. Clinical Impact of an Antibiotic Stewardship Program at a Children's Hospital. Infect Dis Ther 2017;6(1):103–13.

52. Tamma PD, Miller MA, Cosgrove SE. Rethinking how antibiotics are prescribed: incorporating the 4 moments of antibiotic decision making into clinical practice. JAMA 2019;321(2):139–40.

53. Satterfield J, Miesner AR, Percival KM. The role of education in antimicrobial stewardship. J Hosp Infect 2020;105(2):130–41.

54. Luther VP, Shnekendorf R, Abbo LM, et al. Antimicrobial Stewardship Training for Infectious Diseases Fellows: Program Directors Identify a Curriculum Need. Clin Infect Dis 2018;67(8):1285–7.

55. Pediatric Committee on Antimicrobial Stewardship. Antimicrobial stewardship experience for pediatric infectious diseases fellow. Pediatric Infectious Diseases Society. Available at: https://pids.org/wp-content/uploads/2021/04/106969-PIDS-Flyer-ASP-Experience_v2.pdf. November 27, 2021.

56. Leyenaar JK, Ralston SL, Shieh M-S, et al. Epidemiology of pediatric hospitalizations at general hospitals and freestanding children's hospitals in the United States. J Hosp Med 2016;11(11):743–9.

57. Stenehjem E, Hersh AL, Buckel WR, et al. Impact of implementing antibiotic stewardship programs in 15 small hospitals: a cluster-randomized intervention. Clin Infect Dis 2018;67(4):525–32.

Targets and Methods to Improve Outpatient Antibiotic Prescribing for Pediatric Patients

Nicole M. Poole, MD, MPH, Assistant Professor[a],*,
Holly Frost, MD, Assistant Professor[b]

KEYWORDS

- Acute respiratory tract infection • Antibacterial agents • Antibiotic stewardship
- Ambulatory care • Child • Drug prescriptions • Drug utilization review
- Health Services research

KEY POINTS

- Antibiotics are overprescribed to children in outpatient settings, most commonly for acute respiratory tract infections (eg, acute otitis media and pharyngitis).
- High-yield antibiotic stewardship efforts should focus on establishing the correct diagnosis and observing children without an antibiotic prescription. When an antibiotic is indicated, clinicians should prescribe a narrow-spectrum antibiotic agent (eg, amoxicillin) for shorter durations (eg, 5 days) for most outpatient bacterial illnesses in children.
- Clinicians can use existing features in the electronic medical record to measure and trend relatively easy-to-attain metrics of antibiotic prescribing quality in outpatient settings.
- The Centers for Disease Control and Prevention has established 4 Core Elements of Outpatient Antimicrobial Stewardship to serve as a guide to improve antibiotic prescribing in outpatient settings, which include action for policy and procedures, commitment, tracking and reporting (ie, audit and feedback), and education.

Most antibiotics prescribed to children occur in outpatient settings, which include pediatric and family medicine clinics, emergency departments (EDs), urgent care centers, retail clinics, telehealth, and dentist offices.[1] Although the volume of antibiotics prescribed for children has decreased over the past 20 years, antibiotics continue

[a] Department of Pediatrics, Division of Pediatric Infectious Diseases and Epidemiology, University of Colorado School of Medicine, Children's Hospital Colorado, 13123 East 16th Avenue, Aurora, CO 80045, USA; [b] Department of Pediatrics, Center for Health Systems Research, Denver Health and Hospital Authority, University of Colorado School of Medicine, 601 Bannock Street, Denver, CO 80204, USA
* Corresponding author.
E-mail address: Nicole.Poole@ChildrensColorado.org

to be overprescribed for common pediatric illnesses.[2] A conservative estimate is that at least 30% of antibiotic use in outpatient settings is unnecessary, prescribed for infections that do not warrant antibiotics, such as viral infections.[3] Although more than 55% of bacterial acute otitis media (AOM) cases self-resolve, antibiotics are prescribed in greater than 95% of patients diagnosed with AOM.[4] Clinicians prescribe first-line antibiotics in just about 60% of the most common bacterial acute respiratory tract infections (ARTIs [AOM, pharyngitis, and sinusitis]), and 55% of antibiotics are prescribed for durations longer than needed.[5,6] National academic societies, such as the American Academy of Pediatrics and American Academy of Family Practice, recognize the growing body of epidemiologic evidence surrounding the consequences of overprescribing antibiotics and the importance of dedicating efforts to address this problem to improve the quality of care for children in outpatient settings.[7]

Decreasing inappropriate antibiotics prescribed to children in outpatient settings is a national patient and public safety priority.[8] Outpatient antibiotic stewardship efforts have been shown to decrease inappropriate antibiotic prescribing and improve the quality of patient care in a variety of settings.[9] The Centers for Disease Control and Prevention (CDC) has established Core Elements of Outpatient Antimicrobial Stewardship to guide organizations in the development of an outpatient antibiotic stewardship program.[10] The Joint Commission now has specific requirements for outpatient health care organizations to establish an outpatient antibiotic stewardship program, which include outlining annual goals to improve antibiotic prescribing, implementing efforts to improve prescribing, and reporting data on antibiotic prescribing.[11] In this article, the authors describe the burden of antibiotic prescribing to children in outpatient settings, identify targets for improvement, and use the CDC Core Elements of Outpatient Stewardship as a framework to describe pragmatic methods to measure and improve antibiotic prescribing in outpatient settings.

RISKS ASSOCIATED WITH ANTIBIOTIC USE
Adverse Drug Events

Prescribers must consider the risks associated with the use of antibiotics, as they would any medication prescribed to patients. Antibiotics are the most common drug class responsible for ED visits for an adverse drug event (ADE) in children, accounting for nearly 60% of visits for ADEs in children ages 0 to 5 years old.[12] ADEs occur in 25% of children with ARTI who receive narrow-spectrum antibiotics and 36% of patients who receive broader-spectrum antibiotics.[13] The most frequently reported ADEs include diarrhea (70%), rash (40%), and vomiting/upset stomach (21%), with nearly 30% of patients experiencing more than one ADE with a course of antibiotics.[13] Importantly, most adverse events experienced by children prescribed antibiotics are not reported or documented by a clinician.[13]

For the most commonly cited indications for antibiotics in children, including AOM and group A *Streptococcus* (GAS) pharyngitis, the number of children needed to harm approaches or exceeds the number of children needed to treat for symptomatic improvement.[14] For patients with GAS nasopharyngeal carriage but without active GAS pharyngitis, there is no benefit from antibiotic treatment. For every 1000 patients treated for GAS pharyngitis, antibiotics will shorten the duration of symptoms for 270 patients by 16 hours.[15] Data primarily studying rates of acute rheumatic fever in US military troops in the 1950s showed that 53 patients needed to be treated to prevent one episode of acute rheumatic fever.[16] However, cases of acute rheumatic fever are now more rare. When the current rates of acute rheumatic fever are considered in pediatric populations in low-risk countries, the number of children needed to treat nears

10,000 to prevent one case of acute rheumatic fever.[17] The risks of antibiotics are important to consider when developing improvement targets in outpatient settings.

Antibiotic Resistance

The development of antibiotic-resistant organisms is a growing global threat to health.[18] Antibiotic consumption is directly associated with the development of antibiotic resistance at the individual and community level.[19] Children increasingly present to care with community-acquired (CA) antibiotic-resistant urinary tract, skin and soft tissue, and respiratory infections.[20–22] The use of common oral antibiotics (eg, amoxicillin) in children is a significant risk factor for carriage of, or infection by, drug-resistant bacteria in children.[23,24] In addition, cohabiting families and people in close social environments are often colonized with the same bacterial flora, highlighting the need to decrease inappropriate antibiotic prescribing to both children and adults.[25]

Clostridium difficile Infections

More than 70% of *C difficile* infections (CDI) in children are acquired in the community.[26,27] CA-CDI is associated with use of cephalosporin and broad-spectrum penicillin antibiotics within the prior 30 days.[27,28] It is estimated that reducing outpatient antibiotic prescribing rates by 10% would decrease CA-CDI rates by 17%, highlighting the importance of decreasing unnecessary antibiotic courses to decrease the incidence of CA-CDI in children.[29]

Chronic Disease

The use of antibiotics has been linked to dysbiosis of the microbiota of the gut.[30] Epidemiologic studies have linked antibiotic use early in life to chronic diseases later in life, including autoimmune diseases (eg, inflammatory bowel disease and juvenile idiopathic arthritis) and atopic diseases (eg, allergy and asthma).[31,32] The cumulative effect of repeat antibiotic exposures is associated with higher risk of developing these chronic diseases, highlighting the importance of judicious antibiotic prescribing, particularly early in life.[31]

CHARACTERISTICS OF ANTIBIOTICS PRESCRIBED

The selection of an appropriate antibiotic requires making the right diagnosis and prescribing the right drug at the right dose for the right duration. Antibiotics are most frequently prescribed to children for ARTI.[6,33] Many ARTIs are caused by viruses, but even most bacterial ARTIs will self-resolve without antibiotics.[34] Observation with treatment of symptoms is therefore the preferred initial treatment course for most childhood infections.

When antibiotics are indicated, national guidelines for ARTI most commonly recommend a narrow-spectrum penicillin, such as amoxicillin.[35,36] Despite national recommendations, nearly half of antibiotics prescribed to children are broad-spectrum agents, including macrolides and broad-spectrum cephalosporins, frequently prescribed for ARTI but rarely indicated for these conditions.[6,37] Broad-spectrum antibiotics provide no additional clinical benefit for the treatment of most ARTI and are associated with increased ADEs and lower reported quality-of-life scores compared with narrow-spectrum antibiotics.[13] Guideline-concordant narrow-spectrum antibiotic prescribing is therefore an important target for improvement in outpatient settings.

Macrolides (eg, azithromycin) are commonly overprescribed to children, with at least 15 million courses prescribed to children annually in outpatient settings.[6,38,39] Azithromycin is a suboptimal choice for most diagnoses given the high rates of macrolide resistance among the most common bacterial pathogens causing childhood respiratory illnesses: *Streptococcus pneumoniae* and GAS.[38] High rates of azithromycin prescribing are also correlated with higher rates of penicillin and multidrug-resistant *S pneumoniae* strains in children, likely because of the long half-life of azithromycin.[40] In addition, a growing number of studies have correlated azithromycin consumption in children with the development of obesity later in life.[41,42] Azithromycin prescribing in children is a high-yield target for improvement given the relatively poor efficacy of azithromycin in treating common bacterial diagnoses and the associated risks of use.

When antibiotics are necessary, a growing body of literature suggests that shorter durations of antibiotics (eg, 5–7 days) are equally effective as longer durations for the most common diagnoses, including AOM, sinusitis, urinary tract infection, CA pneumonia, and skin and soft tissue infection.[36,43,44] However, the median duration of therapy of antibiotics for common bacterial illnesses in outpatient settings is 10 days.[45] Prolonged durations of therapy have been shown to be one of the greatest risk factors for the selection of antibiotic-resistant organisms.[43] Longer durations of antibiotics are also significantly associated with an increase in gastrointestinal ADEs.[46] Decreasing the duration of therapy of antibiotics for common illnesses is therefore an important target to decrease the selective pressure for resistant bacterial organisms and unnecessary ADEs from antibiotics in children.

VARIABILITY IN ANTIBIOTIC PRESCRIBING AND TARGETS FOR IMPROVEMENT

When controlling for patient-level factors, there is marked variability in the appropriateness of antibiotics prescribed to children at a national and local level.[3,47] Unintended variation in medical management helps identify opportunities for improvement in the quality of health care provided.[48]

Antibiotic prescribing to children varies by region and outpatient setting. Regionally, when controlling for patient-level factors, southern regions of the United States have higher prescribing rates at 553 antibiotic prescriptions per 1000 population compared with the prescribing rates of western regions of the United States at 423 antibiotic prescriptions per 1000 population.[3] Pediatricians prescribe the highest volume of antibiotics to children in the United States.[37] However, children are often cared for by nonpediatric providers. Family medicine providers care for 1 in 3 children nationwide, which is higher in regions with higher density of children and in rural regions where there are fewer pediatric clinics.[49] Children in the United States also increasingly receive medical care from advanced practice providers (nurse practitioners and physician assistants), a trend expected to continue with increased presence of advanced practice providers in outpatient settings.[37] Finally, nearly 90% of the almost 29 million visits by children to EDs in the United States annually occur at nonpediatric EDs, which are less likely to be staffed by pediatric-trained clinicians compared with pediatric EDs.[50,51]

There is variability in the appropriateness of antibiotic prescribing across the diverse group of outpatient settings where children receive their medical care. Pediatricians are an important target for improvement efforts given the volume of antibiotics they prescribe. Nonpediatric providers and clinicians at acute care centers (eg, ED and urgent care centers) have been found to prescribe antibiotics more frequently for ARTI and use off-guideline agents, such as azithromycin, more frequently in children compared with pediatric centers.[38,50,52,53] The differences in antibiotic prescribing practices seen between provider and outpatient setting types could reflect differences in training, competing priorities, or less awareness of changing guidelines for children.

There are disparities in antibiotic prescribing for children from different insurance types, which is often used as a proxy for socioeconomic status, and for children from different races. Compared with White children, Black children are less likely to be prescribed antibiotics overall (29.0% vs 23.5%; adjusted odds ratio [aOR], 0.75), broad-spectrum antibiotics (36.9% vs 34.0%; aOR, 0.88), and/or antibiotics for upper respiratory infection (URI) and AOM.[54–57] Children with private insurance are 15% to 20% more likely to be prescribed azithromycin and broad-spectrum antibiotics compared with those with public insurance.[6,38] These findings suggest that there are drivers of antibiotic prescribing based on factors independent of the diagnosis, such as implicit bias and health care plan reimbursement. There is a need to better understand and target improvement efforts toward the drivers of regional, provider, and patient-level variations in antibiotic prescribing to promote health equity.

Sociobehavioral Factors

Inappropriate antibiotic prescribing is influenced by sociobehavioral factors and human behavior. The perception of parent expectations for antibiotics is frequently reported by providers as a primary driver for inappropriate antibiotic prescribing in children.[58,59] However, clinicians accurately predict parent expectations for antibiotics about half of the time.[58,60] Clinicians perceive an expectation for antibiotics from parents that might actually be seeking reassurance surrounding the severity of their child's illness.[60] Clinicians prescribe antibiotics unnecessarily in response to perceived parent expectations because they wish to provide something that seems "valuable" during the clinic visit, prefer to avoid negative repercussions from denying antibiotics, and believe that efforts to refuse antibiotics are futile, leading to wasted time and energy.[61]

Concern over patient satisfaction scores drives inappropriate antibiotic prescribing.[59] However, research has shown that patient satisfaction is not driven by the receipt of an antibiotic, but rather by strong communication during the visit.[62,63] The personal perception of risk by a clinician and diagnostic uncertainty also drives inappropriate prescribing.[64] Finally, time pressures increase inappropriate prescribing. Inappropriate antibiotics are prescribed more frequently toward the end of a clinic shift and work week, suggesting that decision fatigue plays a role in the appropriateness of antibiotics.[65]

PRACTICAL STRATEGIES FOR OUTPATIENT STEWARDSHIP

Outpatient stewardship efforts must span a breadth of practice environments ranging from small private practices to large integrated health systems and EDs. Because 40% to 60% of antibiotics for children are prescribed by nonpediatrician providers (including family medicine, ED, and advanced practice providers), organizations should strongly consider interventions that span specialties and disciplines to improve antibiotic prescribing for children and assure there is consistency in prescribing practices.[3,6,53] Given the global diversity in outpatient practice settings, a one-size-fits-all approach is unlikely to be feasible or effective for all organizations.

Low-Hanging Fruit

The most commonly cited indications for antibiotics in children are AOM (24%), pharyngitis (14%), sinusitis (10%), and viral URI (7%).[3,6,37] Thus, focusing on these diagnoses will have the greatest impact on overall antibiotic use. Considerable attention has been given to improving outpatient prescribing for CA pneumonia, urinary tract infections, and skin and soft tissue infections; however, combined, these diagnoses account for fewer than 13% of total antibiotics prescribed to children.[3,6,37]

Interventions for bacterial infections should focus on the correct diagnosis, drug, dose, and/or antibiotic duration. In addition, for many ARTIs such as AOM and sinusitis, the use of observation or delayed antibiotic prescribing, where a family is given a prescription to fill only if the child worsens or does not improve, is recommended by national guidelines. Observation or delayed prescribing for ARTIs may significantly reduce antibiotic utilization (utilization: 93%–98% immediate; 27%–39% delayed; 10%–12% observation) and does not result in worse patient outcomes.[34,36,66–68]

Table 1 shows potential high-yield antibiotic stewardship metrics, targets, and difficulty rating for common outpatient infections for children. For each diagnosis, the denominator can be obtained by using either International Classification of Diseases (ICD) codes, selected indication in antibiotic prescription fields, or query of the electronic health record (EHR) by diagnosis text or category. Although the accuracy of these methodologies is not well described, anecdotal experience indicates that of

Table 1
High-yield outpatient antibiotic stewardship metrics and targets for children

Diagnosis/Drug	Metric	Target	Difficulty
Total prescribing	% Patients seen who are prescribed an antibiotic	Varies	Easy
Viral upper respiratory infection	% No antibiotics	100%	Easy
Amoxicillin index	% Antibiotics prescribed that are amoxicillin	[a]	Easy
Acute respiratory tract infection	% Prescribed an antibiotic	[a]	Easy
Acute otitis media	% First-line antibiotic: amoxicillin	80%[b]	Easy
	% Delayed antibiotic or observation	30%[c]	Difficult
	% Children ≥2 y of age who receive 5–7 d of therapy	80%[d]	Moderate
Pharyngitis	% First-line antibiotic: amoxicillin or penicillin	90%[e]	Easy
	% Patients treated that had a positive test (rapid test or culture) for group A streptococcus	100%	Easy
	% Tests ordered that were appropriate (patient ≥3 y, no congestion or cough documented)	80%	Difficult
Sinusitis	% First-line antibiotic: amoxicillin or amoxicillin-clavulanate	90%[f]	Easy
Azithromycin	% Patients with AOM, pharyngitis, or sinusitis prescribed azithromycin	<5%[g]	Easy
All diagnoses prescribed an antibiotic	% Antibiotics prescribed with prescription duration of ≥7 d	[a]	Moderate

[a] National benchmarking metrics are needed to set a definitive target.
[b] Accounts for 10% penicillin allergy and patients with recurrent or recent AOM.
[c] Based on American Academy of Pediatrics/CDC collaborative target achievable in clinic practices.
[d] Assumes up to 20% of children will have recurrence, severity, or complications that necessitate a longer duration. Consider removing patients who received azithromycin from the denominator. Based on achievable target in pediatric clinics.
[e] Assumes a 10% patient-reported penicillin allergy.
[f] Accounts for 10% patient-reported penicillin allergy.
[g] Accounts for patient-reported severe penicillin allergy.

these methods, use of ICD codes tends to be the most accurate and easiest to use if available. Laboratory test results can be obtained by searching for Current Procedure Technology codes or query of the EHR by laboratory test text or category. The metrics associated with viral URI and laboratory testing for GAS can be particularly important for organizations because they are publicly reported Healthcare Effectiveness Data and Information Set measures and can affect reimbursement rates.[69]

Effective Interventions

The CDC has outlined 4 Core Elements of Outpatient Stewardship to guide program development, including action for policy and procedures, commitment, tracking and reporting (ie, audit and feedback), and education.[10] Generally, multifaceted interventions have been shown to be the most effective.[9,70–74] Here, the authors provide practical strategies for program implementation in alignment with the CDC Core Elements of Outpatient Stewardship.

Commitment

Establishing a clinician champion at each clinical site or for the organization is important to help direct changes, answer questions, and monitor progress. A clinical champion could be a physician, pharmacist, advanced practice provider, or nurse that has direct contact with clinical staff. Although data on the effectiveness of clinician champions for stewardship in outpatient settings are lacking, there is a small but growing body of evidence that this approach is effective in inpatient stewardship programs and for general implementation of quality improvement programs.[10,75,76] Ideally, clinician champions would have antibiotic stewardship tasks incorporated into their job descriptions; however, the authors have found that in practice this can be challenging, particularly within larger health care systems.[10,77]

Commitment posters are likely the least expensive strategy to reduce inappropriate prescribing. A study by Meeker and colleagues[78] found that putting a poster in examination rooms describing commitment to not prescribing antibiotics unless needed decreased prescribing by 20% compared with controls. The CDC and many state health departments have free templates for commitment posters that can be downloaded and modified.[79] In the authors' experience, printing logistics, finding photographs, and formatting can be barriers to the use of commitment posters.[77] Therefore, practices should prioritize prompt use of posters over insertion of signatures and photographs or large-size printing that cannot be completed in-house. In larger health care systems, needing administrative approval to hanging posters can be a challenge. Some practices have circumvented this by displaying commitment posters as a screen saver on computers in examination rooms.[77]

Action for Policy and Procedures

The key element of action for policy and procedures is to make the "right" choice the easy choice for providers and staff. Easy-to-read, evidence-based clinical care pathways that are readily accessible to providers from all specialties that care for children are critically important.[80–82] Although most professional societies publish guidelines, these are not always easily identified and accessible to providers from other specialties. Furthermore, they are typically too lengthy to read while directly caring for patients. For practices that do not have internal clinical care pathways, numerous free resources from children's hospitals are available online and can be linked to directly from the EHR tool bar, prescription fields, or provider desktop with permission from the hosting organization.[83–85] These pathways are evidence-based, are updated regularly by teams of experts, are viewable on mobile devices, and can reduce the burden on practices to develop their own pathways. The pathways also provide key information on diagnostic testing, antibiotic choice, dosage, and duration. Providers should be aware that local epidemiology and antibiotic susceptibilities may differ between organizations for certain infections, such as skin and soft tissue infections and urinary tract infections, and they should consider local susceptibility patterns when determining antibiotic choice. The authors highly recommend that practices that do not have internal clinical pathways use these free public resources so they can more wholly devote internal resources to other components of stewardship.

Requiring providers to associate the antibiotic with a diagnostic code or indication before signing the order can also reduce inappropriate prescribing.[86,87] Although most inpatient antibiotic stewardship programs use indication categories (eg, skin and soft tissue infection, urinary tract infection) within the prescription field, association with ICD codes rather than selecting an indication can often reduce clicks for outpatient providers because they are also required for outpatient billing. Most major EHR have this setting available, and it can simply be turned on rather than requiring a major EHR change.[88,89]

Changes to prescription fields for the most common antibiotics prescribed to children can substantially improve prescribing (Frost H, Lou Y, Keith A, et al. Increasing guideline-concordant durations of antibiotic therapy for acute otitis media. 2021, unpublished data). These changes can include additional guidance, such as a hyperlink to clinical care pathways directly from the prescription or "help" text that describes the appropriate dosage and duration for each diagnosis. Minor changes to the default order can be highly effective, such as adjusting the "quick select" buttons so the correct dose and duration are easy to select and inappropriate options are not readily available or have to be manually typed in (eg, quick select button for 5 and 10 days of amoxicillin with the 14-day button removed), and providing a quick method to select if the prescription is an immediate or delayed prescription so it is sent to the pharmacy correctly and displays accurate patient instructions.[70] Similarly, clinical decision support can be provided within the text of laboratory results.[90] Finally, diagnosis-specific order sets can facilitate appropriate antibiotic selection and reduce time for providers by incorporating patient education, billing codes, and documentation.[89,91]

Diagnostic stewardship can be critical to reducing antibiotic utilization. This is particularly true for GAS because pharyngeal carriage rates are high among children.[92] Often, pharyngeal swabs are collected and tested for GAS by medical assistants or nurses before the provider seeing the patient. If the test is positive, most providers will treat with antibiotics even if testing was not indicated and infection is unlikely.[93] Clinical algorithms for medical assistants that provide guidance on who to test for GAS can be easily created and hung in clinical practice locations to guide collection and testing. A study by Norton and colleagues found that a simple algorithm for medical assistants combined with provider education decreased testing for GAS by 24%.[72] EHR laboratory decision support can also be created such that laboratory tests that may be inappropriate are flagged for providers (eg, GAS test in a patient <3 years of age).

Tracking and Reporting

Tracking and reporting (also known as audit and feedback) is one of the most effective strategies to improve antibiotic prescribing.[71,86] A variety of effective approaches can be taken, including (1) individualized provider feedback with blinded peer comparison; (2) individualized provider feedback with nonblinded peer comparison; and (3) individualized provider feedback that informs providers if the prescribers "are a top prescriber" or "are not a top prescriber."[86] Some practices have chosen to only provide feedback to poor prescribers (eg, 10% highest prescribers), whereas others provide feedback to everyone. Studies have shown that tracking and reporting likely needs to be continued after an initial intervention to sustain lower prescribing rates.[87,94] It is not clear how often continued feedback should be provided.

Unfortunately, tracking and reporting is often found to be the most laborious and logistically challenging Core Element to implement.[77] To simplify tracking and reporting, practices can identify easy metrics (**Table 2**) that allow data to be pulled completely electronically. If accessing data or producing reports is a major limitation or manual chart review will be needed to obtain data, consider providing feedback less often (eg, quarterly) or use a point-prevalence approach.[95,96] To use a point-prevalence approach, select a small number of random dates during each time period and only analyze data from those dates. This substantially reduces the time needed for abstraction and can provide a good estimate of prescribing trends. Reports can be discussed at provider meetings, posted on clinic bulletin boards, or e-mailed to providers. E-mail and provider meetings offer the advantage that you can clearly document who has reviewed reports, which is useful for stewardship, but also typically required for American Board of Pediatrics Maintenance of Certification programs.

Table 2	
Practical strategies for outpatient pediatric antibiotic stewardship	
Core Element	**Strategy**
Overall guidance	CDC Core Elements of Outpatient Stewardship web page[75] MITIGATE toolkit (available on CDC Web site)[99] American Academy of Pediatrics: Improving antibiotic prescribing for children change package[100]
Commitment	Clinician champions Include stewardship activities in job descriptions Commitment posters Commitment screen saver

Action for policy and procedures	Clinical care guidelines
	 Accountable justification- link diagnostic code with antibiotic
	 order in EHR
	 Prescription field prompts
	   Hyperlink to clinical care guidelines
	   Brief "help text"
	   Correct easy select buttons for dosage and duration
	   Quick check box for immediate vs delayed prescription
	 Laboratory result "help text"
	 Order sets for specific diagnoses
	 Clinical algorithms for diagnostic testing for ancillary staff
	 Clinical algorithms for diagnostic testing for providers built into
	 the EHR

Tracking and reporting	If resource limited:
	   Choose an easy metric that can be pulled electronically
	   Reduce frequency (quarterly)
	   Point-prevalence approach
	   Automate feedback reporting

Education	Diagnosis specific
	 Dialogue Around Respiratory Illness Treatment modules[95]
	 CDC outpatient antibiotic stewardship training[75]
	 American Board of Pediatrics or American Board of Family Medicine
	   Maintenance of Certification or Performance Improvement credit
	   programs

Finally, consider automating tracking and reporting. Tracking can be automated by setting up a recurring report in your EHR or asking your informational technology department to send you reports at predefined intervals. To fully automate tracking and reporting or for complex metrics, consider using an external statistical software code that accesses the EHR data warehouse.[88] This free method can be set up once by a data analyst or biostatistician and will e-mail reports out at predefined intervals for as long as desired with no additional labor or cost. Once set up, the code can be easily expanded to other provider groups, shared or borrowed from other organizations, or modified for different metrics.

Education and Expertise

Education is an important component of any stewardship program. It is often the easiest Core Element for practices to implement, although it is unlikely to sustain reduced prescribing without the addition of other stewardship activities. In addition to education on appropriate prescribing by diagnosis, dedicated education on communicating with patients and families has been shown to significantly change prescribing behavior and improve patient satisfaction.[97,98] The Dialogue Around Respiratory Illness Treatment education videos are evidence-based and freely available online.[99] In addition, the CDC offers free training on antibiotic stewardship in outpatient settings that provides continuing medical education credits.[100] These tools are not specialty specific and are relevant and available to providers who care for children across specialties. Finally, American Board of Pediatrics Part 4 Maintenance of Certification, American Board of Family Medicine Performance Improvement activities, and continuing medication education programs can be easily and inexpensively created by practices to encourage provider engagement.[101,102]

SUMMARY

In summary, antibiotic overprescribing in outpatient settings causes increased CA antibiotic-resistant infections and high rates of ADEs, which threatens the health of children globally. Variations in antibiotic prescribing by medical setting, provider type, and diagnosis identify opportunities to improve the quality of antibiotic prescribing in children. Antibiotic prescribing metrics should be used to measure antibiotic prescribing in order to identify high-yield targets for improvement, trend antibiotic prescribing over time, and provide feedback to prescribers. Clinicians and outpatient health care organizations can use resources, such as the CDC Core Elements of Outpatient Stewardship, to aid in the implementation of antibiotic stewardship efforts.

CLINICS CARE POINTS

- When deciding whether to prescribe an antibiotic, clinicians should weigh the harm caused by antibiotics, including diarrhea, rash, increased risk of drug resistant infections, and increased risk for developing chronic diseases.
- Most bacterial upper respiratory infections (eg acute otitis media or sinusitis) will self-resolve; therefore, clinicians should strongly consider observation or delayed prescribing for these diagnoses.
- Avoid using azithromycin for pediatric respiratory infections given the high national rates of macrolide resistance and the risk of drug-resistant bacterial colonization after azithromycin use.

- If an antibiotic is warranted, select the most narrow-spectrum antibiotic (eg amoxicillin or cephalexin) for the shortest duration possible (eg 5 days) to treat most pediatric outpatient infections.
- Utilize clinical care pathways as a reference for diagnostic testing, antibiotic choice, dosage, and duration of antibiotic therapy for common pediatric outpatient infections.
- The CDCs four Core Elements of Outpatient Stewardship outlines key components of successful programs to improve outpatient antibiotic use.

DISCLOSURE

The authors have no conflicts of interest to disclose.

REFERENCES

1. Suda KJ, Hicks LA, Roberts RM, et al. A national evaluation of antibiotic expenditures by healthcare setting in the United States, 2009. J Antimicrob Chemother 2013;68(3):715–8.
2. Finkelstein JA, Raebel MA, Nordin JD, et al. Trends in outpatient antibiotic use in 3 health plans. Pediatrics 2019;143(1):e20181259.
3. Fleming-Dutra KE, Hersh AL, Shapiro DJ, et al. Prevalence of inappropriate antibiotic prescriptions among US ambulatory care visits, 2010-2011. JAMA 2016; 315(17):1864–73.
4. Frost HM, Gerber JS, Hersh AL. Antibiotic recommendations for acute otitis media and acute bacterial sinusitis. Pediatr Infect Dis J 2019;38(2):217.
5. King LM, Hersh AL, Hicks LA, et al. Duration of outpatient antibiotic therapy for common outpatient infections, 2017. Clin Infect Dis 2020;72(10):e663–6.
6. Hersh AL, Shapiro DJ, Pavia AT, et al. Antibiotic prescribing in ambulatory pediatrics in the United States. Pediatrics 2011;128(6):1053–61.
7. Gerber JS, Jackson MA, Tamma PD, et al, AAP Committee on Infectious Diseases and Pediatric Infectious Diseases Society. Policy statement: antibiotic stewardship in pediatrics. J Pediatr Infect Dis Soc 2021;10(5):641–9.
8. The White House. National action plan for combating antibiotic-resistant bacteria, 2020-2025, Federal Task Force on Combating Antibiotic-Resistant Bacteria. Washington D.C: U.S. Department of Health & Human Services; 2020.
9. Drekonja DM, Filice GA, Greer N, et al. Antimicrobial stewardship in outpatient settings: a systematic review. Infect Control Hosp Epidemiol 2015;36(2):142–52.
10. Sanchez GV, Fleming-Dutra KE, Roberts RM, et al. Core elements of outpatient antibiotic stewardship. MMWR Recomm Rep 2016;65(6):1–12.
11. The Joint Commission. Antimicrobial Stewardship in Ambulatory Health Care. Requirement, Rationale, Reference Report (R3), Issue 23. June 20, 2019.
12. Shehab N, Lovegrove MC, Geller AI, et al. US emergency department visits for outpatient adverse drug events, 2013-2014. JAMA 2016;316(20):2115–25.
13. Gerber JS, Ross RK, Bryan M, et al. Association of broad- vs narrow-spectrum antibiotics with treatment failure, adverse events, and quality of life in children with acute respiratory tract infections. JAMA 2017;318(23):2325–36.
14. Venekamp RP, Burton MJ, van Dongen TM, et al. Antibiotics for otitis media with effusion in children. Cochrane Database Syst Rev 2016;6:CD009163.
15. Spinks A, Glasziou PP, Del Mar CB. Antibiotics for sore throat. Cochrane Database Syst Rev 2013;11:CD000023.

16. Robertson KA, Volmink JA, Mayosi BM. Antibiotics for the primary prevention of acute rheumatic fever: a meta-analysis. BMC Cardiovasc Disord 2005;5(1):11.

17. McMurray K, Garber M. Taking chances with strep throat. Hosp Pediatr 2015; 5(10):552–4.

18. Bryce A, Hay AD, Lane IF, et al. Global prevalence of antibiotic resistance in paediatric urinary tract infections caused by Escherichia coli and association with routine use of antibiotics in primary care: systematic review and meta-analysis. BMJ 2016;352:i939.

19. Bell BG, Schellevis F, Stobberingh E, et al. A systematic review and meta-analysis of the effects of antibiotic consumption on antibiotic resistance. BMC Infect Dis 2014;14:13.

20. Edlin RS, Shapiro DJ, Hersh AL, et al. Antibiotic resistance patterns of outpatient pediatric urinary tract infections. J Urol 2013;190(1):222–7.

21. Kaur R, Pham M, Yu KOA, et al. Rising pneumococcal antibiotic resistance in the post-13-valent pneumococcal conjugate vaccine era in pediatric isolates from a primary care setting. Clin Infect Dis 2021;72(5):797–805.

22. Khamash DF, Voskertchian A, Tamma PD, et al. Increasing clindamycin and trimethoprim-sulfamethoxazole resistance in pediatric staphylococcus aureus infections. J Pediatr Infect Dis Soc 2019;8(4):351–3.

23. Koliou MG, Andreou K, Lamnisos D, et al. Risk factors for carriage of Streptococcus pneumoniae in children. BMC Pediatr 2018;18(1):144.

24. Paschke AA, Zaoutis T, Conway PH, et al. Previous antimicrobial exposure is associated with drug-resistant urinary tract infections in children. Pediatrics 2010;125(4):664–72.

25. Brito IL, Gurry T, Zhao S, et al. Transmission of human-associated microbiota along family and social networks. Nat Microbiol 2019;4(6):964–71.

26. Antonara S, Leber AL. Diagnosis of Clostridium difficile infections in children. J Clin Microbiol 2016;54(6):1425–33.

27. Wendt JM, Cohen JA, Mu Y, et al. Clostridium difficile infection among children across diverse US geographic locations. Pediatrics 2014;133(4):651–8.

28. Crews JD, Anderson LR, Waller DK, et al. Risk factors for community-associated Clostridium difficile-associated diarrhea in children. Pediatr Infect Dis J 2015; 34(9):919–23.

29. Dantes R, Mu Y, Hicks LA, et al. Association between outpatient antibiotic prescribing practices and community-associated Clostridium difficile infection. Open Forum Infect Dis 2015;2(3):ofv113.

30. Vangay P, Ward T, Gerber JS, et al. Antibiotics, pediatric dysbiosis, and disease. Cell Host Microbe 2015;17(5):553–64.

31. Horton DB, Scott FI, Haynes K, et al. Antibiotic exposure and juvenile idiopathic arthritis: a case-control study. Pediatrics 2015;136(2):e333–43.

32. Kronman MP, Zaoutis TE, Haynes K, et al. Antibiotic exposure and IBD development among children: a population-based cohort study. Pediatrics 2012;130(4): e794–803.

33. Hersh AL, King LM, Shapiro DJ, et al. Unnecessary antibiotic prescribing in US ambulatory care settings, 2010-2015. Clin Infect Dis 2021;72(1):133–7.

34. Mas-Dalmau G, Villanueva Lopez C, Gorrotxategi Gorrotxategi P, et al. Delayed antibiotic prescription for children with respiratory infections: a randomized trial. Pediatrics 2021;147(3):e20201323.

35. Shulman ST, Bisno AL, Clegg HW, et al. Clinical practice guideline for the diagnosis and management of group A streptococcal pharyngitis: 2012 update by

the Infectious Diseases Society of America. Clin Infect Dis 2012;55(10): 1279–82.

36. Lieberthal AS, Carroll AE, Chonmaitree T, et al. The diagnosis and management of acute otitis media. Pediatrics 2013;131(3):e964–99.
37. King LM, Bartoces M, Fleming-Dutra KE, et al. Changes in US outpatient antibiotic prescriptions from 2011-2016. Clin Infect Dis 2020;70(3):370–7.
38. Sanchez GV, Shapiro DJ, Hersh AL, et al. Outpatient macrolide antibiotic prescribing in the United States, 2008-2011. Open Forum Infect Dis 2017;4(4): ofx220.
39. Hicks LA, Bartoces MG, Roberts RM, et al. US outpatient antibiotic prescribing variation according to geography, patient population, and provider specialty in 2011. Clin Infect Dis 2015;60(9):1308–16.
40. Hicks LA, Chien YW, Taylor TH Jr, et al, Active Bacterial Core Surveillance Team.. Outpatient antibiotic prescribing and nonsusceptible Streptococcus pneumoniae in the United States, 1996-2003. Clin Infect Dis 2011;53(7):631–9.
41. Kenyon C, Laumen J, Manoharan-Basil SS, et al. Strong association between adolescent obesity and consumption of macrolides in Europe and the USA: an ecological study. J Infect Public Health 2020;13(10):1517–21.
42. Block JP, Bailey LC, Gillman MW, et al. Early antibiotic exposure and weight outcomes in young children. Pediatrics 2018;142(6):e20183555.
43. Spellberg B, Rice LB. Duration of antibiotic therapy: shorter is better. Ann Intern Med 2019;171(3):210–1.
44. American Academy of Pediatrics, Committee on Infectious Diseases, ed: Kimberlin, D. Red Book: 2021–2024 Report of the Committee on Infectious Diseases. Itasca, IL. 2021.
45. King LM, Hersh AL, Hicks LA, et al. Duration of outpatient antibiotic therapy for common outpatient infections, 2017. Clin Infect Dis 2021;72(10):e663–6.
46. Kozyrskyj A, Klassen TP, Moffatt M, et al. Short-course antibiotics for acute otitis media. Cochrane Database Syst Rev 2010;2010(9):CD001095.
47. Gerber JS, Prasad PA, Russell Localio A, et al. Variation in antibiotic prescribing across a pediatric primary care network. J Pediatr Infect Dis Soc 2015;4(4): 297–304.
48. Tomson CR, van der Veer SN. Learning from practice variation to improve the quality of care. Clin Med (Lond) 2013;13(1):19–23.
49. Makaroff LA, Xierali IM, Petterson SM, et al. Factors influencing family physicians' contribution to the child health care workforce. Ann Fam Med 2014; 12(5):427–31.
50. Poole NM, Shapiro DJ, Fleming-Dutra KE, et al. Antibiotic prescribing for children in United States emergency departments: 2009-2014. Pediatrics 2019; 143(2):e20181056.
51. Vu TT, Hampers LC, Joseph MM, et al. Job market survey of recent pediatric emergency medicine fellowship graduates. Pediatr Emerg Care 2007;23(5): 304–7.
52. Saleh EA, Schroeder DR, Hanson AC, et al. Guideline-concordant antibiotic prescribing for pediatric outpatients with otitis media, community-acquired pneumonia, and skin and soft tissue infections in a large multispecialty healthcare system. Clin Res Infect Dis 2015;2(1):1010.
53. Frost HM, McLean HQ, Chow BDW. Variability in antibiotic prescribing for upper respiratory illnesses by provider specialty. J Pediatr 2018;203:76–85.e8.
54. Raman J, Johnson TJ, Hayes K, et al. Racial differences in sepsis recognition in the emergency department. Pediatrics 2019;144(4):e20190348.

55. Fleming-Dutra KE, Shapiro DJ, Hicks LA, et al. Race, otitis media, and antibiotic selection. Pediatrics 2014;134(6):1059–66.

56. Gerber JS, Prasad PA, Localio AR, et al. Racial differences in antibiotic prescribing by primary care pediatricians. Pediatrics 2013;131(4):677–84.

57. Goyal MK, Johnson TJ, Chamberlain JM, et al. Racial and ethnic differences in antibiotic use for viral illness in emergency departments. Pediatrics 2017; 140(4):e20170203.

58. Mangione-Smith R, McGlynn EA, Elliott MN, et al. The relationship between perceived parental expectations and pediatrician antimicrobial prescribing behavior. Pediatrics 1999;103(4 Pt 1):711–8.

59. Szymczak JE, Feemster KA, Zaoutis TE, et al. Pediatrician perceptions of an outpatient antimicrobial stewardship intervention. Infect Control Hosp Epidemiol 2014;35(Suppl 3):S69–78.

60. Stivers T, Mangione-Smith R, Elliott MN, et al. Why do physicians think parents expect antibiotics? What parents report vs what physicians believe. J Fam Pract 2003;52(2):140–8.

61. Kohut MR, Keller SC, Linder JA, et al. The inconvincible patient: how clinicians perceive demand for antibiotics in the outpatient setting. Fam Pract 2020;37(2): 276–82.

62. Mangione-Smith R, McGlynn EA, Elliott MN, et al. Parent expectations for antibiotics, physician-parent communication, and satisfaction. Arch Pediatr Adolesc Med 2001;155(7):800–6.

63. Poole NM. Judicious antibiotic prescribing in ambulatory pediatrics: communication is key. Curr Probl Pediatr Adolesc Health Care 2018;48(11):306–17.

64. Dempsey PP, Businger AC, Whaley LE, et al. Primary care clinicians' perceptions about antibiotic prescribing for acute bronchitis: a qualitative study. BMC Fam Pract 2014;15:194.

65. Linder JA, Doctor JN, Friedberg MW, et al. Time of day and the decision to prescribe antibiotics. JAMA Intern Med 2014;174(12):2029–31.

66. Stuart B, Hounkpatin H, Becque T, et al. Delayed antibiotic prescribing for respiratory tract infections: individual patient data meta-analysis. BMJ 2021;373: n808.

67. Spurling GK, Del Mar CB, Dooley L, et al. Delayed antibiotic prescriptions for respiratory infections. Cochrane Database Syst Rev 2017;9:Cd004417.

68. Little P, Moore M, Kelly J, et al. Delayed antibiotic prescribing strategies for respiratory tract infections in primary care: pragmatic, factorial, randomised controlled trial. BMJ 2014;348:g1606.

69. National Committee for Quality Assurance. HEDIS and performance measurement. National Committee for Quality Assurance. 2021. Available at: https://www.ncqa.org/hedis/. Accessed May 21, 2021.

70. Frost H, Monti J, Andersen L, et al. Improving delayed antibiotic prescribing for acute otitis media. Pediatrics 2021;147(6). e2020026062.

71. Gerber JS, Prasad PA, Fiks AG, et al. Effect of an outpatient antimicrobial stewardship intervention on broad-spectrum antibiotic prescribing by primary care pediatricians: a randomized trial. JAMA 2013;309(22):2345–52.

72. Norton LE, Lee BR, Harte L, et al. Improving guideline-based streptococcal pharyngitis testing: a quality improvement initiative. Pediatrics 2018;142(1): e20172033.

73. Santarossa M, Kilber EN, Wenzler E, et al. BundlED Up: a narrative review of antimicrobial stewardship initiatives and bundles in the emergency department. Pharmacy (Basel) 2019;7(4):145.

74. Hamdy RF, Katz SE. The key to antibiotic stewardship is combining interventions. Pediatrics 2020;146(3). e2020012922.

75. Miech EJ, Rattray NA, Flanagan ME, et al. Inside help: an integrative review of champions in healthcare-related implementation. SAGE Open Med 2018;6. 2050312118773261.

76. Pollack LA, Srinivasan A. Core elements of hospital antibiotic stewardship programs from the Centers for Disease Control and Prevention. Clin Infect Dis 2014; 59(Suppl 3):S97–100.

77. Frost HM, Andersen LM, Fleming-Dutra KE, et al. Sustaining outpatient antimicrobial stewardship: do we need to think further outside the box? Infect Control Hosp Epidemiol 2020;41(3):382–4.

78. Meeker D, Knight TK, Friedberg MW, et al. Nudging guideline-concordant antibiotic prescribing: a randomized clinical trial. JAMA Intern Med 2014;174(3): 425–31.

79. Centers for Disease Control and Prevention. Core elements of outpatient antibiotic stewardship. Centers for Disease Control and Prevention. 2021. Available at: https://www.cdc.gov/antibiotic-use/core-elements/outpatient.html. Accessed May 12, 2021.

80. Jenkins TC, Irwin A, Coombs L, et al. Effects of clinical pathways for common outpatient infections on antibiotic prescribing. Am J Med 2013;126(4): 327–35.e2.

81. Donà D, Zingarella S, Gastaldi A, et al. Effects of clinical pathway implementation on antibiotic prescriptions for pediatric community-acquired pneumonia. PLoS One 2018;13(2):e0193581.

82. Dona D, Baraldi M, Brigadoi G, et al. The impact of clinical pathways on antibiotic prescribing for acute otitis media and pharyngitis in the emergency department. Pediatr Infect Dis J 2018;37(9):901–7.

83. Childrens Hospital of Colorado. Clinical Pathways. Available at: https://www.childrenscolorado.org/health-professionals/clinical-resources/clinical-pathways/ , 2022. Accessed January 10, 2022 84. Seattle Children's Hospital. Clinical standard work pathways and tools. Available at: https://www.seattlechildrens.org/healthcare-professionals/gateway/clinical-resources/pathways/, 2022. Accessed June 9, 2021.

84. Hospital SCs. Clinical standard work pathways and tools. 2021. Available at: https://www.seattlechildrens.org/healthcare-professionals/gateway/clinical-resources/pathways/. Accessed June 9, 2021.

85. Children's Hospital of Philadelphia. Clinical Pathways Program. Available at: https://www.chop.edu/pathways-library. 202w. Accessed January 10, 2022.

86. Meeker D, Linder JA, Fox CR, et al. Effect of behavioral interventions on inappropriate antibiotic prescribing among primary care practices: a randomized clinical trial. JAMA 2016;315(6):562–70.

87. Linder JA, Meeker D, Fox CR, et al. Effects of behavioral interventions on inappropriate antibiotic prescribing in primary care 12 months after stopping interventions. JAMA 2017;318(14):1391–2.

88. Frost HM, Munsiff SS, Lou Y, et al. Simplifying outpatient antibiotic stewardship. Infect Control Hosp Epidemiol 2021;1:1–2.

89. Forrest GN, Van Schooneveld TC, Kullar R, et al. Use of electronic health records and clinical decision support systems for antimicrobial stewardship. Clin Infect Dis 2014;59(Suppl 3):S122–33.

90. Sutton RT, Pincock D, Baumgart DC, et al. An overview of clinical decision support systems: benefits, risks, and strategies for success. NPJ Digital Med 2020; 3:17.

91. May A, Hester A, Quairoli K, et al. Impact of clinical decision support on azithromycin prescribing in primary care clinics. J Gen Intern Med 2021;36(8): 2267–73.

92. Shaikh N, Leonard E, Martin JM. Prevalence of streptococcal pharyngitis and streptococcal carriage in children: a meta-analysis. Pediatrics 2010;126(3): e557–64.

93. Ebell MH, Smith MA, Barry HC, et al. The rational clinical examination. Does this patient have strep throat? JAMA 2000;284(22):2912–8.

94. Gerber JS, Prasad PA, Fiks AG, et al. Durability of benefits of an outpatient antimicrobial stewardship intervention after discontinuation of audit and feedback. JAMA 2014;312(23):2569–70.

95. Tribble AC, Lee BR, Flett KB, et al. Appropriateness of antibiotic prescribing in United States children's hospitals: a national point prevalence survey. Clin Infect Dis 2020;71(8):e226–34.

96. Frost HM, Knepper BC, Shihadeh KC, et al. A novel approach to evaluate antibiotic utilization across the spectrum of inpatient and ambulatory care and implications for prioritization of antibiotic stewardship efforts. Clin Infect Dis 2020;70(8):1675–82.

97. Kronman MP, Gerber JS, Grundmeier RW, et al. Reducing antibiotic prescribing in primary care for respiratory illness. Pediatrics 2020;146(3):e20200038.

98. Mangione-Smith R, Zhou C, Robinson JD, et al. Communication practices and antibiotic use for acute respiratory tract infections in children. Ann Fam Med 2015;13(3):221–7.

99. interactive Medical Training Resources (iMTR). Dialogue around respiratory illness treatment. Seattle, WA: University of Washington; 2019. Available at: https://www.uwimtr.org/dart/. Accessed January 10, 2022.

100. Centers for Disease Control and Prevention. Continuing education and informational resources. Centers for Disease Control and Prevention. 2020. Available at: https://www.cdc.gov/antibiotic-use/training/continuing-education.html.   Accessed May 12, 2021.

101. The American Board of Pediatrics. Your own QI project. The American Board of Pediatrics. 2021. Available at: https://www.abp.org/content/your-own-qi-project. Accessed May 12, 2021.

102. The American Board of Family Medicine. Performance improvement (PI). The American Board of Family Medicine. 2021. Available at: https://www.theabfm. org/continue-certification/performance-improvement. Accessed May 12, 2021.

Diagnostic Stewardship in the Pediatric Intensive Care Unit

Anna C. Sick-Samuels, MD, MPH[a,b,]*,
Charlotte Woods-Hill, MD, MSHP[c,d]

KEYWORDS

- Diagnostic stewardship • Pediatric intensive care • Sepsis
- Ventilator-associated infection • Urinary tract infection

KEY POINTS

- Diagnostic stewardship is a complimentary approach to antibiotic stewardship to improve microbiology diagnostic test practices, reduce avoidable testing, improve the validity of test results, and reduce antibiotic use.
- Blood cultures are commonly obtained for the evaluation of sepsis, and studies have shown safe reductions in the use of blood cultures in patients with low likelihood of bacteremia.
- Endotracheal cultures cannot distinguish infection from bacteria colonizing invasive airway devices and should be reserved for patients with clinical suspicion for ventilator-associated infection.
- Diagnostic stewardship of urine cultures using results from urinalysis has led to safe reductions in treatment of asymptomatic bacteriuria in other settings and may also apply to pediatric intensive care unit (PICU) patients.
- Clinicians should consider 3 questions applying diagnostic stewardship: (1) Does the patient have signs or symptoms of an infectious process? (2) What is the optimal diagnostic test available to evaluate for this infectious process? (3) How should the diagnostic specimen be collected to optimize results?

Funding sources: National Institutes of Health grant KL2TR003099 (A.C. Sick-Samuels) and K23HL151381 (C. Woods-Hill). The content is solely the responsibility of the authors and does not necessarily represent the official views of the National Institutes of Health.
[a] Division of Infectious Diseases, Department of Pediatrics, The Johns Hopkins University School of Medicine, Baltimore, MD, USA; [b] Department of Hospital Epidemiology and Infection Control, The Johns Hopkins Hospital, Baltimore, MD, USA; [c] Division of Critical Care Medicine, The Children's Hospital of Philadelphia, University of Pennsylvania Perelman School of Medicine, Philadelphia, PA, USA; [d] The Leonard Davis Institute of Health Economics, University of Pennsylvania, Philadelphia, PA, USA
* Corresponding author. 200 N. Wolfe Street, Office 3153, Baltimore, MD 21287.
E-mail address: asick1@jhmi.edu

Infect Dis Clin N Am 36 (2022) 203–218
https://doi.org/10.1016/j.idc.2021.11.003
0891-5520/22/© 2021 Elsevier Inc. All rights reserved.

id.theclinics.com

WHAT IS DIAGNOSTIC STEWARDSHIP AND WHY HAS IT EMERGED AS A NEW STRATEGY TO COMBAT ANTIBIOTIC RESISTANCE?

Diagnostic stewardship is the promotion of judicious microbiology testing practices to inform safe, effective, and efficient patient management and treatment decisions.[1,2] Diagnostic stewardship interventions can target various steps of the diagnostic-treatment decision process, such as clinical decision support tools to optimize the selection of diagnostic tests or strategies to improve sample collection and handling practices (preanalytic), optimizing laboratory processing (analytical), and modifications in how test results are reported (postanalytic).[3,4] These strategies aim to support clinicians in appropriately deciding when to send which diagnostics, accurately interpreting test results, and making well-informed treatment decisions. Diagnostic stewardship may be considered an extension of antimicrobial stewardship, a well-recognized strategy to combat antibiotic resistance by optimizing antimicrobial selection and reducing antibiotic over-use.[5] In comparison to antimicrobial stewardship, diagnostic stewardship targets an earlier step of the clinical management process that can occur before a patient is prescribed antibiotics (**Fig. 1**).

In pediatrics, antibiotic resistance is rising with up to 10% of gram-negative bacteria resistant to carbapenems,[6–8] particularly among healthcare-associated infections (HAIs).[9] This a troublesome trend when antibiotic-resistant infections increase the odds of death, prolong duration of hospitalization and increase health care costs.[10–12] Concurrently, advances in technology and medical care have improved survival of children leading to a growing population of children with complex chronic conditions who may require prolonged and recurrent admissions.[13–15] These complex patients are vulnerable to morbidity from health care-associated infections (HAIs) such as such catheter-associated bloodstream infections, urinary tract infections, or pneumonia.[16,17] Not surprisingly, most pediatric intensive care unit (PICU) patients are treated with antibiotics, but there is also variability in use.[18,19] Therefore, there is a need to use multi-faceted and interdisciplinary strategies to optimize the management of both diagnostics and antimicrobials in critically ill children. Diagnostic stewardship can help reduce avoidable testing among patients with a low pretest probability of infection, which may help reduce avoidable antibiotic treatment.

WHAT ARE PITFALLS OF COMMON MICROBIOLOGY TESTING APPROACHES AND WHY CAN THEY LEAD TO OVER-DIAGNOSIS AND TREATMENT OF INFECTIONS?

Microbiology testing, either traditional culture-based methods or molecular testing, has limited ability to definitively identify infection. However, positive test results can

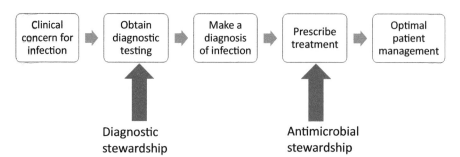

Fig. 1. Diagnostic stewardship supplements antibiotic stewardship to optimize patient management of infectious processes.

be misinterpreted by clinicians as definitive evidence of infection, which drives antibiotic treatment. In reality, detection or growth of bacteria can reflect one of the 3 scenarios:

- Pathogen: bacteria causing active infection
- Contamination: bacteria that accidentally were incorporated into the specimen during collection or processing
- Colonization: bacteria present on the tissues but not involved in the infectious process

This issue may be even more pronounced with increasingly sensitive molecular testing. For example, *Clostridium difficile (C. difficile)* nucleic acid amplification testing has high sensitivity to detect the presence of genetic material but does not confirm infection.[20] Especially if tests are obtained in the absence of clinical signs and symptoms of an infectious process, treatment of positive microbiology tests leads to possible harm with avoidable antibiotic treatment. Therefore, the decision to obtain a diagnostic test and the interpretation of results must be considered within the clinical context of the patient and supportive clinical data rather than relying on the test as confirmative evidence of infection.

WHAT ARE THE BENEFITS OF DIAGNOSTIC STEWARDSHIP AS A STRATEGY TO IMPROVE THE QUALITY AND VALUE OF HEALTH CARE?

There are multiple downstream benefits of improving microbiology testing practices. The benefit of diagnostic stewardship is well established in the case of *C. difficile* whereby reductions in testing among patients with low clinical suspicion for *C. difficile* colitis has led to reductions in *C. difficile* diagnoses[21,22] and antibiotic treatment of *C. difficile* colonization[23] without detrimental impacts to patient well-being. Beyond antibiotic resistance, avoiding unnecessary antibiotic treatment can improve patient outcomes by preventing unintended adverse reactions to antibiotics such as acute kidney injury, disruption to the microbiome, secondary fungal infections, and secondary *C. difficile* infections.[24–26] Mindful testing can also reduce the risk of cognitive biases and diagnostic errors. In particular, anchoring bias can happen if a clinician focuses on an early piece of information when determining a diagnosis and prematurely concludes a diagnostic work-up, which can lead to missing the true diagnosis and possible patient harm.[27] For example, if a clinician obtained a urine culture from a patient when they had a fever and interpreted a positive urine culture as a UTI and therefore failed to recognize the patient had developed appendicitis. In addition, reductions in unnecessary *C. difficile* testing has demonstrated that reducing false-positive results may improve the accuracy of HAI reporting, which in turn impacts hospital reimbursement and public perceptions of the hospitals quality and safety.[28] Diagnostic stewardship aligns with concepts of deimplementation[29] and the national "Choosing Wisely" campaign to reduce unnecessary or potentially harmful medical testing, improve health care value and reduce health care costs.[30,31] Lastly, diagnostic stewardship often aims to standardize diagnostic approaches, thereby reducing the risk of unconscious biases around patient racial or ethnic demographics and supporting more equitable health care delivery.

HOW DOES DIAGNOSTIC STEWARDSHIP EMBRACE INTERDISCIPLINARY COLLABORATION, AND WHAT IS THE ROLE OF THE CLINICIAN?

Diagnostic stewardship requires interdisciplinary partnership among the gamut of front-line health care workers. The primary team caring for the patient may be responsible for the decision to order a test, but other clinicians involved in the patient's care also play important roles in testing decisions. Some aspects of diagnostic stewardship may lie beyond the clinician's prevue and include optimally obtaining specimens (preanalytic), processing (analytical), and reporting the results (postanalytic).[3] For example, nurses or technicians may obtain specimens from patients; ancillary medical staff may help transport specimens; the microbiology laboratory processes specimens; and both the microbiology laboratory and electronic medical reporting system are involved in the display and communication of testing results.

For the remainder of this review, we will focus on diagnostic stewardship from the perspective of the bedside clinician, and the decision *to obtain or not obtain a test* among hospitalized critically ill pediatric patients. Below, we consider the evidence for over-testing and associated over-treatment of blood, urine, and endotracheal cultures and strategies that have been associated with improved testing practices. Though equally important to consider for diagnostic stewardship, we will not discuss molecular pathogen panels (eg, respiratory viral panels or gastrointestinal pathogen panels) in this review.

GENERAL CONSIDERATIONS FOR DIAGNOSTIC STEWARDSHIP IN THE PEDIATRIC INTENSIVE CARE UNIT

Much of the antibiotic use in the PICU reflects the high proportion of PICU patients who are ill with confirmed or suspected bacterial infections, but a significant number of PICU patients likely receive antibiotics in the absence of infection.[32–34] National guidelines and patient safety and quality collaboratives call for rapid recognition and treatment of suspected infection in children.[35,36] However, there is considerable overlap in the clinical presentation of infectious and noninfectious etiologies of fever, shock, and multi-organ failure in critically ill children. No single symptom, test, or biomarker can reliably distinguish the 2.[37–40] Due to this uncertainty, clinicians understandably may choose to start or continue antibiotic therapy without definitive evidence of bacterial infection.[41] PICU clinicians are faced with the complex task of ensuring rapid antibiotic administration to critically ill patients with possible or definite serious bacterial infections, while avoiding or deescalating antibiotics in patients who do not need such treatment. This makes the PICU a challenging, but particularly important, environment for diagnostic and antibiotic stewardship.

Within the PICU setting, diagnostic stewardship strategies can be applied when a clinician is deciding whether or not to order a microbiology test. Specifically, we propose that there are 3 questions the clinical team should ask:

1) Does the patient have signs and symptoms consistent with a particular infectious disease process?
2) What is the optimal diagnostic test available to the clinician to evaluate for this infectious process?
3) How should the diagnostic specimen be collected to optimize the accuracy of the results?

Below, we provide a more in-depth review of current literature evaluating blood cultures, respiratory cultures, and urine cultures in the pediatric hospital setting. **Fig. 2** summarizes these questions with example applications to clinical practice.

BLOOD CULTURES

Blood cultures are fundamental in the diagnosis and treatment of bacteremia, a primary cause of sepsis and associated morbidity and mortality in PICU patients.[42]

		Bacteremia Patient with a CVC has a new fever to 38.5C	Urinary tract infection Patient with a urine catheter has a new fever to 38.5C	Pneumonia An intubated patient has a new fever to 38.5C
1 Does the patient have signs or symptoms of an infectious process?	**YES**	AND is hypotensive, lethargic, with cold, mottled extremities	AND has dysuria and suprapubic pain	AND has increased oxygen requirement, increased need for suctioning of secretions from the endotracheal tube, or new infiltrate on chest x-ray
	NO The patient has symptoms explained by a non-infectious or non-bacterial process.	Received general anesthesia 4 hours ago; is normotensive, awake, and well perfused. Culture deferred, continue to monitor.	Has elevated withdrawal assessment scores after recent wean of sedative infusions. Culture deferred, continue to monitor.	Was diagnosed with RSV bronchiolitis day prior. Has thicker secretions, with stable ventilator settings and no focal infiltrate on chest x-ray. Culture deferred, continue to monitor.
2 What is the best diagnostic test available to evaluate for this infectious process?		Blood culture	Urinalysis and Urine culture	Endotracheal aspirate culture
3 How should the sample be collected to optimize results?		Optimal blood volume collected with clean technique to reduce risk of contamination.	Urinalysis obtained first and demonstrates pyuria with WBC>10 per high power field. A new urine catheter is placed and fresh urine sent for culture.	A new sterile suction catheter is used to obtain endotracheal secretions. Saline instillation is not recommended.
Example practices inconsistent with diagnostic stewardship		Automatic blood cultures for all patients with fever and a CVC Drawing blood culture from an existing peripheral intravenous catheter	Automatic urine culture for all patients with fever and a urine catheter Urine culture without preceding urinalysis	Automatic endotracheal culture for transient changes in secretions without other signs of pneumonia Expectorated sputum culture from a child unable to expectorate

Fig. 2. Applying 3 steps of clinical diagnostic stewardship when assessing for bacterial infections commonly considered in the Pediatric Intensive Care Unit (PICU).

National guidelines call for rapid recognition and empiric broad-spectrum antibiotics for suspected sepsis because delayed treatment of sepsis is associated with worse outcomes.[36] Compared with the failure to diagnose and treat bacteremia, blood cultures are perceived as a low-risk test. However, blood cultures are used excessively in PICU patients even when the pretest probability of bacteremia is low.[42–45] For example, in a review of blood cultures obtained in a PICU, only 72% and 57% of cases met the criteria for systemic inflammatory response syndrome or sepsis, respectively.[45] Importantly, performing blood cultures on patients with a very low likelihood of bacteremia increases the chance of obtaining a false-positive result, making proper selection of patients for testing critical.[46] False-positive blood cultures cause patient harm and strain on health care resources: repeat testing, unnecessary antibiotics, longer length of stay, exposure to additional procedures and consultations, and increased cost.[47,48]

There is growing evidence suggesting that blood culture use can be safely reduced using a diagnostic stewardship approach in the PICU setting without an associated increase in mortality, readmissions, or change in the frequency of blood cultures from patients with suspected infection or septic shock.[49,50] National consensus recommendations describe clinical scenarios that can be targeted for blood culture reduction.[51] For example, avoidable cultures include surveillance blood cultures in asymptomatic patients, blood cultures in stable patients with an identified noninfectious or nonbacteremia explanation for a new fever, and repeat blood cultures in stable patients with persistent fever in whom bacteremia has already been ruled out. Of paramount importance is the bedside clinician assessment of the patient to ensure there is no suspicion for sepsis or clinical worsening that would warrant a diagnostic evaluation for bacteremia. Reflexive practices (eg, always ordering a blood culture from a patient with fever and a central venous catheter), the local unit culture, and fear of missing sepsis have emerged as potential drivers of blood culture overuse; targeting these factors may be important in further successful reduction of excess blood cultures.[52] It is not yet clear what the potential impact of blood culture stewardship on PICU antibiotic use may be, although an initial study suggested that it did not lead to unanticipated increase in empiric broad-spectrum antibiotic treatment.[53]

RESPIRATORY CULTURES

Children requiring invasive mechanical ventilation are at risk for developing ventilator-associated infections (VAI)[9,16,17] due to the poor clearance of secretions and aspirations containing bacteria that have colonized the airways.[54–57] The term VAI encompasses ventilator-associated pneumonia (VAP) and tracheobronchitis because these diagnoses can be difficult to distinguish and are commonly treated interchangeably.[58–61] In contrast to blood, the respiratory tract is not a sterile environment. Bacteria colonize and quickly form biofilms on artificial airways, which is the primary reason endotracheal cultures have a low specificity for infection.[55–57,62] Even after targeted antibiotic therapy, bacteria such as *Staphylococcus aureus* and *Pseudomonas aeruginosa* persist in the airway.[63,64]

Clinicians may consider the density of white blood cells or bacteria in an endotracheal specimen to inform a diagnosis of VAI. Unfortunately, neither white blood cells on Gram-stains nor bacterial growth or quantity in endotracheal cultures can reliably distinguish bacterial colonization from invasive infection.[65–69] In neonatal, pediatric and adult patients, endotracheal cultures can have evidence of inflammation and growth of potentially pathogenic bacteria irrespective of clinical signs or symptoms.[66,67,70] Sample collection practices (eg, using an existing instead of a new sterile catheter) greatly affect bacterial growth in cultures.[67,71] Furthermore, sample processing, including specimen rejection criteria, institutional definitions of "normal respiratory flora," and how microbiology results are displayed to clinicians, vary widely across clinical laboratories, all of which may impact the clinical interpretation of the results.[72]

Despite the diagnostic limitations, clinicians having a low threshold to obtain endotracheal cultures (eg, after isolated fever)[73,74] and are likely to treat ventilated patients with antibiotics if the gram stain or culture has purulence or bacterial growth.[69,74–76] Strikingly, treatment of suspected VAIs may account for as much as 50% of antibiotic use in the PICU, emphasizing the potential impact of overtesting.[18] This finding is likely a result of clinical uncertainty in the absence of a gold standard and variability in the diagnosis of VAI among providers and institutions[75,76] coupled with the desire to minimize morbidity from treatable infection among medically complex children.[13,14,77] Treatment of VAI is critical to prevent excess mortality and morbidity related to mechanical ventilation among adult patients.[78] Interestingly, in a multicenter prospective cohort of invasively ventilated children, antibiotic treatment of clinician-suspected VAI did not improve clinical outcomes of mortality, length of stay or ventilator duration for the overall cohort, though a sub-analysis of patients with endotracheal tubes suggested reduced mortality if treated with antibiotics.[76] This finding underscores the potential significance of distinguishing patients with nonspecific clinical changes from those with infection.

In contrast to blood cultures, there are not yet consensus-based recommendations to inform specific indications to obtain an endotracheal culture in the evaluation of suspected VAIs. Two groups have explored the drivers of endotracheal culture use in their PICUs (eg, fever or change in secretion characteristics), and used the existing evidence to develop and implement clinical decision support tools to standardize indications for endotracheal cultures.[79,80] Implementation of these algorithms led to 35% to 41% declines in the rates of endotracheal cultures and reduction of antibiotic treatment of VAIs by 59% to 71% without changes in mortality, length of stay, readmissions,[80] or number of ventilator-associated events.[79] Clinical decision support tools that recommend obtaining endotracheal cultures only from patients with signs and symptoms of a VAI, rather than isolated fever or changes in secretions, thus far seems to be a safe approach to reduce avoidable testing and treatment while supporting the antibiotic treatment of true infections. Further research is needed to understand the scope of endotracheal culturing practices, define optimal indications for these cultures, and examine the impact on antibiotic prescribing.

URINE CULTURES

In the ICU setting, fever in a patient with an indwelling urinary catheter may prompt testing for urinary tract infection (UTI). Patients with urinary catheters certainly can develop clinically significant UTI, and these catheter-associated UTIs (CAUTI) contribute to poor patient outcomes and increased cost.[81,82] The risk of bacteriuria increases 3% to 10% with each additional catheter day, while only about 1 in 4 patients with bacteriuria will develop a symptomatic UTI and only 3.6% developed secondary bacteremia.[83] Therefore, positive urine cultures may reflect asymptomatic bacteriuria or catheter colonization that clinicians may inappropriately treat with antibiotics.[84] Diagnostic stewardship strategies, such as discouraging reflexive urinary testing for patients with fever but no other symptoms of UTI and only sending urine cultures if urinalysis results are abnormal with evidence of pyuria, have been successfully applied in adult ICUs and effectively reduced antibiotic treatment of asymptomatic bacteriuria.[84–88] To date, work to facilitate similar stewardship strategies for urinary cultures in the PICU is limited, despite the significant burden of CAUTI and its associated negative consequences on critically ill children.[81,89,90] Standardized care bundles for catheter maintenance and efforts to remove urinary catheters as soon as they are no longer needed have been associated with improvement in pediatric CAUTI rates, but specific attention to decision strategies around urinary cultures in the PICU is needed to reduce unnecessary antibiotic use for patients with bacteriuria or colonization without true infection of the urinary tract.[91]

SPECIAL POPULATIONS
ONCOLOGY PATIENTS IN THE PEDIATRIC INTENSIVE CARE UNIT

Critically ill children with malignancies undergoing chemotherapy present unique challenges to diagnostic stewardship efforts. Clinicians are understandably hesitant to reduce diagnostic testing for infection because of their high risk of morbidity and mortality from infections.[47,92–94] However, such patients may also be at higher risk of poor outcomes from the events that diagnostic stewardship seeks to prevent (ie, excessive entry into central venous catheters for frequent blood cultures and adverse effects of unnecessary antibiotics such as kidney injury and antimicrobial resistance).[95] Examples of diagnostic stewardship efforts in pediatric oncology patients (in any clinical setting) are limited, but include investigations demonstrating low yield of repeat blood cultures beyond 48 hours for children with persistent febrile neutropenia, and safe outcomes for febrile, non-neutropenic children who did not receive empiric antibiotics.[96,97] Pediatric oncology patients were included in a multi-center quality improvement collaborative that safely standardized and reduced use of blood cultures in the PICU.[58] Recent Delphi consensus work from that same collaborative also developed 2 recommendations focused on blood culture reduction in this population: for immunocompromised PICU patients with persistent fever without signs of sepsis or infection and initial negative blood cultures: (1) to avoid repeat blood cultures if antibiotics will not be changed and (2) if blood cultures are obtained, to avoid repeatedly culturing more than one lumen of the central venous catheter.[51] Concerns about limited safety data in this population prevented consensus on additional recommendations.[51] Efforts to include pediatric oncology patients in diagnostic stewardship initiatives and research remain important.

CARDIAC SURGICAL PATIENTS

Children with congenital heart disease are at increased risk of infections, including higher severity of illness in the setting of infection owing to the frequent occurrence of multi-system comorbidities and underlying genetic or immune system abnormalities.[98] Nosocomial infections in the perioperative period, in particular, are associated with higher mortality rates in these patients, and the use of perioperative extracorporeal membrane oxygenation (ECMO) support is an independent risk factor for infection.[99] As with pediatric oncology patients, specific work in diagnostic stewardship for infections in children in the cardiac ICU setting is limited. However, there are national society guidelines for infection detection in patients on ECMO that notably do not recommend routine surveillance cultures.[100] Pediatric cardiac ICU patients have also been successfully included in collaborative work to reduce unnecessary use of blood cultures and respiratory cultures.[49,50,80] Thus there is a precedent for diagnostic stewardship work in pediatric cardiac ICU patients that can be expanded with further study in this population.

NEONATAL INTENSIVE CARE UNIT PATIENTS

Antibiotics are the most commonly used medications in the neonatal intensive care unit (NICU),[101] but significant variation in prescribing patterns and duration of therapy suggest an opportunity for improvement.[102] Antimicrobial stewardship efforts are increasingly implemented in the NICU setting.[103] The physiologic and logistical complexities of caring for critically ill neonates may make diagnostic stewardship particularly challenging; neonates are at higher risk of infection and manifest infection in nonspecific ways.[103,104] There have been significant efforts to improve the assessment and management of early onset neonatal sepsis,[105] which has demonstrated the feasibility of diagnostic stewardship in the NICU and we encourage future study in this population as there may be a significant benefit for fragile critically ill neonates to limit adverse effects of avoidable antibiotics.

IMPLEMENTATION OF DIAGNOSTIC STEWARDSHIP STRATEGIES IN THE PEDIATRIC INTENSIVE CARE UNIT

The success of a diagnostic stewardship initiative will depend, to a large degree, on the implementation plan. It is not enough to simply create a new testing algorithm and hope that clinicians adhere to it. Specific attention to implementation strategies for diagnostic stewardship clinical guidelines will facilitate their successful translation into clinical practice.[106] Consideration of local context, stakeholder perspectives, and potential barriers to widespread adoption of a diagnostic stewardship project is of paramount importance. We, therefore, encourage the early use of elements of *implementation science*, a field dedicated to the study of methods to promote the systematic uptake of evidence-based or consensus-based practice into widespread clinical care.[107] Additionally, concepts from human factors engineering and quality improvement can offer useful insight and provide structure to the implementation process. For example, the Systems Engineering Initiative for Patient Safety (SEIPS) model[108] was applied to study the work system around and drivers of blood culture overuse in the

PICU.[52,109] And an integrated approach of the "Translating evidence into Practice" (TRIP) model[110] was used in an endotracheal culture stewardship initiative.[80] Other quality improvement tools may be helpful to guide diagnostic stewardship programs, such as driver diagrams and Plan-Do-Study-Act cycles.[111] While a detailed discussion of how to implement diagnostic stewardship in the ICU setting is beyond the scope of this article, we have outlined the basic recommended steps before, during, and after the implementation of a diagnostic stewardship project in the ICU environment (**Table 1**).

FUTURE RESEARCH RECOMMENDATIONS

Considering the ever-growing threat of antimicrobial resistance and the finite limitations of health care resources, it is increasingly clear that we must take definitive action to optimize the use of microbiologic diagnostic tests and antimicrobial treatments for patients. Diagnostic stewardship is a critically important tool in our armamentarium. For critically ill children, data is emerging that the use of blood and respiratory

Table 1 Suggested implementation approach for diagnostic stewardship initiatives in the pediatric intensive care unit	
Before Implementation	Identify key personnel: a dedicated project champion and a core project team; recommend both infectious disease and critical care clinician
	Identify required data elements (ex: monthly number of endotracheal aspirate cultures)
	Examine the unit's baseline performance of the metric of interest before implementation and establish a system for how to analyze that data in each phase of the project
	Understand the current/baseline approach to the test of interest in the unit (the current drivers of testing use, and potential barriers or facilitators to changing practice), via survey, focus groups, or interviews
	Reach out to key stakeholders whose perspectives and buy-in will be important for your new approach (eg, leadership, relevant consultants, nurses, respiratory therapists, advance practice providers).
	Create the new tool/algorithm for your stewardship initiative that reflects key drivers/barriers/facilitators and stakeholder perspectives
	Establish the balancing metrics and unintended consequences of your practice change and how to monitor for those after implementation
Implementation	Develop one or more strategies for disseminating the new tool/algorithm to the appropriate end-users (ie, clinicians, laboratory personnel, etc.) in your ICU (eg, emails, posters, checklists, educational seminars)
After Implementation	Analyze the use of the test of interest on a weekly or monthly basis to monitor progress, using a run or control chart if possible
	Share this data with the appropriate end-users that your tool/algorithm targeted, using feedback to help drive behavior change
	Monitor for adherence to the new guidelines and for unintended consequences of the practice change
	Revise the clinical approach or implementation plan if initial results are suboptimal

cultures can be safely reduced, and urine cultures are ripe for similar attention. More work is needed to understand the impact on patient outcomes and on antibiotic use. Specific focus is needed among neonates and children with cardiac or oncologic diseases to understand how to best apply diagnostic stewardship principles to these particularly vulnerable populations. Finally, evidence regarding optimal strategies to implement diagnostic stewardship for impactful and sustained practice change is lacking, and implementation science may offer important insights.

CLINICS CARE POINTS

- Temperature instability can have many causes in the critical care setting. Consider both infectious and non-infectious sources of fever prior to obtaining microbiology testing.
- The frontline healthcare team can reduce the likelihood of misleading positive culture results by optimizing how specimens are collected.
- Diagnostic stewardship has been done safely in the pediatric critical care setting by employing principles from quality improvement, human factors engineering and implementation science.

DISCLOSURE

The authors have no financial or commercial disclosures.

REFERENCES

1. World Health Organization. Diagnostic stewardship: a guide to implementation in antimicrobial resistance surveillance sites. 2016; 27. Available at: https://www.who.int/glass/resources/publications/diagnostic-stewardship-guide/en/. Accessed May 21, 2021.
2. World Health Organization. Global Antimicrobial Resistance Surveillance System: Manual for Early Implementation. 2015. Available at: http://www.who.int/antimicrobial-resistance/publications/surveillance-system-manual/en/. Accessed May 21, 2021.
3. Morgan DJ, Malani P, Diekema DJ. Diagnostic stewardship-leveraging the laboratory to improve antimicrobial use. JAMA 2017;318(7):607–8.
4. Kenaa B, Richert ME, Claeys KC, et al. Ventilator-associated pneumonia: diagnostic test stewardship and relevance of culturing practices. Curr Infect Dis Rep 2019;21(12):50.
5. Centers for Disease Control and Prevention. Antibiotic resistance threats in the United States, 2019. Atlanta, GA: U.S. Department of Health and Human Services; 2019.
6. Logan LK, Renschler JP, Gandra S, et al. Carbapenem-resistant enterobacteriaceae in children, United States, 1999-2012. Emerging Infect Dis 2015;21(11):2014–21.
7. Logan LK, Gandra S, Mandal S, et al. Multidrug- and carbapenem-resistant pseudomonas aeruginosa in children, United States, 1999-2012. J Pediatr Infect Dis Soc 2016;6(4):352–9.
8. Lake JG, Weiner LM, Milstone AM, et al. See I. Pathogen distribution and antimicrobial resistance among pediatric healthcare-associated infections reported to the National Healthcare Safety Network, 2011-2014. Infect Control Hosp Epidemiol 2018;39(1):1–11.

9. Weiner-Lastinger LM, Abner S, Benin AL, et al. Antimicrobial-resistant pathogens associated with pediatric healthcare-associated infections: Summary of data reported to the National Healthcare Safety Network, 2015-2017. Infect Control Hosp Epidemiol 2020;41(1):19–30.

10. Foglia EE, Fraser VJ, Elward AM. Effect of nosocomial infections due to antibiotic-resistant organisms on length of stay and mortality in the pediatric intensive care unit. Infect Control Hosp Epidemiol 2007;28(3):299–306.

11. Giske CG, Monnet DL, Cars O, et al. ReAct-Action on Antibiotic R. Clinical and economic impact of common multidrug-resistant gram-negative bacilli. Antimicrob Agents Chemother 2008;52(3):813–21.

12. Mauldin PD, Salgado CD, Hansen IS, et al. Attributable hospital cost and length of stay associated with health care-associated infections caused by antibiotic-resistant gram-negative bacteria. Antimicrob Agents Chemother 2010;54(1): 109–15.

13. Cohen E, Kuo DZ, Agrawal R, et al. Children with medical complexity: an emerging population for clinical and research initiatives. Pediatrics 2011; 127(3):529–38.

14. Edwards JD, Houtrow AJ, Lucas AR, et al. Children and young adults who received tracheostomies or were initiated on long-term ventilation in PICUs. Pediatr Crit Care Med 2016;17(8):e324–34.

15. Paulides FM, Plotz FB, Verweij-van den Oudenrijn LP, et al. Thirty years of home mechanical ventilation in children: escalating need for pediatric intensive care beds. Intensive Care Med 2012;38(5):847–52.

16. Grohskopf LA, Sinkowitz-Cochran RL, Garrett DO, et al. A national point-prevalence survey of pediatric intensive care unit-acquired infections in the United States. J Pediatr 2002;140(4):432–8.

17. Raymond J, Aujard Y. Nosocomial infections in pediatric patients: a European, multicenter prospective study. European Study Group. Infect Control Hosp Epidemiol 2000;21(4):260–3.

18. Fischer JE, Ramser M, Fanconi S. Use of antibiotics in pediatric intensive care and potential savings. Intensive Care Med 2000;26(7):959–66.

19. Brogan TV, Thurm C, Hersh AL, et al. Variability in antibiotic use across PICUs. Pediatr Crit Care Med 2018;19(6):519–27.

20. Boly FJ, Reske KA, Kwon JH. The role of diagnostic stewardship in clostridioides difficile testing: challenges and opportunities. Curr Infect Dis Rep 2020;22(3).

21. Sperling K, Priddy A, Suntharam N, et al. Optimizing testing for Clostridium difficile infection: A quality improvement project. Am J Infect Control 2019;47(3): 340–2.

22. Truong CY, Gombar S, Wilson R, et al. Real-time electronic tracking of diarrheal episodes and laxative therapy enables verification of clostridium difficile clinical testing criteria and reduction of clostridium difficile infection rates. J Clin Microbiol 2017;55(5):1276–84.

23. Christensen AB, Barr VO, Martin DW, et al. Diagnostic stewardship of C. difficile testing: a quasi-experimental antimicrobial stewardship study. Infect Control Hosp Epidemiol 2019;40(3):269–75.

24. Tamma PD, Avdic E, Li DX, et al. Association of adverse events with antibiotic use in hospitalized patients. JAMA Intern Med 2017;177(9):1308–15.

25. Luther MK, Timbrook TT, Caffrey AR, et al. Vancomycin plus piperacillin-tazobactam and acute kidney injury in adults: a systematic review and meta-analysis. Crit Care Med 2018;46(1):12–20.

26. Belkaid Y, Hand TW. Role of the microbiota in immunity and inflammation. Cell 2014;157(1):121–41.

27. Hayes MM, Chatterjee S, Schwartzstein RM. Critical thinking in critical care: five strategies to improve teaching and learning in the intensive care unit. Ann Am Thorac Soc 2017;14(4):569–75.

28. Rock C, Pana Z, Leekha S, et al. National Healthcare Safety Network laboratory-identified Clostridium difficile event reporting: A need for diagnostic steward-ship. Am J Infect Control 2018;46(4):456–8.

29. Norton WE, Chambers DA. Unpacking the complexities of de-implementing inappropriate health interventions. Implement Sci 2020;15(1):2.

30. Morgan DJ, Croft LD, Deloney V, et al. Choosing wisely in healthcare epidemi-ology and antimicrobial stewardship. Infect Control Hosp Epidemiol 2016; 37(7):755–60.

31. Cassel CK, Guest JA. Choosing wisely: helping physicians and patients make smart decisions about their care. JAMA 2012;307(17):1801–2.

32. Weiss SL, Fitzgerald JC, Pappachan J, et al. Global epidemiology of pediatric severe sepsis: the sepsis prevalence, outcomes, and therapies study. Am J Re-spir Crit Care Med 2015;191(10):1147–57.

33. Blinova E, Lau E, Bitnun A, et al. Point prevalence survey of antimicrobial utiliza-tion in the cardiac and pediatric critical care unit. Pediatr Crit Care Med 2013; 14(6):e280–8.

34. Hartman ME, Linde-Zwirble WT, Angus DC, et al. Trends in the epidemiology of pediatric severe sepsis. Pediatr Crit Care Med 2013;14(7):686–93.

35. Children's Hospital Association. Improving Pediatric Sepsis Outcomes (IPSO) is successfully challenging sepsis. Available at: https://www.childrenshospitals. org/programs-and-services/quality-improvement-and-measurement/ collaboratives/sepsis. Accessed April 6, 2021.

36. Weiss SL, Peters MJ, Alhazzani W, et al. Surviving sepsis campaign international guidelines for the management of septic shock and sepsis-associated organ dysfunction in children. Pediatr Crit Care Med 2020;21(2):e52–106.

37. Lautz AJ, Dziorny AC, Denson AR, et al. Value of procalcitonin measurement for early evidence of severe bacterial infections in the pediatric intensive care unit. J Pediatr 2016;179:74–81 e72.

38. Nijman RG, Moll HA, Vergouwe Y, et al. C-reactive protein bedside testing in febrile children lowers length of stay at the emergency department. Pediatr Emerg Care 2015;31(9):633–9.

39. Hsiao AL, Baker MD. Fever in the new millennium: a review of recent studies of markers of serious bacterial infection in febrile children. Curr Opin Pediatr 2005; 17(1):56–61.

40. Milcent K, Faesch S, Gras-Le Guen C, et al. Use of procalcitonin assays to pre-dict serious bacterial infection in young febrile infants. JAMA Pediatr 2016; 170(1):62–9.

41. Chiotos K, Tamma PD, Gerber JS, et al. Antibiotic stewardship in the intensive care unit: Challenges and opportunities. Infect Control Hosp Epidemiol 2019; 40(6):693–8.

42. Darby JM, Linden P, Pasculle W, et al. Utilization and diagnostic yield of blood cultures in a surgical intensive care unit. Crit Care Med 1997;25(6):989–94.

43. Kiragu AW, Zier J, Cornfield DN. Utility of blood cultures in postoperative pedi-atric intensive care unit patients. Pediatr Crit Care Med 2009;10(3):364–8.

44. Bates DW, Goldman L, Lee TH. Contaminant blood cultures and resource utilization. The true consequences of false-positive results. JAMA 1991;265(3): 365–9.

45. Tran CA, Zschaebitz JV, Spaeder MC. Epidemiology of blood culture utilization in a cohort of critically ill children. J Pediatr Intensive Care 2019;8(3):144–7.

46. Doern GV, Carroll KC, Diekema DJ, et al. Practical guidance for clinical microbiology laboratories: a comprehensive update on the problem of blood culture contamination and a discussion of methods for addressing the problem. Clin Microbiol Rev 2019;33(1).

47. Elward AM, Hollenbeak CS, Warren DK, et al. Attributable cost of nosocomial primary bloodstream infection in pediatric intensive care unit patients. Pediatrics 2005;115(4):868–72.

48. Alahmadi YM, Aldeyab MA, McElnay JC, et al. Clinical and economic impact of contaminated blood cultures within the hospital setting. J Hosp Infect 2011; 77(3):233–6.

49. Woods-Hill CZ, Fackler J, Nelson McMillan K, et al. Association of a clinical practice guideline with blood culture use in critically ill children. JAMA Pediatr 2017;171(2):157–64.

50. Woods-Hill CZ, Lee L, Xie A, et al. Dissemination of a novel framework to improve blood culture use in pediatric critical care. Pediatr Qual Saf 2018; 3(5):e112.

51. Woods-Hill CZ, Koontz DW, Voskertchian A, et al. Consensus recommendations for blood culture use in critically ill children using a modified Delphi approach. Pediatr Crit Care Med 2021;22(9):774–84.

52. Woods-Hill CZ, Koontz DW, King AF, et al. Practices, perceptions, and attitudes in the evaluation of critically ill children for bacteremia: a national survey. Pediatr Crit Care Med 2020;21(1):e23–9.

53. Sick-Samuels AC, Woods-Hill CZ, Fackler JC, et al. Association of a blood culture utilization intervention on antibiotic use in a pediatric intensive care unit. Infect Control Hosp Epidemiol 2019;40(4):482–4.

54. Chiang J, Amin R. Respiratory care considerations for children with medical complexity. Children (Basel) 2017;4(5).

55. Danin PE, Girou E, Legrand P, et al. Description and microbiology of endotracheal tube biofilm in mechanically ventilated subjects. Respir Care 2015; 60(1):21–9.

56. Diaconu O, Siriopol I, Polosanu LI, et al. Endotracheal tube biofilm and its impact on the pathogenesis of ventilator-associated pneumonia. J Crit Care Med (Targu Mures) 2018;4(2):50–5.

57. Vandecandelaere I, Coenye T. Microbial composition and antibiotic resistance of biofilms recovered from endotracheal tubes of mechanically ventilated patients. Adv Exp Med Biol 2015;830:137–55.

58. Fayon MJ, Tucci M, Lacroix J, et al. Nosocomial pneumonia and tracheitis in a pediatric intensive care unit: a prospective study. Am J Respir Crit Care Med 1997;155(1):162–9.

59. Gauvin F, Dassa C, Chaibou M, et al. Ventilator-associated pneumonia in intubated children: comparison of different diagnostic methods. Pediatr Crit Care Med 2003;4(4):437–43.

60. Craven DE, Chroneou A, Zias N, et al. Ventilator-associated tracheobronchitis: the impact of targeted antibiotic therapy on patient outcomes. Chest 2009; 135(2):521–8.

61. Alves AE, Pereira JM. Antibiotic therapy in ventilator-associated tracheobronchitis: a literature review. Rev Bras Ter Intensiva 2018;30(1):80–5.

62. Yan XX, Li S, Qi TJ, et al. [The characteristics of biofilm formation in endotracheal tubes in ventilated patients]. Zhonghua Jie He He Hu Xi Za Zhi 2008; 31(7):501–4.

63. Dennesen PJ, van der Ven AJ, Kessels AG, et al. Resolution of infectious parameters after antimicrobial therapy in patients with ventilator-associated pneumonia. Am J Respir Crit Care Med 2001;163(6):1371–5.

64. Thorarinsdottir HR, Kander T, Holmberg A, et al. Biofilm formation on three different endotracheal tubes: a prospective clinical trial. Crit Care (London, England) 2020;24(1):382.

65. Hill JD, Ratliff JL, Parrott JC, et al. Pulmonary pathology in acute respiratory insufficiency: lung biopsy as a diagnostic tool. J Thorac Cardiovasc Surg 1976;71(1):64–71.

66. Durairaj L, Mohamad Z, Launspach JL, et al. Patterns and density of early tracheal colonization in intensive care unit patients. J Crit Care 2009;24(1): 114–21.

67. Willson DF, Conaway M, Kelly R, et al. The lack of specificity of tracheal aspirates in the diagnosis of pulmonary infection in intubated children. Pediatr Crit Care Med 2014;15(4):299–305.

68. Klompas M. Does this patient have ventilator-associated pneumonia? JAMA 2007;297(14):1583–93.

69. Yalamanchi S, Saiman L, Zachariah P. Decision-making around positive tracheal aspirate cultures: the role of neutrophil semiquantification in antibiotic prescribing. Pediatr Crit Care Med 2019;20(8):e380–5.

70. Langston SJ, Pithia N, Sim MS, et al. Lack of utility of tracheal aspirates in the management of suspected pneumonia in intubated neonates. Infect Control Hosp Epidemiol 2020;41(6):660–5.

71. Morris AJ, Tanner DC, Reller LB. Rejection criteria for endotracheal aspirates from adults. J Clin Microbiol 1993;31(5):1027–9.

72. Prinzi AM, Parker SK, Curtis DJ, et al. The Pediatric Endotracheal Aspirate Culture Survey (PETACS): examining practice variation across pediatric microbiology laboratories in the United States. J Clin Microbiol 2021;59(3).

73. Sick-Samuels AC, Fackler JC, Berenholtz SM, et al. Understanding reasons clinicians obtained endotracheal aspirate cultures and impact on patient management to inform diagnostic stewardship initiatives. Infect Control Hosp Epidemiol 2019;1–2.

74. Willson DF, Kirby A, Kicker JS. Respiratory secretion analyses in the evaluation of ventilator-associated pneumonia: a survey of current practice in pediatric critical care. Pediatr Crit Care Med 2014;15(8):715–9.

75. Venkatachalam V, Hendley JO, Willson DF. The diagnostic dilemma of ventilator-associated pneumonia in critically ill children. Pediatr Crit Care Med 2011;12(3): 286–96.

76. Willson DF, Hoot M, Khemani R, et al. Pediatric ventilator-associated infections: the ventilator-associated infection study. Pediatr Crit Care Med 2017;18(1): e24–34.

77. Benneyworth BD, Gebremariam A, Clark SJ, et al. Inpatient health care utilization for children dependent on long-term mechanical ventilation. Pediatrics 2011;127(6):e1533–41.

78. Nseir S, Favory R, Jozefowicz E, et al. Antimicrobial treatment for ventilator-associated tracheobronchitis: a randomized, controlled, multicenter study. Crit Care (London, England) 2008;12(3):R62.
79. Ormsby J, Conrad P, Blumenthal J, et al. Practice improvement for standardized evaluation and management of acute tracheitis in mechanically ventilated children. Pediatr Qual Saf 2021;6(1):e368.
80. Sick-Samuels AC, Linz M, Bergmann J, et al. Diagnostic stewardship of endotracheal aspirate cultures in a PICU. Pediatrics 2021;147(5).
81. Umscheid CA, Mitchell MD, Doshi JA, et al. Estimating the proportion of healthcare-associated infections that are reasonably preventable and the related mortality and costs. Infect Control Hosp Epidemiol 2011;32(2):101–14.
82. Yi SH, Baggs J, Gould CV, et al. Medicare reimbursement attributable to catheter-associated urinary tract infection in the inpatient setting: a retrospective cohort analysis. Med Care 2014;52(6):469–78.
83. Saint S. Clinical and economic consequences of nosocomial catheter-related bacteriuria. Am J Infect Control 2000;28(1):68–75.
84. Page S, Hazen D, Kelley K, et al. Changing the culture of urine culturing: Utilizing Agile Implementation to improve diagnostic stewardship in the ICU. Am J Infect Control 2020;48(11):1375–80.
85. Epstein L, Edwards JR, Halpin AL, et al. Evaluation of a novel intervention to reduce unnecessary urine cultures in intensive care units at a tertiary care hospital in Maryland, 2011-2014. Infect Control Hosp Epidemiol 2016;37(5):606–9.
86. Mullin KM, Kovacs CS, Fatica C, et al. A multifaceted approach to reduction of catheter-associated urinary tract infections in the intensive care unit with an emphasis on "Stewardship of Culturing". Infect Control Hosp Epidemiol 2017; 38(2):186–8.
87. Stagg A, Lutz H, Kirpalaney S, et al. Impact of two-step urine culture ordering in the emergency department: a time series analysis. BMJ Qual Saf 2018;27(2): 140–7.
88. Keller SC, Feldman L, Smith J, et al. The use of clinical decision support in reducing diagnosis of and treatment of asymptomatic bacteriuria. J Hosp Med 2018;13(6):392–5.
89. Reilly L, Sullivan P, Ninni S, et al. Reducing foley catheter device days in an intensive care unit: using the evidence to change practice. AACN Adv Crit Care 2006;17(3):272–83.
90. Sonmez Duzkaya D, Bozkurt G, Uysal G, et al. The effects of bundles on catheter-associated urinary tract infections in the pediatric intensive care Unit. Clin Nurse Spec 2016;30(6):341–6.
91. Schiessler MM, Darwin LM, Phipps AR, et al. Don't have a doubt, get the catheter out: a nurse-driven CAUTI prevention protocol. Pediatr Qual Saf 2019;4(4): e183.
92. Pittet D, Tarara D, Wenzel RP. Nosocomial bloodstream infection in critically ill patients. Excess length of stay, extra costs, and attributable mortality. JAMA 1994;271(20):1598–601.
93. Kelly M, Conway M, Wirth K, et al. Moving CLABSI prevention beyond the intensive care unit: risk factors in pediatric oncology patients. Infect Control Hosp Epidemiol 2011;32(11):1079–85.
94. Simon A, Ammann RA, Bode U, et al. Healthcare-associated infections in pediatric cancer patients: results of a prospective surveillance study from university hospitals in Germany and Switzerland. BMC Infect Dis 2008;8:70.

95. Karandikar MV, Milliren CE, Zaboulian R, et al. Limiting vancomycin exposure in pediatric oncology patients with febrile neutropenia may be associated with decreased vancomycin-resistant enterococcus incidence. J Pediatr Infect Dis Soc 2020;9(4):428–36.

96. Haeusler GM, De Abreu Lourenco R, Clark H, et al. Diagnostic yield of initial and consecutive blood cultures in children with cancer and febrile neutropenia. J Pediatr Infect Dis Soc 2021;10(2):125–30.

97. Allaway Z, Phillips RS, Thursky KA, et al. Nonneutropenic fever in children with cancer: A scoping review of management and outcome. Pediatr Blood Cancer 2019;66(6):e27634.

98. Murni IK, MacLaren G, Morrow D, et al. Perioperative infections in congenital heart disease. Cardiol Young 2017;27(S6):S14–21.

99. Herrup EA, Yuerek M, Griffis HM, et al. Hospital-acquired infection in pediatric subjects with congenital heart disease postcardiotomy supported on extracorporeal membrane oxygenation. Pediatr Crit Care Med 2020;21(11):e1020–5.

100. Extracorporeal Life Support Organization Infectious Disease Task Force. Infection Control and Extracorporeal Life Support. 2008. https://www.elso.org/Portals/0/Files/Infection-Control-and-Extracorporeal-Life-Support.pdf. Accessed May 21, 2021.

101. Hsieh EM, Hornik CP, Clark RH, et al. Medication use in the neonatal intensive care unit. Am J Perinatol 2014;31(9):811–21.

102. Willis Z, de St Maurice A. Strategies to improve antibiotic use in the neonatal ICU. Curr Opin Pediatr 2019;31(1):127–34.

103. Gkentzi D, Dimitriou G. Antimicrobial stewardship in the neonatal intensive care unit: an update. Curr Pediatr Rev 2019;15(1):47–52.

104. Mukhopadhyay S, Sengupta S, Puopolo KM. Challenges and opportunities for antibiotic stewardship among preterm infants. Arch Dis Child Fetal Neonatal Ed 2019;104(3):F327–32.

105. Achten NB, Klingenberg C, Benitz WE, et al. Association of use of the neonatal early-onset sepsis calculator with reduction in antibiotic therapy and safety: a systematic review and meta-analysis. JAMA Pediatr 2019;173(11):1032–40.

106. Gagliardi AR, Marshall C, Huckson S, et al. Developing a checklist for guideline implementation planning: review and synthesis of guideline development and implementation advice. Implement Sci 2015;10:19.

107. Eccles MP, Mittman BS. Welcome to implementation science. Implementation Sci 2006;1(1):1.

108. Holden RJ, Carayon P, Gurses AP, et al. Seips 2.0: A human factors framework for studying and improving the work of healthcare professionals and patients. Ergonomics 2013;(56):1669–86.

109. Xie A, Woods-Hill CZ, King AF, et al. Work system assessment to facilitate the dissemination of a quality improvement program for optimizing blood culture use: a case study using a human factors engineering approach. J Pediatr Infect Dis Soc 2019;8(1):39–45.

110. Pronovost PJ, Berenholtz SM, Needham DM. Translating evidence into practice: a model for large scale knowledge translation. BMJ 2008;337:a1714.

111. Institute for Healthcare Improvement. Resources. 2021. http://www.ihi.org/resources. Accessed May 21, 2021.

Management of Children with Reported Penicillin Allergies

Tracy N. Zembles, PharmD[a],*, David E. Vyles, DO, MS[b],
Michelle L. Mitchell, MD[c]

KEYWORDS

• Penicillin • Allergy • Challenge • Children

KEY POINTS

- Penicillin (PCN) allergy is the most commonly reported medication allergy.
- Most of the patients are at low risk for true PCN allergy, and the determination of allergy risk level is paramount to determine the best method to test for allergy.
- Among patients deemed low risk for PCN allergy, multiple studies have shown that an oral challenge is safe and effective.
- Locations outside of the allergy clinic, such as primary care clinics, inpatient units, and emergency departments, may be ideal places to delabel patients with PCN allergy.
- Multi-faceted approaches are needed to ensure the adherence and endurance of the removal of a PCN allergy.

INTRODUCTION

Penicillin (PCN) is the most prevalent reported drug allergy, with about 10% of all people reporting a PCN allergy.[1] However, 95% of those are not truly allergic when formally evaluated and are able to tolerate this class of drugs.[2] Frequently, symptoms of reported "allergy" are actually nonallergic adverse effects, or are a result of viral/antibiotic interactions that lead to a rash and a patient being falsely labeled as allergic.[3,4] Additionally, 90% of people with a true PCN allergy lose their sensitivity after 10 years rendering them no longer allergic.[5]

[a] Department of Enterprise Safety, Children's Wisconsin, Children's Corporate Center, Suite C450, 999 North 92nd Street, Milwaukee, WI 53226, USA; [b] Department of Pediatrics, Section of Pediatric Emergency Medicine, Medical College of Wisconsin, Children's Corporate Center, Suite C550, 999 North 92nd Street, Milwaukee, WI 53226, USA; [c] Department of Pediatrics, Division of Infectious Diseases, Pediatric Infectious Diseases, Medical College of Wisconsin, Children's Corporate Center, Suite C450, 999 North 92nd Street, Milwaukee, WI 53226, USA
* Corresponding author.
E-mail address: tzembles@chw.org

Infect Dis Clin N Am 36 (2022) 219–229
https://doi.org/10.1016/j.idc.2021.11.001
0891-5520/22/© 2021 Elsevier Inc. All rights reserved.

id.theclinics.com

Hypersensitivity reactions are classified into immediate-type reactions mediated by drug-specific IgE antibodies, cytotoxic reactions mediated by drug-specific IgG or IgM antibodies, immune complex reactions, and delayed-type hypersensitivity reactions mediated by cellular immune mechanisms.[6] Most symptoms attributed to PCN allergy are due to acute and subacute reactions mediated by IgE and IgG antibodies respectively.[7] IgE-mediated reactions typically occur within 1 hour of exposure. Characteristics of this type of reaction include hives, angioedema, wheezing and shortness of breath, and anaphylaxis.[5] IgG-mediated reactions occur 7 to 10 days after treatment or 1 to 2 days after a repeat exposure.[7] While many patients report a PCN allergy, few correspond with an anaphylactic reaction. In fact, among 100 million people exposed to oral amoxicillin between 1972 and 2007 in the United Kingdom, the risk of true anaphylaxis was 0.015%. Furthermore, only 1 death after anaphylaxis was identified.[8]

The consequences of being labeled with a PCN allergy include the use of alternative antibiotic regimens that may be less effective, more toxic, and/or more expensive than preferred agents.[9–12] The use of alternative, often overly broad-spectrum, antimicrobials increases the risk of developing *Clostridioides difficile* infection, methicillin-resistant *Staphylococcus aureus*, or vancomycin-resistant enterococcus.[9,13] In theory, the ability to prescribe narrow-spectrum antibiotics following PCN allergy evaluation should decrease the development of antimicrobial resistance, though this has not been formally evaluated. Studies evaluating the impact of a PCN allergy are limited to adults or not specified in the methods. A PCN allergy label has been associated with a 14% increased risk of mortality.[14] Furthermore, being labeled with a PCN allergy increases the risk of surgical site infections, with a reported odds ratio of 1.51 (95% confidence interval 1.02–2.22).[15] Finally, a PCN allergy label has been associated with a 28% increase in antibiotic costs and 6% longer hospital stay when compared with patients without a reported PCN allergy.[16]

The significant burden on patient outcomes and the low rate of true IgE-mediated PCN allergy makes it essential to reconcile a reported allergy and expand future antibiotic options for patients found not to have a true allergy. Formal evaluation of patients reporting a PCN allergy has been recommended by several large clinical societies, including the Centers for Disease Control and Prevention, the Infectious Diseases Society of America, and the American Academy of Allergy, Asthma, and Immunology.[17–19] This review summarizes risk categorization, current evidence for delabeling PCN allergy, and approaches to implementation.

RISK CATEGORIZATION

When a clinician is presented with a patient who reports a PCN allergy, it is important to identify and classify symptoms by risk level to choose the optimal testing strategy. This method has gained traction over the past several years. Risk level in the literature has ranged from identifying high and low-risk patients to levels including a medium-risk category as well.[20,21] High-risk symptoms are generally easily categorized and include symptoms of anaphylaxis, throat tightness, shortness of breath, wheezing, and angioedema. More scrutiny is required when assessing how to categorize low-risk symptoms.

There are multiple different pathways for identifying a patient as low risk based on reported symptoms.[20–23] Shenoy and colleagues identifies both intolerance histories (isolated gastrointestinal (GI) upset, chills, headache, and fatigue) and low-risk histories (family history, itching, unknown remote, and denying of allergy).[21] Castells and colleagues identify low-risk histories that are defined as nausea/diarrhea or other single symptoms not suggestive of allergy. They provide additional allergy categorization with symptoms that include "unknown" reaction and isolated rash. Within this classification, rash is defined as low risk based on a time component that identifies individuals with rash occurring less than 6 hours from medication administration as high, and greater than 6 hours as low risk.[22] Vyles and colleagues had a similar classification with regards to rash; however, their designation listed rash as high risk only when it occurred within 1 hour of medication administration.[20] Lastly, Banks and colleagues defined low-risk history as patients with any benign rash, GI symptoms, headaches, or other benign somatic symptoms occurring greater than 12 months ago.[23] Previously described low-risk criteria share common themes in qualifying symptomatology including nausea/diarrhea, unknown reactions, family history, and benign somatic symptoms. The main area of disagreement is with regards to the designation of rash as a low or high-risk symptom. However, despite inconsistencies, these different pathways provide a useful guide toward the best way to approach the patient in the context of the clinical picture (**Fig. 1**).

CURRENT EVALUATION EVIDENCE

Once an appropriate risk categorization level has been assigned, it is important to choose the optimal testing strategy. For patients with truly nonallergic symptoms

1) What age was your child at the time of diagnosis?

2) What symptoms did your child have to the penicillin medication?

LOW risk symptoms	HIGH risk symptoms
Cough	Blisters (mouth)
Diarrhea	Blood pressure drop
Dizziness	Difficulty breathing
Family history of penicillin allergy	Seizures
Headache	Skin peeling
Itching (isolated)	Syncope
Nausea	Swelling (face)
Runny nose	Swelling (lips)
Vomiting (single episode)	Swelling (throat)
	Wheezing

3) Did any of these symptoms occur **within one hour** of giving the medication?

Symptom	No	Unsure	Yes
Abdominal pain			
Itching (with rash)			
Rash			
Vomiting (multiple episodes)			

4) Is this patient low or high risk? (*One or more high risk symptoms = high risk*)

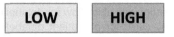

5) Document in the medical record.

Fig. 1. Assessment of penicillin allergy risk level.

such as diarrhea, it may be appropriate to remove the allergy without testing. In patients with low-risk symptoms, proceeding to a direct oral drug challenge (ODC) without preceding skin tests is slowly becoming the standard of care.[20,24,25] Over the past several years, the safety of this approach has been highlighted in several studies that include both children and adults.[20,24–27] These studies have included a mix of single dose and graded oral challenges, different clinic settings/sites, and dosing that has ranged from fixed to weight-based. Mill and colleagues completed 818 graded oral challenges on children with reported amoxicillin allergy and 94.1% of patients tolerated the medication without an allergic reaction.[24] The remaining patients that reacted had nonserious mild reactions. Vyles and colleagues completed 100 oral challenges on children with reported low-risk PCN allergy and every child tolerated the medication without having an allergic reaction.[20] Additionally, these patients were followed up 1 year later, and many PCN derivatives were prescribed to this cohort without any serious allergic reactions.[28] Lastly, in a study completed by Labrosse and colleagues, 130 children with a history of amoxicillin allergy underwent a graded drug provocation test and 122 had no symptoms of allergy with challenge.[25] The other patients all had minor symptoms that resolved without difficulty. Clearly, single dose oral challenge in low-risk patients is safe and trending toward the standard of care.

Patients who report high-risk symptoms of allergy should be approached with a tiered skin testing process. These patients include those with symptoms more typical of IgE-mediated reaction such as angioedema, bronchospasm, GI symptoms in conjunction with other signs of IgE-mediated reaction, and anaphylaxis. Typical skin tests consist of 2 steps before the oral challenge. The first step is an epicutaneous test followed by intradermal skin testing. Most patients that have negative results from skin tests do not have allergy after subsequent oral challenge. In prior studies, the percentage of patients that developed apparent IgE-mediated reactions to PCN following negative skin test ranged from 1.2% to 2.9%.[29,30] The combination of negative skin testing with an oral challenge has more than a 99% negative predictive value in excluding an IgE-mediated PCN allergy.[5,31]

The common theme with all testing strategies is to first perform an appropriate history. In some instances, the historical reaction may preclude the need for any testing at all. Systemic reactions in which a patient should not undergo a drug challenge due to the likelihood of a repeat serious reaction include: drug reaction with eosinophilia and systemic symptoms/drug-induced hypersensitivity syndrome (DRESS/DiHS), Stevens-Johnson syndrome (SJS) or toxic epidermal necrolysis (TEN), and serum sickness-like reactions.

Approach to Implementation

With over 30 million people in the United States with a PCN allergy label, and many more worldwide, referring them all to an allergy clinic for testing is not a viable option. A multifaceted approach that meets patients whereby they are in the health care system is needed to efficiently delabel these patients and ensure they receive optimal antibiotic therapy when necessary.[32]

Many hospitals and institutions have initiated programs to remove PCN allergies on patients admitted to the hospital. This allows for optimizing antimicrobial therapy when patients potentially need it the most. The inpatient setting can also allow for delabeling of patients that might not otherwise visit an allergy clinic for outpatient delabeling whether due to additional cost, transportation challenges, or other issues. To date, the published predominant approach for hospitalized patients, namely in adults, has consisted of skin testing followed by direct oral challenge in patients who could not otherwise have the allergy removed based on history alone. These programs have been facilitated by infectious diseases (ID) physicians, allergy nurses, pharmacists, and ID or allergy fellows, often in coordination with an antimicrobial stewardship program to help identify patients and/or facilitate the PCN skin test.[33–37] Published studies of this approach demonstrate efficacy in delabeling patients who otherwise would have retained an allergy label, including patients who are not conventionally considered to have a low-risk allergy. Some studies have also shown this approach to be safe and effective in particularly vulnerable patients like those in intensive care or with a cancer diagnosis.[38–40]

The additional comorbidities present in hospitalized adults likely contribute to the propensity to use the traditional 3 step testing method as opposed to direct oral challenge that several pediatric institutions have initiated. In one multi-center study of an allergy delabeling program in adults, 48.3% of patients were immunocompromised, 47% required hospitalization or were already hospitalized during their inciting adverse drug reaction (ADR), and 51% required specific therapy for the ADR.[33] This is in contrast to one study showing over three-quarters of children with PCN allergies reported exclusively low-risk reactions, most of which occurred before 3 years of age.[41]

However, skin testing is inherently more labor intensive and requires specialized training to perform the procedure, which can be limiting factors to implementation at some institutions. Rapidly expanding data have shown the safety of direct oral challenges in patients with low-risk PCN allergies in both adults and children.[20,26,42–47] As a result, an increasing number of hospitals have begun to use direct oral challenges on inpatients stratified as low risk with success in delabeling without significant adverse events.[48–52] One study also performed a cost analysis between direct oral challenges and PCN skin testing on inpatients and demonstrated significant financial savings with direct oral challenges ($206.18/patient vs $419.63/patient).[48] Without the technical challenges of a skin test and the lower risk stratification of patients, an additional potential advantage demonstrated from this approach is allowing more of the process to be in the hands of the primary providers, and thus perhaps aiding in the sustainability of this method.[51,52]

There is still a paucity of published studies examining direct oral challenges in higher risk or more vulnerable patients, whether due to history that is more consistent with an IgE-mediated reaction or due to comorbidities such as cancer, other immunocompromised states, critical illness, or even pregnancy. Though research in this area continues to evolve, initial experience shows the potential for successful direct oral challenges for these patients as well, when determined to have a low-risk PCN allergy. One study reported successful delabeling in all of 23 patients with cancer with low-risk PCN allergy who also met additional inclusion criteria (no history of idiopathic urticaria or anaphylaxis, no recent medical emergency team call, and hemodynamically stable) who were administered a direct oral challenge.[53] In pregnant women, there has historically been reluctant to implement any kind of PCN allergy delabeling method. This is despite the potential benefits of reducing maternal morbidity by using a more narrow-spectrum agent (ie, PCN) while possibly improving coverage for Group B *Streptococcus* (GBS) versus an alternative such as clindamycin. One retrospective study even discovered that GBS-positive women with an unconfirmed PCN allergy had significantly higher rates of adverse drug reactions and cesarean deliveries along with a prolonged hospital stay.[54] More recent published studies have demonstrated the safety of PCN skin testing during pregnancy.[55–57] Though the current inclination is still to avoid direct challenges in favor of skin testing except in particularly low-risk pregnant women (ie, reaction reported as headache, nausea, vomiting, or itching, or a family history of allergy), Blumenthal and colleagues did not exclude pregnant women in their health care system-wide guideline for oral challenges, though it is unclear how many or if any pregnant women may have received an oral challenge.[51,58] Similarly, in patients with a reported PCN allergy with multiple drug allergy syndrome (defined by more than 2 allergies to unrelated drugs), PCN skin testing remains commonplace.

Outpatient clinics, aside from functioning as a referral source for allergy clinic, have largely remained an untapped resource for widely addressing PCN allergy labels in children or adults. Aside from the many demands already placed on the primary care physician with significant time constraints, studies show there is also a lack of comfort and knowledge regarding PCN allergy risk assessment.[59,60] However, one study has demonstrated the feasibility of direct oral challenges for pediatric patients in a primary care setting with the use of available telehealth consultation with an allergist which could serve as a potential model for other practices.[61]

Another study, conducted in a surgical preassessment clinic, showed the feasibility and success of integrating direct oral challenges in low-risk adults into an already existing surgical pathway.[62] Several pediatric subspecialty clinics stand to benefit from similar approaches whether it be presurgical evaluations, oncology clinic before chemotherapy, or in solid organ transplant evaluations among others. Even if practical or logistical issues preclude outpatient providers from performing skin testing or direct oral challenges in pediatric clinics, additional opportunities for innovation in this area include standardizing correct categorization and detailed descriptions of new allergic reactions, streamlining allergy specialist referrals when needed, dedicated penicillin allergy clinics at/near the primary care location, and modifications to the electronic medical record that may prompt and/or aid the practitioner in these and other related endeavors.[32]

Finally, PCN allergy delabeling has even been shown to be possible in the emergency department (ED). The first study to demonstrate feasibility occurred in a convenience sample of 150 adults with self-reported PCN allergy who had skin testing performed; 137 (91.3%) had a negative PCN skin test.[63] Unfortunately, the nature and fast-paced environment of the ED can easily be prohibitive to skin testing. However, a study by Vyles and colleagues demonstrated the feasibility of oral challenges in a pediatric ED by testing 100 children with low-risk penicillin allergy symptoms who were easily identified by a risk-stratifying allergy questionnaire (see **Fig. 1**). All 100 children were found to be negative for true penicillin allergy.[20]

COMPLICATIONS OF IMPLEMENTATION

The process of delabeling requires more than determining the results of allergy skin testing and/or oral drug challenge; the removal of an allergy is only as good as the communication to and buy-in from the patient and their other providers and pharmacists. A whole body of literature has now emerged in trying to ensure the endurance and adherence to the PNC allergy delabel.[52,64–66] After a patient has successfully shown they can tolerate PCN or related beta-lactam drugs, the next step is for the provider to document this process and update the medical record including removal of the allergy as applicable. One study demonstrated the potential utility of a best practice advisory (BPA) alert to prompt providers to appropriately modify or remove the allergy label in the medical record.[64]

Reliable and effective communication to the patient/family, the primary care provider, other practitioners, and pharmacists is important to maintain the delabeled status. Standardized order sets within an electronic medical record may aid in this process; they can be programmed to automatically populate "after visit summaries" and discharge summaries with standardized language regarding the allergy removal and appropriate education to both the patient/family and other medical providers of the patient respectively.[52] Optimization of the method and relevant language may require multiple iterations. In a follow-up survey of patients that were delabeled in an outpatient allergy testing clinic, Bourke and colleagues found only 68% of patients were following modifications made to their allergy label due to reservations by the patient/family and/or their provider.[65] After several changes in the communication process (including simplification and wider distribution of the clinic discharge letter with a summary table containing details of each investigated drug), they observed an improvement to 85% adherence to the allergy label modification. Even still, they noted several patients who reported self or provider reservation regarding the modified allergy label leading to failure to adhere to it. This finding is similar to a pediatric study that surveyed parents approximately 1 year following PCN allergy delabeling and found 73% of parents reported they would be "comfortable" or "very comfortable" for their child to receive a PCN antibiotic.[28] Another 24% and 4% were "somewhat comfortable" and "not comfortable" respectively, with the majority citing fear their child would have a repeat allergic reaction with reexposure to the inciting drug. Unfortunately, 52% of study patients still had a PCN allergy label in the primary care medical record.

Multifaceted, preventive measures against an illegitimate "relabel" for a PCN allergy are needed. This was shown by Lutfeali and colleagues, who used educational interventions, a BPA alert notifying providers of prior PCN allergy testing results if relabeling was attempted, and a wallet card given to patients documenting their negative allergy testing; together, this achieved a 12.9% relabel rate as opposed to 9% to 51% in other studies.[66] With the addition of a manual chart review of all relabeled patients by a pharmacist, identified by the BPA, the relabel rate was further decreased to 2.5%.

Future Directions

Health care providers frequently encounter patients with a reported PCN allergy, which interferes with the ability to prescribe first-line antibiotics. Appropriate assessment of the allergy, followed by oral drug challenge or skin testing as appropriate is essential, though delabeling (and subsequent relabeling) can be challenging. Multiple medical records may exist for a single patient (eg, different health care systems, pharmacies, clinics), making consistency throughout a patient's entire electronic medical record difficult. A frequently reported issue is difficulty with cross-talk among electronic medical records, meaning a patient may be delabeled in one system, but then the allergy label is reimported from another. A universal electronic medical record could help with keeping the patient delabeled. Another area requiring additional study includes determining how PCN allergy delabeling impacts overly broad-spectrum antibiotic prescriptions, total durations of therapy, and potential cost-implications to both families and health care systems. Lastly, the authors believe the development of genetic testing with the ability to predict drug allergy before it occurs could be another exciting approach to help tackle PCN allergies.

SUMMARY

Many children have a parent-reported PCN allergy, but few are clinically significant. Formal evaluation of PCN allergy labels is critical to efforts to optimize antibiotic use and prevent the emergence of antimicrobial resistance. A reported PCN allergy has serious implications for patient care. Therefore, PCN allergy assessment and management are important for antimicrobial stewardship in both inpatient and outpatient venues. Many tools exist to categorize patients by risk level based on reported symptoms. Optimal testing strategies include oral drug challenge approaches for low-risk patients and skin testing for high-risk patients. Ample evidence exists for these strategies and both are supported by national societies within Allergy and Immunology and Infectious Diseases. Systematic approaches to identifying and testing patients with a PCN allergy label can help meet the needs of patients whereby they present, maximize impact, and increase the sustainability of the removal of an allergy.

CLINICS CARE POINTS

- Oral drug challenge is a reasonable strategy to delabel low risk patients with reported penicillin allergy.
- Skin testing should be administered to high risk patients.
- Strategies are need to ensure patients understand the results and remain delabeled.

DISCLOSURE

The authors have nothing to disclose.

REFERENCES

1. Zhou L, Dhopeshwarkar N, Blumenthal KG, et al. Drug allergies documented in electronic health records of a large healthcare system. Allergy 2016;71:1305–13.
2. Sacco KA, Bates A, Brigham TJ, et al. Clinical outcomes following inpatient penicillin allergy testing: a systematic review and meta-analysis. Allergy 2017;72(9):1288–96.
3. Miller LE, Knoderer CA, Cox EG, et al. Assessment of the validity of reported antibiotic allergic reactions in pediatric patients. Pharmacotherapy 2011;31(8):736–41.
4. Marom T, Nokso-Koivisto J, Chonmaitree T. Viral-bacterial interactions in acute otitis media. Curr Allergy Asthma Rep 2012;12(6):551–8.
5. Joint Task Force on Practice Parameters representing the American Academy of Allergy, Asthma and Immunology, American College of Allergy, Asthma and Immunology, Joint Council of Allergy, Asthma and Immunology. Drug allergy: an updated practice parameter. Ann Allergy Asthma Immunol 2010;105(4):259–73.
6. Pichler WJ. Delayed drug hypersensitivity reactions. Ann Intern Med 2003;139:683–93.
7. Bhattacharya S. The facts about penicillin allergy: a review. J Adv Pharm Technol Res 2010;1(1):11–7.
8. Lee P, Shanson D. Results of a UK survey of fatal anaphylaxis after oral amoxicillin. J Antimicrob Chemother 2007;60(5):1172–3.
9. Macy E, Contreras R. Health care use and serious infection prevalence associated with penicillin "allergy" in hospitalized patients: a cohort study. J Allergy Clin Immunol 2014;133(3):790–6.
10. Al-Hasan MN, Acker EC, Kohn JE, et al. Impact of penicillin allergy on empirical carbapenem use in gram-negative bloodstream infections: an antimicrobial stewardship opportunity. Pharmacotherapy 2018;38(1):42–50.
11. Lee CE, Zembower TR, Fotis MA, et al. The incidence of antimicrobial allergies in hospitalized patients: implications regarding prescribing patterns and emerging bacterial resistance. Arch Intern Med 2000;160(18):2819–22.

12. Jeffres MN, Narayanan PP, Shuster JE, et al. Consequences of avoiding beta-lactams in patients with beta-lactam allergies. J Allergy Clin Immunol 2016; 137(4):1148–53.

13. Blumenthal KG, Lu N, Zhang Y, et al. Risk of methicillin resistant Staphylococcus aureus and Clostridium difficile in patients with a documented penicillin allergy: population based matched cohort study. BMJ 2018;361:k2400.

14. Blumenthal KG, Lu N, Zhang Y, et al. Recorded penicillin allergy and risk of mortality: a population-based matched cohort study. J Gen Intern Med 2019;34(9):1685–7.

15. Blumenthal KG, Ryan EE, Li Y, et al. The impact of reported penicillin allergy on surgical site infection risk. Clin Infect Dis 2018;66(3):329–36.

16. Powell N, Honeyford K, Sandoe J. Impact of penicillin allergy records on antibiotic costs and patient length of hospital say: a single centre observational retrospective cohort. J Hosp Infect 2020;106(1):35–42.

17. Centers for Disease Control and Prevention. Is it really a penicillin allergy? Evaluation and diagnosis of penicillin allergy for healthcare professionals. 2018. Available at: https://www.cdc.gov/antibiotic-use/community/pdfs/penicillin-factsheet.pdf. Accessed March 23, 2021.

18. Barlam TF, Cosgrove SE, Abbo LM, et al. Implementing an antimicrobial stewardship program: guidelines by the Infectious Diseases Society of America and the Society for Healthcare Epidemiology of American. Clin Infect Dis 2016;62(10): e51–77.

19. American Academy of Asthma, Allergy, and Immunology. Position statement: penicillin allergy. Available at: https://www.aaaai.org/Aaaai/media/MediaLibrary/PDF%20Documents/Practice%20and%20Parameters/Penicillian-Allergy-Testing-Febraury-17.pdf. Accessed March 23, 2021.

20. Vyles D, Adams J, Chiu A, et al. Allergy testing in children with low-risk penicillin allergy symptoms. Pediatrics 2017;140(2):e20170471.

21. Shenoy ES, Macy E, Rowe T, et al. Evaluation and management of penicillin allergy: a review. JAMA 2019;321(2):188–99.

22. Castells M, Khan DA, Phillips EJ. Penicillin allergy. N Engl J Med 2019;381(24): 2338–51.

23. Banks TA, Tucker M, Macy E. Evaluating penicillin allergies without skin testing. Curr Allergy Asthma Rep 2019;19:27.

24. Mill C, Primeau MN, Medoff E, et al. Assessing the diagnostic properties of a graded oral provocation challenge for the diagnosis of immediate and nonimmediate reactions to amoxicillin in children. JAMA Pediatr 2016;170(6):e160033.

25. Labrosse R, Paradis L, Lacombe-Barrios J, et al. Efficacy and safety of 5-day challenge for the evaluation of nonsevere amoxicillin allergy in children. J Allergy Clin Immunol Pract 2018;6(5):1673–80.

26. Tucker MH, Lomas CM, Ramchandar N, et al. Amoxicillin challenge without penicillin skin testing in evaluation of penicillin allergy in a cohort of Marine recruits. J Allergy Clin Immunol Pract 2017;5(3):813–5.

27. Confino-Cohen R, Rosman Y, Meir-Shafrir K, et al. Oral challenge without skin testing safely excludes clinically significant delayed-onset penicillin hypersensitivity. J Allergy Clin Immunol Pract 2017;5(3):669–75.

28. Vyles D, Chiu A, Routes J, et al. Antibiotic use after removal of penicillin allergy label. Pediatrics 2018;141(5):e20173466.

29. Sogn DD, Evans R 3rd, Shepherd GM, et al. Results of the National Institute of Allergy and Infectious Diseases Collaborative Clinical Trial to test the predictive value of skin testing with major and minor penicillin derivatives in hospitalized adults. Arch Intern Med 1992;152(5):1025–32.

30. Gadde J, Spence M, Wheeler B, et al. Clinical experience with penicillin skin testing in a large inner-city STD clinic. JAMA 1993;270(20):2456–63.
31. Blumenthal KG, Peter JG, Trubiano JA, et al. Antibiotic allergy. Lancet 2019; 393(10167):183–98.
32. Staicu ML, Vyles D, Shenoy ES, et al. Penicillin allergy delabeling: a multidisciplinary opportunity. J Allergy Clin Immunol Pract 2020;8(9):2858–68.e16.
33. Trubiano JA, Thursky KA, Stewardson AJ, et al. Impact of an integrated antibiotic allergy testing program on antimicrobial stewardship: a multicenter evaluation. Clin Infect Dis 2017;65(1):166–74.
34. du Plessis T, Walls G, Jordan A, et al. Implementation of a pharmacist-led penicillin allergy de-labelling service in a public hospital. J Antimicrob Chemother 2019;74(5):1438–46.
35. Leis JA, Palmay L, Ho G, et al. Point-of-care β-lactam allergy skin testing by antimicrobial stewardship programs: a pragmatic multicenter prospective evaluation. Clin Infect Dis 2017;65(7):1059–65.
36. Heil EL, Bork JT, Schmalzle SA, et al. Implementation of an infectious disease fellow-managed penicillin allergy skin testing service. Open Forum Infect Dis 2016;3(3):ofw155.
37. Blumenthal KG, Wickner PG, Hurwitz S, et al. Tackling inpatient penicillin allergies: Assessing tools for antimicrobial stewardship. J Allergy Clin Immunol 2017;140(1):154–61.e6.
38. Arroliga ME, Wagner W, Bobek MB, et al. A pilot study of penicillin skin testing in patients with a history of penicillin allergy admitted to a medical ICU. Chest 2000; 118(4):1106–8.
39. Arroglia ME, Radojicic C, Gordon SM, et al. A prospective observational study of the effect of penicillin skin testing on antibiotic use in the intensive care unit. Infect Control Hosp Epidemiol 2003;5:347–50.
40. Taremi M, Artau A, Foolad F, et al. Safety, efficacy, and clinical impact of penicillin skin testing in immunocompromised cancer patients. J Allergy Clin Immunol Pract 2019;7(7):2185–91.e1.
41. Vyles D, Chiu A, Simpson P, et al. Parent-reported penicillin allergy symptoms in the pediatric emergency department. Acad Pediatr 2017;17(3):251–5.
42. Macy E, Ensina LF. Controversies in allergy: is skin testing required prior to drug challenges? J Allergy Clin Immunol Pract 2019;7(2):412–7.
43. Li J, Shahabi-Sirjani A, Figtree M, et al. Safety of direct drug provocation testing in adults with penicillin allergy and association with health and economic benefits. Ann Allergy Asthma Immunol 2019;123(5):468–75.
44. Kuruvilla M, Shih J, Patel K, et al. Direct oral amoxicillin challenge without preliminary skin testing in adult patients with allergy and at low risk with reported penicillin allergy. Allergy Asthma Proc 2019;40(1):57–61.
45. Abrams EM, Ben-Shoshan M. Delabeling penicillin allergy: Is skin testing required at all? J Allergy Clin Immunol Pract 2019;7(4):1377.
46. Iammatteo M, Alvarez Arango S, Ferastraoaru D, et al. Safety and outcomes of oral graded challenges to amoxicillin without prior skin testing. J Allergy Clin Immunol Pract 2019;7(1):236–43.
47. Stevenson B, Trevenen M, Klinken E, et al. Multicenter Australian study to determine criteria for low- and high-risk penicillin testing in outpatients. J Allergy Clin Immunol Pract 2020;8(2):681–9.e3.
48. Ramsey A, Mustafa SS, Holly AM, et al. Direct challenges to penicillin-based antibiotics in the inpatient setting. J Allergy Clin Immunol Pract 2020;8(7):2294–301.

49. Chua KYL, Vogrin S, Bury S, et al. The penicillin allergy delabeling program: a multicenter whole-of-hospital health services intervention and comparative effectiveness study. Clin Infect Dis 2020;ciaa653.

50. Ham Y, Sukerman ES, Lewis JS 2nd, et al. Safety and efficacy of direct two-step penicillin challenges with an inpatient pharmacist-driven allergy evaluation. Allergy Asthma Proc 2021;42(2):153–9.

51. Blumenthal KG, Li Y, Hsu JT, et al. Outcomes from an inpatient beta-lactam allergy guideline across a large US health system. Infect Control Hosp Epidemiol 2019; 40(5):528–35.

52. Bauer ME, MacBrayne C, Stein A, et al. A multidisciplinary quality improvement initiative to facilitate penicillin allergy delabeling among hospitalized pediatric patients. Hosp Pediatr 2021;11(5):427–34.

53. Trubiano JA, Smibert O, Douglas A, et al. The safety and efficacy of an oral penicillin challenge program in cancer patients: a multicenter pilot study. Open Forum Infect Dis 2018;5(12):ofy306.

54. Desai SH, Kaplan MS, Chen Q, et al. Morbidity in pregnant women associated with unverified penicillin allergies, antibiotic use, and group b streptococcus infections. Perm J 2017;21:16–080.

55. Macy E. Penicillin skin testing in pregnant women with a history of penicillin allergy and group B Streptococcus colonization. Ann Allergy Asthma Immunol 2006;97:164–8.

56. Kuder MM, Lennox MG, Li M, et al. Skin testing and oral amoxicillin challenge in the outpatient allergy and clinical immunology clinic in pregnant women with penicillin allergy. Ann Allergy Asthma Immunol 2020;125(6):646–51.

57. Desravines N, Waldron J, Venkatesh KK, et al. Outpatient penicillin allergy testing in pregnant women who report an allergy. Obstet Gynecol 2021;137(1):56–61.

58. Blumenthal KG, Shenoy ES. Penicillin allergy in pregnancy. JAMA 2020;323(12): 1216.

59. Stukus DR, Green T, Montandon SV, et al. Deficits in allergy knowledge among physicians at academic medical centers. Ann Allergy Asthma Immunol 2015; 115:51–5.e1.

60. Vyles D, Mistry RD, Heffner V, et al. Reported knowledge and management of potential penicillin allergy in children. Acad Pediatr 2019;19(6):684–90.

61. Allen HI, Vazquez-Ortiz M, Murphy AW, et al. De-labeling penicillin-allergic children in outpatients using telemedicine: Potential to replicate in primary care. J Allergy Clin Immunol Pract 2020;8(5):1750–2.

62. Savic L, Gurr L, Kaura V, et al. Penicillin allergy de-labelling ahead of elective surgery: feasibility and barriers. Br J Anaesth 2019;123(1):e110–6.

63. Raja AS, Lindsell CJ, Bernstein JA, et al. The use of penicillin skin testing to assess the prevalence of penicillin allergy in an emergency department setting. Ann Emerg Med 2009;54(1):72–7.

64. Wright A, Rubins D, Shenoy ES, et al. Clinical decision support improved allergy documentation of antibiotic test dose results. J Allergy Clin Immunol Pract 2019; 7(8):2919–21.

65. Bourke J, Pavlos R, James I, et al. Improving the effectiveness of penicillin allergy de-labeling. J Allergy Clin Immunol Pract 2015;3(3). 365-34.e1.

66. Lutfeali S, DiLoreto FF, Alvarez KS, et al. Maintaining penicillin allergy delabeling: A quality improvement initiative. J Allergy Clin Immunol Pract 2021;9(5): 2104–6.e2.

Moving?

Make sure your subscription moves with you!

To notify us of your new address, find your **Clinics Account Number** (located on your mailing label above your name), and contact customer service at:

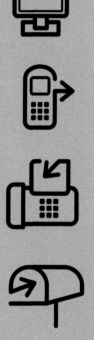

Email: journalscustomerservice-usa@elsevier.com

800-654-2452 (subscribers in the U.S. & Canada)
314-447-8871 (subscribers outside of the U.S. & Canada)

Fax number: 314-447-8029

Elsevier Health Sciences Division
Subscription Customer Service
3251 Riverport Lane
Maryland Heights, MO 63043

*To ensure uninterrupted delivery of your subscription, please notify us at least 4 weeks in advance of move.